Bipolar for Psychotherapists and Their Clients

C. Raymond Lake

Bipolar for Psychotherapists and Their Clients

Springer

C. Raymond Lake
Department of Psychiatry and Behavioral Sciences
University of Kansas Health System
Kansas City, KS, USA

ISBN 978-3-031-38749-4 ISBN 978-3-031-38750-0 (eBook)
https://doi.org/10.1007/978-3-031-38750-0

This Springer imprint is published by the registered company Springer Nature Switzerland AG
The registered company address is: Gewerbestrasse 11, 6330 Cham, Switzerland

This book is dedicated to psychotherapists who have some interest in Bipolar and Bipolar clients and their families who are questioning the Bipolar diagnosis, and to Departments of Psychology, Social Work, and other psychotherapy training programs who can benefit those noted above.

Preface

This book is written for psychotherapists, potential Bipolar clients, and their families. The ideas presented may also be of interest to academic departments of psychology, social work, and other psychotherapy teaching institutions.

Bipolar is a neurogenetic disease of the brain that is not under voluntary control and is unique in psychology because, despite being a lifelong severe mental illness, it associates with success, accomplishments, leadership, and fame. Despite success, chaos is not rare in the Bipolar's day-to-day life while in either manic or depressive episodes. Psychotherapy can be lifesaving.

Medications alone, without psychotherapy, in the treatment of Bipolar are associated with disappointingly low rates of remission, high rates of recurrence, residual symptoms, and psychosocial impairment. Psychotherapy is mandatory in the effective management of Bipolar. The question is who is going to do it and how.

Achieving remission in cases with active symptoms is no longer the only goal of treatment. Preventing or delaying the next episode after remission is essential for successful lifetime management. This requires knowledge about Bipolar and frequent contact with clients to recognize the early onset of an oncoming episode.

Both therapists and clients are responsible for recognizing and managing this complicated disease. Because better management is needed, this book addresses at least four significant issues upon which better management depends: formal student education about Bipolar; early recognition; appropriate treatment with psychoeducation, psychotherapy, and medications when needed; and client acceptance. A source for therapists' and clients' education is this book, *Bipolar for Psychotherapists and Their Clients*.

Over the past decade, there has been a substantial increase in the number of articles on Bipolar in both the lay and academic literatures. As a result, although still substantial, the stigma and shame associated with having Bipolar have diminished as the recognition of Bipolar has expanded. These factors have prompted a redoubling of the numbers of Bipolar cases. Some have estimated that at some point in their lives, as many as 5% or 16 million people in the United States will have recognized or unrecognized Bipolar.

Such growth has resulted in underserved clients with Bipolar, primarily due to the shortage of Bipolar-knowledgeable mental health providers. The number of knowledgeable treaters has not kept up. A relevant challenge now is to develop a source of mental health workers able to recognize and manage such Bipolar clients. There is an opportunity for psychotherapists. They get to know their clients well, can treat with psychotherapy, and substantially outnumber psychiatrists.

For the past century, the management of Bipolar has been the responsibility of psychiatrists. At least three factors now inhibit adequate care for Bipolar clients by psychiatrists. First, there are not enough psychiatrists to care for the expanding Bipolar populations. Second, the time limitations and managed care restraints have discouraged psychiatrists spending more than 10–15 minutes with their clients; there is enough time for a chat and writing prescriptions but not enough to thoroughly know their clients as is the case for psychotherapists. Third, few psychiatrists do psychotherapy…making it necessary for Bipolar clients to hire a second mental health worker for psychotherapy. Having two mental health providers does not allow adequate focus and collaboration on Bipolar.

A further flaw in this system of psychiatrists managing Bipolar clients is that psychiatrists typically reschedule clients for follow-up visits in one to six months. This scheduling system inadequately serves Bipolar clients because some cycle faster than others and episodes could be missed. In clients who have experienced four lifetime episodes going forward, the anticipated frequency is at least one episode every year; the more episodes, the faster they come and the worse they get. Missing an episode is a detriment to the client's welfare.

Psychotherapists usually take 50 minutes with each client on a weekly basis. They have the opportunity to get to know their clients' personalities and potential mood swings. Since Bipolar is usually a lifetime, and certainly a cycling disorder, contact more frequent than one to six months is necessary to effectively manage. Psychotherapists are in a good position to help more Bipolars.

There are barriers to therapists managing Bipolar clients despite their being in a good position to do so, given their 50-minute weekly sessions. Training for psychologists, social workers, and other psychotherapists does not emphasize Bipolar because traditionally training for medical doctors has done so and prescriptions may be needed, requiring a medical doctor or nurse practitioner. For the benefit of the growing population of Bipolar clients, and for therapists with the opportunity to expand their practices, training programs for psychotherapists must adapt to this need of Bipolar clients with a greater focus on Bipolar education.

Although therapists cannot prescribe medications, often necessary for moderate to severe Bipolar clients, they can become familiar with the most useful medications, their dosages, their adverse effects, and how they should be prescribed. Therapists who become trained in Bipolar must solicit a mutually beneficial collaboration with a vetted Bipolar-knowledgeable prescriber to assist in care without the therapist giving up the overall management of such clients.

Such a change in the increased education of psychotherapists about Bipolar would require the recognition by academic departments and other psychotherapy training programs of this opportunity. Altering academic curriculum is a barrier but full of reward in this case. Further, a major responsibility for psychotherapists in their treatment role is the continuing psychoeducation of their Bipolar clients. Bipolar clients must also self-educate. Recognition and acceptance then start the treatment process. Psychotherapists can fill this need for care of more Bipolar clients.

Bipolar is usually a lifetime condition of cycling episodes of depression and mania. There is a wide range in its symptom severity, degree of life destruction, and the frequency of episode recurrence. Cycles vary from monthly to several decades. Such variations obscure recognition. This book promotes the understanding of Bipolar across its wide ranges of variabilities.

Useful to this book is a table of abbreviations, a guide to 70 case reports, and tables of 37 tables and 9 figures that are included in the front matter for easy reference. These tables give the locations of each case, table, and figure in the text and contribute considerable information that expands the text. Further, there is extensive cross-referencing between chapters to link themes across varied topics. *Bipolar for Psychotherapists and Their Clients* offers discussions of how to differentiate medical, non-mood psychological, and Substance Use Disorders sometimes confused with Bipolar. There is emphasis on recognition and treatment of Bipolar among therapists' current case load and new clients.

Additional topics addressed in the book include the following:

- A history of Bipolar spanning 2,000 years of consistent recordings of classic cycling of mood confirm its scientific grounding.
- Bipolar is under-recognized especially in children where more traditional childhood disorders are used instead of Bipolar, to such clients' detriment since misdiagnosed Bipolars can be given medicines that can make them worse.
- *Bipolar for Psychotherapists and Their Clients* helps conceptualize how the disease fits into the group of Mood Disorders.
- Bipolar is a common, costly disorder fiscally and emotionally.
- In adults, misdiagnoses of Major Depressive Disorder (MDD), Attention-Deficit Hyperactivity Disorder (ADHD), "Schizophrenia," and "Schizoaffective Disorder" in Bipolar clients lead to below standard-of-care treatment.
- Surprisingly, pharmacological treatment for Bipolar and MDD is the same; three mood-stabilizing drugs at once.
- Academic departments of psychology, social work, and other programs of psychotherapy are asked to give more time and emphasis to Bipolar in the teaching curriculum.
- The new concept of a spectrum between Bipolar and Unipolar Disorders ends the traditional binary concept and moves many cases from Unipolar to Bipolar based on the presence of non-manic Bipolar features.
- An important, unrecognized source of diagnosing and managing new cases of Bipolar, especially Type II and Cyclothymia, is non-MD psychotherapists during their weekly sessions in contrast to the typical 10-minute medication checks conducted monthly to six-monthly by psychiatrists.

- Clients with severe to psychotic Bipolar Disorders are at greater risk for violence, suicide, murder, and mass murder compared to non-Bipolar individuals. One of this book's goals is to help identify those at such risk and potentially prevent bad outcomes.

Kansas City, KS, USA C. Raymond Lake

Acknowledgments

Martha Breckenridge, PhD, worked on technical editing, research, bibliography, and typing for this book. Without her untiring dedication…no book.

Anita swisher was outstanding in producing 37 tables and 9 figures and also organizing the case reports.

Alexis Banegas, graphic designer, provided the complex graphics.

Contents

About the Author

C. Raymond Lake, MD, PhD is Professor Emeritus of Psychiatry, The University of Kansas Health System, Kansas City, KS.

Dr. Lake graduated from Tulane University, New Orleans, LA, in 1965. He received an MS in Insect Physiology, also from Tulane, in 1966. He graduated from Duke University, School of Medicine and Duke Graduate School (Department of Physiology and Pharmacology), Durham, NC, in 1971 and 1972. He studied at Oxford University with Professor Peter Brunet, PhD, and at St. Bartholomew's Hospital, London, with Professor Mike Besser, MD. His residency in Psychiatry was completed at Duke and at the National Institute of Mental Health (NIMH). As a research associate and staff psychiatrist at the NIMH, Laboratory of Clinical Sciences, he worked under Irv Kopin and alongside Mike Ziegler, Mike Ebert, Fred Goodwin, Dennis Murphy, Richard Wyatt, Julie Axelrod, and Bob Post. In 1979 he moved across the pike to take a professorship of Psychiatry and Pharmacology at the then-new Uniformed Services University of the Health Sciences (USUHS), School of Medicine. He secured two NIH RO1s continuing his research on the regulation of the sympathetic nervous system in patients with neuropsychiatric and cardiovascular disorders.

In 1993 he accepted the chairmanship of Psychiatry at the University of Kansas School of Medicine and remained chair for three years after which he continued on the full-time faculty until his recent partial retirement. As Professor Emeritus he continues to publish, teach about Mood Disorders, and follow his long-term patients. He has over 250 publications including two recent 400-plus page textbooks. He has achieved life-fellowship status in the American Psychiatric Association and the American College of Neuropsychopharmacology. His current interests are the misdiagnosis of Schizophrenia, a more effective strategy for teaching Psychiatry in medical schools, and violence among Mood-Disordered individuals. He believes Bipolar clients are underserved and that psychotherapists are in a good position to undertake their overall management once psychotherapy training departments educate their students about Bipolar. His most recent single-authored books are titled *Schizophrenia Is a Misdiagnosis* published by Springer in 2012, *Bipolar*, published by Elsevier in 2021, and *Bipolar for Psychotherapists and Their Clients*, to be published by Nature, 2023.

List of Figures

List of Tables

List of Cases

Chapter 1
The Management of Bipolar by Psychotherapists

> "In summary, once knowledgeable about Bipolar, psychotherapists are best positioned to both diagnose and manage Bipolar clients because of their time investment in learning about their clients' lives during weekly therapy." (Lake 2022)

1.1 Psychotherapists Are Best Positioned to Recognize, Diagnose, and Manage Bipolar

Throughout its history, Bipolar has been managed not by psychotherapists but by MD psychiatrists, because their psychiatric training emphasizes severe mental illnesses including Bipolar and the medications needed to treat them. More than medications is required for effective treatment of Bipolar, however (Sects. 6.1, 6.4, and 6.5). Long-term psychotherapy is mandatory for the best chance for effective management. This book encourages psychotherapists to endeavor to recognize, diagnose, and manage new Bipolar clients and to reassess long-term clients who may have been misdiagnosed.

Psychotherapists may initially avoid caring for even mild to moderate Bipolars due to uncertainty about their management. Assuredly, moderate to severe cases must also be referred to a psychiatrist, a primary care physician (PCP), or a nurse practitioner for medications. However, such a referral does not mean the psychotherapist must give up the lead management of these cases, but rather that the psychotherapist will collaborate with a well-vetted prescriber.

Initially psychiatrists were trained in both psychotherapy and medication management, but from the 1980s, insurance and managed care companies have discouraged psychiatrists from conducting psychotherapy because of time and cost. As a result, many psychiatry residency training programs have de-emphasized teaching psychotherapy. Psychiatrists are now trained to prescribe medicines in 10- to 15-minute sessions with follow-up typically every one to six months, even in individuals with rapid cycling or histories of severe episodes.

C. R. Lake, *Bipolar for Psychotherapists and Their Clients*,
https://doi.org/10.1007/978-3-031-38750-0_1

Therefore, as determined by the insurance and managed care industries, Bipolar clients now must have two mental health providers: a prescriber for medications and a psychotherapist for psychotherapy. This arrangement does not work well for clients since often there is inconsistent collaboration between the two mental health professionals because collaboration is time-consuming and not reimbursable.

Psychiatrists' or primary care physicians' sessions with cycling mood-disordered clients every one to six months afford inadequate opportunity to recognize mild to moderate mood changes that may come and go between visits. Rapid recognition of such cycles allows treatment adjustments such as increased therapy sessions. Clients may not recognize such mood changes either, and even if they do, they may have difficulty getting an interim appointment with an MD. Client options are not good: they might choose to go to the ED, endure their symptoms until their next scheduled prescriber appointment, or suffer the consequences from poor decisions during mania or depression. Episodes of mania or depression cause life-altering disruptions that deserve more rapid recognition and treatment adjustments. A paradigm shift to management of Bipolar by therapists is in order, as advocated in this book.

Since to date there is no cure for Bipolar, the overriding goal in treatment is to postpone future episodes and minimize their severity. Bipolar tends to get worse with each episode and the rate of cycling increases, so the next episode will come faster, the symptoms will become more severe, and treatment resistance may occur (Fig. 1.1). After only four episodes, Bipolar clients will suffer an average of one episode every 12 months.

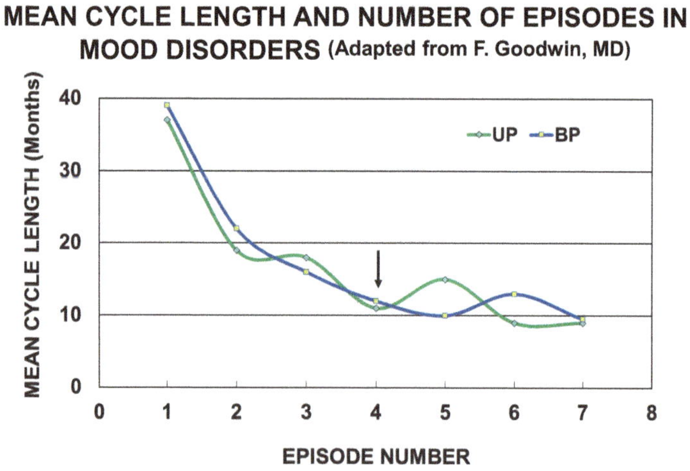

Fig. 1.1 Mean cycle length and number of episodes in Mood Disorders. (Adapted from F. Goodwin, MD)

For both Unipolar and Bipolar Mood Disorders, each episode of either mania or depression causes the next episode of either mania or depression to come faster. By the fourth episode as denoted by the arrow, clients suffer, on average, an episode of mania or depression every 12 months. Given that the average Major Depressive Episode lasts about six months and a manic episode about three months, one's life is disrupted in a major way with an episode every 12 months. Abbreviations: *UP* Unipolar or Major Depressive Disorder, *BP* Bipolar Disorder

Further, Bipolar clients are less compliant with their medicines and their appointments when not scheduled often, such as weekly. Psychotherapists are in an advantageous position to recognize and manage Bipolar clients because they see their clients for *50 minutes every week* and get to know their lives in detail by following them over months to years.

If a weekly client misses a psychotherapy appointment, the therapist or client is more likely to make contact and reschedule because weekly psychotherapy establishes a close relationship between the psychotherapist and client, in contrast to monthly to six-monthly 10-minute appointments with a prescriber (Sect. 5.2).

Once therapists are aware of the signs and symptoms of cyclical mood changes including persistent mood instability, they can make the diagnosis and manage Bipolar. They collaborate with their client to monitor mood, sleep, and medications, and to discern initial mild mood changes that can herald a major episode and, most importantly, to emphasize compliance. Early appreciation of a mild mood shift is critical to blunt a full episode and is enabled by a therapist's pre-established relationship with a prescriber (Chap. 5). When the therapist suspects an oncoming episode, in collaboration with their Bipolar client, therapists can help schedule an emergency appointment with the prescriber. In addition, therapy sessions can be increased to multiple times per week. Once educated about appropriate medications, therapists' discussions, in collaboration with psychiatrist and client, of dosage and medication changes, as well as adverse effects (AEs), are appropriate (Sects. 6.2 and 6.3).

Most non-MD therapists are not trained or licensed to prescribe medications or to directly admit clients to hospitals. Social work and psychotherapy training programs usually do not address Bipolar medications. However, such instruction is valuable as these future psychotherapists learn to recognize Bipolar in their clients and realize they can more effectively manage them. Many Bipolars benefit from medications, and with more training focused on Bipolar, psychotherapists can assume some input into the oversight of their Bipolar clients' medications through a prescriber. Potential prescribers are MDs, including psychiatrists, family practitioners, and primary care physicians, as well as nurse practitioners and DOs.

The first challenge for psychotherapists is to gain knowledge and understanding of Bipolar in order to make correct diagnostic assessments in their clinic population. Since medication plus psychotherapy gives moderate to severe Bipolar clients the best chance for a good outcome, the psychotherapist can vet, recommend, and collaborate with a prescriber but without giving up primary management of the client (Sect. 5.2).

The psychotherapist works closely with the client regarding referral to a knowledgeable prescriber. Important discussions between therapist and client include diagnoses and medications as well as an exit strategy if the prescriber does not meet expectations. Ideally, the psychotherapist takes charge in recommending a prescribing psychiatrist, PCP, or nurse practitioner after vetting for their diagnostic preferences and choices of mood-stabilizing medications (Sects. 5.2 and 6.2). Mutual agreements between therapists and prescribers to cross-refer Bipolar clients may also ensue.

After an appropriate prescriber is found, a meeting including the client, the psychotherapist, and the prescriber is recommended to confirm the prescriber's diagnostic and prescription practices. The psychotherapist guides the client to the knowledgeable psychiatrist, PCP, or nurse practitioner for prescriptions while maintaining his/her role as person in charge of the client's overall Bipolar care.

If a client has a psychiatrist or PCP before beginning psychotherapy, only after establishing a therapeutic relationship can the psychotherapist begin to evaluate and discuss the prescriber's recommendations. If the psychiatrist or PCP has already made a diagnosis other than Bipolar, such as "Schizophrenia," "Schizoaffective Disorder," ADHD, or has prescribed medications deemed inappropriate by the knowledgeable psychotherapist, a change in prescriber is in order, as soon as feasible. At this point, the therapist and the client together find a different psychiatrist, PCP, or nurse practitioner who is *better vetted for their knowledge of Bipolar*. If Bipolar clients become psychotic, such preparation will also facilitate their referral to hospitals with inpatient units where the psychotherapist knows the psychiatrist's or PCP's Bipolar practice habits (Sects. 5.2 and 6.2).

So much data are available online and in this and other books that clients can themselves become knowledgeable about Bipolar and productively discuss best treatment plans with their psychotherapist and MD.

For clients who have had severe episodes, a model plan for changes in medication or for hospitalization is best outlined in writing with the client's signature early on in treatment, so if there is another moderate to severe episode and the client becomes resistant to verbal input, the psychotherapist can refer to these previously agreed-upon written plans.

In summary, psychotherapists with Bipolar education are best positioned to both diagnose and manage Bipolar clients because of their time investment in learning about their clients' lives during weekly therapy. Such close follow-up enables early recognition of an oncoming episode. Understanding more about Bipolar and its medications, psychotherapists can consider Bipolar diagnoses among their new and ongoing clients. Clients and their therapists must collaborate regarding diagnosis and medication if needed. Both can invest effort toward learning about Bipolar and vetting local psychiatrists or PCPs for their knowledge of Bipolar. For a good outcome, frequent follow-up with weekly psychotherapy and several life changes are critical along with specific medications (Chap. 6).

1.2 Guilt and Shame of Bipolar Inhibit Recognition

> "Celebrities…who publicly address their…illness give Bipolar Disorder a face. Their courage in going public helps reduce fear and ignorance by reminding everyone of our shared humanity." (Fawcett et al. 2007)

Mental illness has always been stigmatized because of stereotypes suggesting that the mentally ill are possessed by the devil or that there are defective genes, weakness in character, lack of self-control, or simply willful immoral behavior

(Sect. 2.1). Such ignorance about mental illness promotes fear of clients with mental illness which in turn increases stigma. First steps to alleviate stigma include educating the public. Schools are a recommended starting point to help combat stigma, especially in the lower grades where teachers can more effectively educate children about mental illness.

Shame, at the core of stigma, affects the mentally ill and also their families. Shame is more profound than guilt; both are painful but the mentally ill respond to their shame by wanting to hide, get away, or die. Stigma and guilt, particularly associated with Bipolar Disorder, promote denial and inhibit recognition and acceptance and therefore effective management of Bipolar. Kitty Dukakis said, "The tragedy is that so many people, particularly people in highly visible positions, don't get the help they need because of concern about what the public will perceive…" Kate Spade is an example of a high-profile personality who never acknowledged her Bipolar (Case 4.18; Sects. 4.1 and 4.3). "Celebrities who publicly address their illness give Bipolar Disorder a face. Their courage in going public helps reduce fear and ignorance by reminding everyone of our shared humanity" (Fawcett et al. 2007). Patty Duke, Richard Dreyfuss, Kay Redfield Jamison, Margot Kidder, Dale Chihuly, and Carrie Fisher are examples of famous individuals who have spoken publicly about their Bipolar, thereby increasing acceptance (Sects. 4.2, 4.3, and 4.4). Throughout history, hundreds of famous and successful individuals have managed their Bipolar (Table 1.1).

Table 1.1 Famous people reportedly diagnosed with Bipolar Disorder ($N = 287$)

Name	Country	Occupation
Alvin Ailey	USA	Choreographer
Sherman Alexie	USA	Poet, Writer, and Filmmaker
Lilly Allen	England	Musician
Louis Althusser	France	Marxist Philosopher
August Ames	Canada	Pornographic Actress
Michael Angelakos	USA	Musician, Frontman of "Passion Pit"
Adam Ant	England	Musician and Actor
Noah Antwiler	USA	Actor
Emilie Autumn	USA	Singer and Violinist
Tyler Baltierra	USA	Reality Television Personality
Maria Bamford	USA	Comedian
Marcel Barbeau	Canada	Artist and Painter
Maria Bello	USA	Producer, Actress, Writer
Helena Belmonte	USA	Model
Max Bemis	USA	Frontman of band "Say Anything"
Maurice Benard	USA	Actor
Benga (Adegbenga Adejumo)	England	Dubstep DJ and Producer
A.C. Benson	England	Essayist, Poet, Author, 28th Master of Magdalene College, Cambridge
Davone Bess	USA	Football Player

(continued)

Table 1.1 (continued)

Name	Country	Occupation
Jayson Blair	USA	Journalist
Paul Boyd	Canada	Classical Animator
Ronald Braunstein	USA	Orchestra Conductor and Cofounder of the ME2/ Orchestra
L. Brent Bozell, Jr	USA	Conservative Activist and Writer
Russell Brand	England	Comedian and Actor
Jeremy Brett	England	Actor
Chris Brown	USA	Singer, Songwriter, Rapper, Dancer, and Actor
Tiffany Lee Brown	USA	Writer, Artist, and Musician
Frank Bruno	England	Boxer
Barney Bubbles	England	Graphic Artist (suicided at age 41)
Art Buchwald	USA	Humorist and Pulitzer Prize Winner
Elbridge Ayer Burbank	USA	Artist and Painter
Eoin Cameron	Australia	Former Mbr Australian House of Rep and Radio Personality
Robert Campeau	Canada	Financier and Real Estate Developer
Cosmo Compoli	USA	Sculptor and Teacher
Georg Cantor	Germany	Mathematician
Mariah Carey	USA	Singer
Quincy Carter	USA	Football Quarterback
Keisha Castle-Hughes	New Zealand	Oscar-nominated Actor
Dick Cavett	USA	Comedian and TV Journalist
Eason Chan	Hong Kong	Popular Music Singer
Changio	South Korea	Singer, Actor, and Dancer
Akio Chiba	Japan	Manga Artist (suicided)
Winston Churchill	England	Prime Minister of United Kingdom, 1940–1945
Rosemary Clooney	USA	Singer and Actress
Neil Cole	Australia	Labor Party Politician
Samuel Taylor Coleridge	England	Romantic Poet
Mary Ellen Copeland	USA	PhD, Author, Educator, and Mental Health Advocate
Francis Ford Coppola	USA	Film Director, Producer, and Screenwriter
Patricia Cornwell	USA	Crime Writer
Robert S Corrington	USA	Philosopher and Professor of Philosophical Theology
Michael Costa	Australia	Labor Party Politician and Treasurer of NSW
Sean Costello	USA	Blues Musician
Vincent Crane	England	Keyboard Player of "Atomic Rooster"
John Curtin	Australia	14th Prime Minister (1941–1945)
Paul Dalio	USA	Writer, Director, and Composer
Ray Davies	England	Composer; Attempted Suicide
Adam Deacon	England	Film Actor, Rapper, Writer, and Director
Swadesh Deepak	India	Playwright, Novelist, and Short-story Writer

(continued)

Table 1.1 (continued)

Name	Country	Occupation
Disco D	USA	Record Producer and Composer
DMX	USA	Rapper and Actor
Gaetano Donizetti	Italy	Composer
Mike Doughty	USA	Singer from Alternative Rock Band "Soul Coughing"
Richard Dreyfuss	USA	Actor
Patty Duke	USA	Actress, Author, and Mental Health Advocate
Thomas Eagleton	USA	Senator from Missouri
David Feherty	Ireland	Professional Golfer
Carrie Fisher	USA	Actress and Writer
Zelda Fitzgerald	USA	American Socialite and Novelist; Wife of Author F. Scott Fitzgerald
Helen Flanagan	England	Model, Actress
Tom Fletcher	England	Singer, Songwriter, Pianist, and Guitarist
Larry Flynt	USA	Publisher
Ellen Forney	USA	Graphic Artist, Cartoonist
Connie Francis	USA	Singer
Jennifer Frey	USA	Journalist
Stephen Fry	England	Actor, Comedian, and Writer
Sia Furler	Australia	Singer, Songwriter, and Producer
Alan Garner	England	Novelist
Paul Gascoigne	England	Footballer, Author
Isa Genzken	Germany	Contemporary Artist
Mel Gibson	USA	Actor and Director
Matthew Good	Canada	Musician
Glenn Gould	Canada	Pianist
Phillip Graham	USA	Publisher and Businessman
Graham Greene	England	Novelist
Charles Haley	USA	Football Linebacker
Terry Hall	England	Lead Singer of "The Specials"
Halsey	India	Pop Singer
Charles Hamilton	USA	Hip Hop Recording Artist
Linda Hamilton	USA	Actress
Suzy Favor Hamilton	USA	Former Middle Distance Runner
Jeff Hammerbacher	USA	Data Scientist, Chief Scientist at Cloudera
David Harbour	USA	Actor
Anthony Hardy	England	Serial Killer
Beth Hart	USA	Singer and Songwriter
Teddy Hart	Canada	Professional Wrestler
Mariette Hartley	USA	Actress, Founder of the American Foundation for Suicide Prevention
Doug Harvey	Canada	Professional Ice Hockey Player
Jonathan Hay	Australia	Rules Footballer

(continued)

Table 1.1 (continued)

Name	Country	Occupation
Ernest Hemingway	USA	Journalist, Writer
Drewe Henley	England	Actor
Kristin Hersh	USA	Musician of Rock Band “Throwing Muses”
Derek Hess	USA	Designer and Visual Artist
Shane Hmiel	USA	NASCAR Driver
Abbie Hoffman	USA	Political Activist, Anarchist
Marya Hornbacher	USA	Writer
Byron Houston	USA	Basketball Player
Cat Hulbert	USA	Card Player
Meg Hutchinson	USA	Folk Singer-Songwriter
Julian Huxley	England	Biologist, Eugenicist, and Internationalist
Jesse Jackson, Jr	USA	Former member of US House of Representatives
Kay Redfield Jamison	USA	Clinical Psychologist, Professor of Psychiatry, Writer
Jang Guen-seok	South Korea	Actor
Jill Janus	USA	Heavy Metal Singer
Alice de Janzé	USA	Heiress
Adam Jasinski	USA	Winner of US series Big Brother 9
Andrew Johns	Australia	Rugby League Player
Daniel Johnston	USA	Musician, Singer-Songwriter, Visual Artist
Lee Joon	Korea	Actor, Musician
Lucia Joyce	Italy	Dancer, Daughter of Writer James Joyce
Sarah Joyce	England	Singer-Songwriter
Helmi Juvonen	USA	Artist, Painter
Krizz Kaliko	USA	Hip Hop Musician
Antonie Kamerling	The Netherlands	Actor
Chris Kanyon	USA	Professional Wrestler
Kerry Katona	England	Television Presenter, Writer, Magazine Columnist, Former Pop Singer
Patrick J Kennedy	USA	Former Member of the US House of Representatives
Margot Kidder	USA	Actress
Morio Kita	Japan	Psychiatrist, Novelist, Essayist
Otto Klemperer	USA	Conductor, Composer
Cassia Kis	Brazil	Actress
John Konrads	Australia	Freestyle Swimmer
David LaChapelle	USA	Commercial Photographer, Fine-Art Photographer, Music Video Director, File Director, Artist
Mary Lambert	USA	Actress, Singer, Writer
Debra LaFave	USA	School teacher (had sexual relations with minor students)
Andrew Lange	USA	Astrophysicist, Goldberger Professor of Physics at California Institute of Technology, Pasadena CA, Awarded Balzan Prize and David Prize; suicided

(continued)

Table 1.1 (continued)

Name	Country	Occupation
René-Robert Cavelier, Sieur De La Salle	France	Explorer, Explored Great Lakes Region and Claimed Mississippi River Basin for France
AJ Lee	USA	Professional Wrestler, Author
Yoon Ha Lee	USA	Science Fiction Writer
Lee Joon	South Korea	Singer, Actor
Vivien Leigh	England	Actress
Jenifer Lewis	USA	Actress
Bill Lichtenstein	USA	Print and Broadcast Journalist, Documentary Filmmaker
Thomas Ligotti	USA	Horror Author
Arthur Lipsett	Canada	Film Director
Bernard Loiseau	France	Chef; suicided
Ellen Joyce Loo	Hong Kong	Singer, Songwriter
Demi Lovato	USA	Actress, Singer, Writer
Ada Lovelace	England	Mathematician
Ris Low	Singapore	Beauty Pageant Titleholder
Gustav Mahler	Czechnia	Composer
Tina Malone	England	Television Actress, Writer, Director, Producer
Elizabeth Manley	Canada	Former Competitive Figure Skater
Johnny Manziel	USA	Football Player
Jessica Marais	Australia	Actress
Emily Martin	USA	Sinologist, Anthropologist, Feminist, Professor at New York University
Karen McCarthy	USA	Former Member of US House of Representatives
Arthur McIntyre	Australia	Artist
Kristy McNichol	USA	Actress
Burgess Meredith	USA	Actor
Randy Meisner	USA	Musician
H.V. Meyerowitz	Russia	Artist, Educator, British Colonial Administrator in Africa
Dimitri Mihalas	USA	Astrophysicist
Liz Miller	England	Physician, Surgeon, Campaigner, Writer
Kate Millet	USA	Artist, Activist, Feminist Writer
Eric Millegan	USA	Actor
Spike Milligan	India	Comedian
Valdemar Schonheyder Moller	Danish	Painter
Melody Moezzi	USA	Activist, Lawyer, Author
Seaneen Molloy	Northern Ireland	Blogger
Ben Moody	USA	Guitarist, Musician
Jonathan Morrell	England	Radio, Television Producer
Charles Mount	USA	Artist

(continued)

Table 1.1 (continued)

Name	Country	Occupation
Allison Moyet	England	New Wave Singer
Petr Muk	Czech Republic	Singer
John A. Mulheren	USA	Financier, Stock and Options Trader, Philanthropist
Edvard Munch	Norway	Painter
Robert Munsch	USA	Author
Craig Murray	England	Former British Ambassador to Uzbekistan, Political Activist
Kim Novak	USA	Actress
Jason Nash	USA	YouTuber
Phil Ochs	USA	Musician
Bill Oddie	England	Writer, Naturalist, Comedian, Television Presenter
Delores O'Riordan	Ireland	Musician, Songwriter
Craig Owens	USA	Singer
Steven Page	Canada	Singer
Nicola Pagett	Egypt	Actor
Chris Palko	Germany	Rapper, Better Known by his Stage Name Cage
Jaco Pastorius	USA	Jazz Musician
Jane Pauley	USA	TV Presenter, Journalist
Ota Pavel	Czech Republic	Writer, Journalist, Sport Reporter
Lynne Perrie	England	Actress, Singer, Comedienne, Presenter, Author
Jimmy Piersall	USA	Baseball Player
William Pitt	England	1st Earl of Chatham, British Statesman
Edgar Allen Poe	USA	Poet, Writer
Benoit Poelvoorde	Belgium	Comedian, Actor
Jackson Pollock	USA	Artist
Odean Pope	USA	Jazz Musician
Gail Porter	England	TV Presenter
Amber Portwood	USA	Reality Television Personality
Emil Post	USA	Mathematician, Logician
Genesis Potini	New Zealand	Chess Player
Heinz Prechter	Germany	Entrepreneur, Philanthropist, Founder of the American Sunroof Company, Suicided
Charley Pride	USA	Country Music Artist
Gabriele Rabel	Austria	Botanist, Physicist
Mauro Ranallo	Canada	Sport Announcer, Commentator
Lou Reed	USA	Musician
Bebe Rexha	USA	Singer, Songwriter
Jason Ricci	USA	Harmonica Player, Singer
Lynn N Rivers	USA	Member of US House of Representatives
Rene Rivkin	China	Stockbroker, Entrepreneur
Barret Robbins	USA	NFL Pro Football Player

(continued)

Table 1.1 (continued)

Name	Country	Occupation
Svend Robinson	Canada	Politician
John Ruskin	England	Art Critic (Victorian Era), Art Patron, Draughtsman, Watercolourist, Prominent Social Thinker, Philanthropist
Rene Russo	USA	Actress, Producer, Former Model
Gary Lee Sampson	USA	Murderer
Francesco Scavullo	USA	Artist, Fashion Photographer
Franz Schubert	Austria	Composer
Robert Schumann	Germany	Composer
Reggie Sears	USA	Recording Artist, Musician, Singer, Songwriter, Composer, Producer
Tommy Lynn Sells	USA	Serial Killer
Anne Sexton	USA	Poet
Frances Ford Seymour	Canada	Mother of Jane and Peter Fonda
Paul Sharits	USA	Visual Artist
Nina Simone	USA	Singer
Naomi Sims	USA	Model, Businesswoman, Author, First African-American Supermodel
Frank Sinatra	USA	Singer, Actor
Yo Yo Honey Singh	India	Rapper, Music Producer, Singer, Film Actor
Amy Sky	Canada	Songwriter
Michael Slater	Australia	International Cricketer
Tony Slattery	England	Actor, Comedian
Christopher Smart	England	Poet
Harry Smith	USA	Olympian
Tim Smith	Australia	Rugby League Player
Charlene Soraia	England	Singer Songwriter, Musician
Alonzo Sellman	USA	Football Player
Dusty Springfield	England	Pop Singer
Scott Stapp	USA	Frontman for "Creed"
Peter Steele	USA	Frontman for "Type O Negative"
Brody Stevens	USA	Comedian
David Strickland	USA	Actor
Michael Strunge	Denmark	Poet, Suicided
Gilbert Stuart	USA	Painter
Poly Styrene	England	Singer (real name Marion Elliot-Said)
Stuart Sutherland	England	Psychologist, Writer
Matthew Sweet	USA	Singer-Songwriter
Mackenzie Taylor	England	Comedian
Michael Thalbourne	Australia	Psychologist, Parapsychologist
Abbott Henderson Thayer	USA	Artist, Painter
Debi Thomas	USA	Olympic Medalist, Figure Skater, Physician

(continued)

Table 1.1 (continued)

Name	Country	Occupation
Steven Thomas	USA	Entrepreneur
Ron Thompson	USA	Politician, Former Member West Virginia House of Delegates
Gene Tierney	USA	Actress
Devin Townsend	Canada	Musician
Nick Traina	USA	Singer, Son of Best-selling Author Danielle Steele
Timothy Treadwell	USA	Environmentalist, Bear Enthusiast
Margaret Trudeau	Canada	Celebrity, Ex-Wife of former Canadian Prime Minister Pierre Elliott Trudeau
Michael Tunn	Australia	Radio Announcer, Television Presenter
Ted Turner	USA	Media Businessman, Founder of CNN
Dimitrius Underwood	USA	Football Player
Jean-Claude Van Damme	Belgium	Actor, Martial Arts Star
Vincent van Gogh	The Netherlands	Artist
Townes Van Zandt	USA	Singer-Songwriter
Joseph Vasquez	USA	Independent Filmmaker
Eric Victorino	USA	Vocalist, Author
Byron Vincent	England	Writer, Performer, Broadcaster
Lars von Trier	Denmark	Filmmaker
Mark Vonnegut	USA	Author
James Wade	England	Professional Darts Player
Ayelet Waldman	USA	Novelist, Essayist
David Williams	England	Actor, Comedian, Author, Charity Fundraiser
Tom G Warrior	Switzerland	Lead Singer, Guitarist (Genre: Heavy Metal Bands)
Ruby Wax	USA	Actress, Mental Health Campaigner, Lecturer, Author
Scott Weiland	USA	Musician
Pete Wentz	USA	Musician
Delonte West	USA	Basketball Player
Kanye West	USA	Musician, Entrepreneur, Fashion Designer
Norman Wexler	USA	Screenwriter
Mark Whitacre	USA	Business Executive
Norbert Wiener	USA	Mathematician, Philosopher, Originator of *Cybernetics*
Brian Wilson	USA	Musician, Founding Member of the *Beach Boys*
Amy Winehouse	England	Singer, Songwriter
Jonathan Winters	USA	Comedian, Actor, Author, Artist
Frank Wisner	USA	OSS Officer
Lee Thompson Young	USA	Actor
Bert Yancey	USA	Professional Golfer
Bruno Zehnder	Sweden	Photographer
Catherine Zeta-Jones	Scotland (Wales)	Actress

From Wikipedia

1.3 The Dangers of Under-Recognition and Misdiagnosis

> "The average Bipolar individual suffers with episodes of mania for 10 years before receiving an accurate diagnosis and proper management." (Lish et al. 1994)

According to Scott (1995), the onset of Bipolar in a client's twenties costs an average of nine years of life, 12 years of normal health, and 14 years of work activity. These losses coupled with the suicide-related mortality and the psychosocial consequences for significant others define Bipolar as a substantial public health problem. "Financial and employment problems are cited by 70% of patients and their partners as the most frequent long-term difficulties" (Targum et al. 1981). It is reported that a year after a manic episode, as many as 23% of clients were continuously unemployed, and 36% showed a clear decline from their premorbid level of functioning at work (Harrow et al. 1990). "Relationships may be lost because of irrevocable damage done by aberrant behavior during a manic episode" (Scott 1995). Bipolar interpersonal relationships are characterized by significantly higher divorce and separation rates and increased conflict in ongoing marriages. One study sample reported a 57% divorce rate, instigated after the first manic episode. Fifty-three per cent of healthy partners said that they would not have married their Bipolar partner and 47% said that they would not have had children if they had known Bipolar would occur. The threat of violence and poor judgment in interpersonal interactions and financial extravagances have dominated concerns about mania (Chap. 4).

Both therapist failure to recognize and client reluctance to accept inhibit the correct diagnosis and effective management of Bipolar. Psychotherapists sometimes under-recognize and misdiagnose Bipolar clients because of a low index of suspicion. Mental health workers are likely to misdiagnose Bipolar as other disorders emphasized in their training, such as those that can be managed with psychotherapy without medications (Sect. 2.7 and 3.6). Some of these misdiagnoses include Attention-Deficit Hyperactivity Disorder (ADHD), Anxiety Disorders, Panic, Major Depressive Disorder (MDD), Intermittent Explosive Disorder (IED), Oppositional Defiant Disorder (ODD), "Schizophrenia," "Schizoaffective Disorder" (SAD), Borderline Personality Disorder (BPD), Antisocial Personality Disorder (APD), and other Personality Disorders—symptoms of all of which overlap with Bipolar (Sect. 3.6; Tables 2.5, 3.7 and 3.11). Clients with such misdiagnoses are usually prescribed antidepressants, second-generation antipsychotics (SGAs), and stimulants by psychiatrists and primary care physicians (PCPs) rather than therapeutic mood-stabilizing drugs (Sect. 6.2). Such often prescribed medications can cause harm in Bipolar clients (Sect. 6.3).

Misdiagnoses in unrecognized Bipolar cases can be initiated during a first health-care encounter conducted by Emergency Department (ED) physicians, psychiatrists, primary care physicians (PCPs), nurse practitioners, or psychotherapists. Such initial misdiagnoses are common and are influential in the later assessments of these clients by subsequent psychotherapists. With the best interests of their clients in mind, psychotherapists should critically evaluate prior diagnoses in their new and ongoing cases. One group of misdiagnosed or undiagnosed adult Bipolar individuals are those with mild symptoms who may be in psychotherapy for moderate life problems not recognized as related to Bipolar (Sect. 3.3).

Especially difficult to recognize are mild Bipolar clients who can achieve substantial *episodic productivity,* so a diagnosis of Bipolar may not be considered even when such individuals have substantial interpersonal conflict—a characteristic sign to stimulate an evaluation specifically for hypomania and therefore Bipolar. Although they have mild symptoms, clients with Cyclothymia and mild Bipolar II suffer more conflict than the non-mentally ill population, with family, friends, at work, and even with law enforcement, but often go unrecognized, unevaluated, misdiagnosed, and untreated. Psychotherapists can help undiagnosed Bipolar clients by adopting a high level of vigilance and seriously considering a diagnosis of Bipolar among their psychotherapy clients with tumultuous episodes of depressions and hypomanias that cause cycles of increased conflict (Sects. 3.2, 3.3, and 3.5).

On the severe end of the spectrum, severe and untreated depression and mania can be dangerous, even life-threatening to self and others, making a misdiagnosis of such a Bipolar client potentially perilous (Sects. 4.4, 4.5, and 4.6). Although the majority of Bipolar individuals are not psychotic, severe episodes of Bipolar with psychotic features might occur for brief periods in about 10–25% of all Bipolar individuals (Sects. 4.4 and 4.5).

Suicide risk figures range as high as 15–25% in both Bipolar and Unipolar depression (Sect. 6.6). The morbidity and mortality of Bipolar in general are high; about 20–25% suffer premature death. Suicide, comorbid medical conditions, accidents, homelessness, conflict with law enforcement, and incarceration account for such early deaths. All-cause mortality and the suicide rate in Bipolars are double that in non-Bipolars, with Bipolars dying eight to nine years younger than non-Bipolars (Ferrari et al. 2016).

Undiagnosed psychotic manic and depressed clients are at risk for inflicting violence on themselves and even mass murder of strangers, friends, children, families, or therapists (Lake 2014a, b) (Sects. 4.5 and 4.6). Such worst-case scenarios seem to be occurring more often than in the past likely due to the increased availability of guns. At a minimum, work and family life are negatively impacted by unrecognized and untreated Bipolar clients.

Clients also directly influence inaccurate diagnoses. The stigma of having a mental illness, especially one considered as severe as Bipolar, generates shame and guilt and may cause clients to deny, resist, and rationalize their symptoms. Likewise, individuals may contribute to the failure to recognize by knowingly or unknowingly misleading themselves and their therapists. Another block to correct diagnosis and treatment of a manic client is their assertiveness, irritability, and aggressiveness, often despite charm and success. The knowledge that Bipolar can be difficult and time-consuming to manage may inhibit some therapists' willingness to follow-up.

Moderate to severe manic clients may be difficult to convince that their thinking is flawed or delusional, that they have Bipolar, or that therapy, medication, and possibly an inpatient intervention are needed. In more severe mania to include psychosis, clients live their psychoses and behave accordingly, which does not include seeking medical help (Sects. 4.2 and 4.3). Even after the episode is over, the swath of destruction may only be partially recognized. As Kay Redfield Jamison stated, "...mania has the benefit of reducing one's memory for some of the most regrettable decisions" (Goodwin and Jamison 2007). Rationalization and denial occur in mild and moderate manias, denial more in severe cases.

Many psychotic Bipolar clients are not seen in the ED or on psychiatric units but remain on the street or incarcerated in jails or prisons. There are more than three times as many mentally ill persons in jails and prisons than in hospitals (Torrey et al. 2010). Some 16% of incarcerated individuals have a severe mental illness, mostly Bipolar. About 40% of severe Bipolars have been in prison. Within 6 months of discharge from a state mental hospital, about half become homeless and 20% are incarcerated.

Psychotherapists can intervene most effectively in such cases by establishing rapport before the client becomes severe. Still, psychotic clients will have difficulty attending to their therapists' input, and correct medication regulation becomes more critical. Therapists can have a positive impact by emphasizing compliance with session attendance and medications.

Episodes of severe depression may also be difficult to recognize as Bipolar rather than Unipolar (MDD) because the client may not remember a past manic or hypomanic episode which has been considered necessary for the Bipolar diagnosis. The evaluator is obligated to attempt to locate significant others in an effort to get the most complete history possible. A screen for the *non-manic Bipolar factors* can help because, when three or more of these factors are present, consideration of a provisional Bipolar diagnosis is appropriate (Sect. 3.5; Table 3.11).

Depressed clients may not voluntarily present for treatment. Without family and friends, severely depressed clients can suffer malnutrition and death, never getting out of their bed or bedroom, called suicide by self-neglect or inanition. They do not care. They are less likely to be as public or as destructive as manic clients except for self-injury because of decreased motivation and increased social isolation. There are exceptions such as cases of filicide and familicide by psychotically depressed individuals (Sect. 4.6). Depressed clients with family may be more pliable than manic clients, allowing themselves to be taken to a health care provider or the hospital. Swartz and Shorter (2007) have emphasized that when severely depressed clients are evaluated, they can be misdiagnosed with "Schizoaffective Disorder" or "Schizophrenia."

Another atypical but tragic outcome for a client and family is when an unrecognized, initially classic Bipolar individual degenerates for life into a non-cycling, persistent, irritable, dysfunctional state without remissions (Sect. 3.3; Case 1.1). Despite the overall dominance of depression and absence of motivation in these chronic cases, there can be subtle grandiosity as seen in Mr. S. T., below. Such chronicity and severity can be confused with "Schizophrenia" or even Dementia. These clients can be medication-resistant but benefit considerably with long-term supportive psychotherapy.

Case 1.1: Mr. S. T.

An example of a chronic course in Bipolar is Mr. S. T.'s tragic transition from successes in law school, a law practice, a family, a house, three cars, and a country club membership to a chronic end-stage non-cycling psychotic Bipolar state. A successful lawyer through his twenties, Mr. S. T. had classic manic episodes in college and law school that slowed his graduation. After graduation, he took a position in the family law firm. After a few years, he was fired as a result of inappropriate behavior induced by another manic episode. He later struggled with both mania and depression which gradually destroyed his private practice. Step by step he lost his law practice, car, house, wife, and children as well as all contact with his large biological family except for one sister. Although he had received some psychiatric treatment with appropriate mood-stabilizing medications, he was not compliant and was lost to follow-up for over 10 years. Then his sister called and made an appointment for him. She drove him to all of his doctor's appointments, looked in on him on a monthly basis, and said that the rest of his family would not speak to him because of his abusive behavior. At follow-up his appearance was shocking as he was skeletal, clothes rumpled, and stained; he appeared not to have changed clothes or bathed in weeks and to be living on the street. His appearance at first glance was consistent with Dementia but he was fully oriented with intact memory.

When asked how he was doing, he said with a smile, "I am doing just fine… I am busy with work and recently received a new case." His sister said that his apartment was "disgusting" and that his refrigerator on last check was empty except for a "rotten hot dog and a hunk of molded cheese." She confirmed that he had not worked in over a decade, had no new cases, rarely left his apartment, and struggled with his activities of daily living (ADLs). She said that when she brought food to him or just came for a visit, he would invariably get angry, accuse her of sabotaging his work, stealing his inheritance, and scream and curse.

In his session, with a flat affect, he said he was "…excited about his new case and did not need any medicine or help." His medical work-up was unremarkable and eliminated medical, surgical, and substance-related causes. He refused follow-up and medications and was not committable. He is lost to follow-up and his prognosis is dismal. If he would invest in psychotherapy, he could be helped to improve his life.

Recognition of Bipolar in cases like these allows more effective treatment with mood stabilizers than when these clients are misdiagnosed with "Schizophrenia" and given second-generation antipsychotics (SGAs) with substantial AEs and no mood-stabilizing medications. The early diagnosis by a psychotherapist can redirect medication through the client's prescriber that may prevent chronic decline and treatment resistance.

In unrecognized mania and depression that is severe, the range of destructiveness varies widely from client to client and from episode to episode in the same client. Acute psychotic mania wrecks lives. The cases presented in Chap. 4 are examples. Even when there are periods of productivity, some resulting in brilliant long-term successes, unrecognized Bipolar clients are usually subject to significantly more life disruptions and dysfunctionality caused by mania-mediated spur-of-the-moment bad decisions and, during depression, more poor choices such as suicide. Note the cases of Robin Williams (Sect. 4.3, Case 4.21), Kate Spade (Sect. 4.3, Case 4.18), and Margot Kidder (Sect. 4.3, Case 4.14).

There are *more breakups and divorces; more new, often short-term, relationships; more job changes; more contact with law enforcement; and more homelessness and prison time among Bipolar clients than in non-Bipolar psychotherapy clients.*

Psychotherapists can take charge of the management of such clients' care including vetting psychiatrists, PCPs, and nurse practitioners knowledgeable about Bipolar and their use of polypharmacy with mood-stabilizing medications.

References

Fawcett J, Golden B, Rosenfeld N. New hope for people with bipolar disorder. New York: Three Rivers Press; 2007.

Ferrari AJ, Stockings E, Khoo JP, Erskine H, Degenhardt L, et al. The prevalence and burden of bipolar disorder: findings from the Global Burden of Disease Study. Bipolar Disord. 2016;18(5):440–50.

Goodwin FK, Jamison KR. Manic-depressive illness: bipolar disorders and recurrent depression. 2nd ed. Oxford: Oxford U Press; 2007.

Harrow M, Grossman LS, Herbener ES, Davies EW. Ten-year outcome: patients with schizoaffective disorders, schizophrenia, affective disorders, and mood-incongruent psychotic symptoms. Br J Psychiatr. 1990;177:421–6.

Lake CR. Psychotic rampage killers: mania, not schizophrenia—psychiatry's role in prevention. Psychiatr Ann. 2014a;44:213–4.

Lake CR. Rampage murderers, part I: psychotic versus non-psychotic and a role for psychiatry in prevention. Psychiatr Ann. 2014b;44(5):217–25.

Lake CR. Bipolar. London: Elsevier Academic Press; 2022.

Lish JD, Dime-Meenan S, Whybrow PC, Price RA, Hirschfield RM. The national depressive and manic-depressive association (DMDA) survey of bipolar members. J Affect Disord. 1994;31:281–94.

Scott J. Psychotherapy for bipolar disorder. Br J Psychiatr. 1995;167:581–8.

Swartz CM, Shorter E. Psychotic depression. New York: Cambridge University Press; 2007.

Targum S, Dibble E, Davenport Y, et al. The family attitude questionnaire. Patients' and spouses' views of bipolar illness. Arch Gen Psychiatry. 1981;38:562–8.

Torrey EF, Kennard A, Eslinger D, Lamb R, Pavie J. More mentally ill persons are in jails and prisons than hospitals: a survey of the states. Treatment Advocacy Center; 2010; On line.

Chapter 2
The Basics of Bipolar

2.1 History of Bipolar

> "…the brain…is the seat of madness and delirium…where lies the cause of insomnia and sleep walking…visual and auditory hallucinations. *So long as the brain is still, a man is in his right mind.*" (Hippocrates 460–370 BCE)

> "…Baillarger (1845) formally and accurately characterized what we now know as classic Bipolar cycling when he said, 'There exists a special type of insanity characterized by two regular periods, the one of depression and the other of excitement…calling it 'la folie à double forme', emphasizing that the manic and depressive episodes were not two different attacks but rather two different stages of the same attack'." (Goodwin and Jamison 1990)

> "Griesinger (1867) described mania as '…*raving madness, recognizable by restlessness, impulsive behavior, and incoherence of ideas…extravagant volitional states with hallucinations and ideas of grandeur…*'" (Goodwin and Jamison 1990).

Societies before the Greeks and later during the Middle Ages (circa 400–1400) attributed illnesses, especially insanity, to the intervention of supernatural forces, such as evil spirits, gods, witches, and magicians. By contrast, Greco-Roman ideas on medicine, considered the beginning of a scientific approach, held for eight centuries that insanity or mental illness was a disease. *Hippocrates (460–370 BCE)* established the "classical" biological theory of disease that the body consists of *four humors: blood, yellow bile, black bile, and phlegm,* which caused diseases when in disequilibrium.

Hippocrates was ahead of his time when he associated behavior and the brain (Healy 2008). He said that the brain "…is the seat of madness and delirium…where lies the cause of insomnia and sleep walking…visual and auditory hallucinations. *So long as the brain is still, a man is in his right mind.*"

We can recognize that much of the early history of mental illness dealt with Manic-Depressive Insanity or Bipolar because the signs and symptoms reported 2,000 years ago comport with those established today for Bipolar Disorder. This

C. R. Lake, *Bipolar for Psychotherapists and Their Clients*,
https://doi.org/10.1007/978-3-031-38750-0_2

conclusion that very early descriptions were indeed Bipolar is supported by the striking and unique repeating cycles of mania and depression in the same individuals (Evans 2000; Goodwin and Jamison 1990, 2007). A summary of Goodwin and Jamison's (1990) chronological history of Manic-Depressive Insanity/Bipolar is given below (Table 2.1). This long and consistent history establishes Bipolar as a specific bona-fide disease of the brain.

An accurate concept of depression, called melancholia, dates to at least 400 BCE when *Hippocrates* described a condition associated with "an aversion to food, despondency, sleeplessness, irritability, restlessness..." An excess of black bile was thought to be the cause of depression, while too much yellow bile or a mixture of yellow and black bile was connected with mania, suggesting an association of mania and depression in 400 BCE. Such case descriptions were accurate despite the miss on causation.

Table 2.1 Bipolar Disorder has a long and consistent history

Approx. date	Author	Quote
ca. 400 BCE	Hippocrates (and his followers)	Described "melancholia as a condition associated with an aversion to food, despondency, sleeplessness, irritability, restlessness and … when prolonged … means melancholia." Health was explained as "equilibrium of the four humors of blood, yellow bile, black bile, and phlegm and illness as a disturbance of the equilibrium." Melancholia means black bile and was thought to be caused by an excess of black bile; mania, by an excess of yellow bile.
ca. 400 BCE	Aristotle	Believed that the heart was the dysfunctional organ in melancholia and that gifted people such as Plato and Socrates were particularly susceptible
ca 100 BCE	Themison	Considered "melancholy a form of the disease of mania."
ca 100 CE	Soranus of Ephesus	Thought that mania involved an impairment of reason with delusions: fluctuating states of anger and merriment, although sometimes of sadness and futility and sometimes "an overpowering fear of things which are quite harmless; continual wakefulness, the veins are distended, cheeks flushed, and body hard and abnormally strong;" and a tendency for there to be "attacks alternating with periods of remission." Melancholia involved being "downcast and prone to anger and….practically never cheerful and relaxed"; "signs …..as follows: mental anguish and distress, dejection, silence, animosity toward members of the household, sometimes a desire to live and at other times a longing for death, suspicion… that a plot is being hatched against him, weeping without reason, meaningless muttering, and again, occasional joviality; and various somatic symptoms, many of them gastrointestinal."
ca 150 CE	Galen of Pergamon	Firmly established that "melancholia was a chronic and recurrent condition."

(continued)

Table 2.1 (continued)

Approx. date	Author	Quote
ca 150 CE	Aretaeus of Cappadocia	"In my opinion melancholia is without any doubt the beginning and even part of the disorder called mania. The melancholic cases tend towards depression and… if, however, respite from this condition… occurs, gaiety and hilarity in the majority of cases follows, and this finally ends in mania. Summer and autumn are the periods of the year most favorable for the production of this disorder, but it may occur in spring." "The patient who previously was gay, euphoric, and hyperactive suddenly has a tendency to melancholy; he becomes, at the end of the attack, languid, sad, taciturn, he complains… about his future, he feels ashamed. When the depressive phase is over, such patients go back to being gay, they laugh, they joke, they sing, they show off in public with crowned heads as if they were returning victorious from the games; sometimes they laugh and dance all day and all night." In serious forms of mania, called furor, the patient "sometimes kills and slaughters the servants; in less severe forms, he often exalts himself: without being cultivated he says he is a philosopher…and the incompetent [say they are] good artisans…others yet are suspicious and they feel that they are being persecuted, for which reasons they are irascible."
ca 575	Alexander of Trallus	"Those affected with such a condition are not suffering from melancholia only, for they tend to become maniacal periodically and in a cycle. Mania is nothing else but melancholia in a more intense form."
ca 1000	Avicenna	"Undoubtedly the material which is the effective producer of mania is of the same nature as that which produces melancholia."
ca 1300	John of Gaddesden	"Mania and melancholia are different forms of the same thing."
ca 1500	Joan Manardus	"[Melancholia] manifestly differs from what is properly called mania; there is no doubt, however, that at some time or other, authorities agree that it replaces melancholia."
ca 1549	Jason Pratensis	"Most physicians associate mania and melancholia (truly dreadful diseases) as one disorder, because they consider that they both have the same origin and cause, and differ only in degree and manifestation. Others consider them to be quite distinct."
ca 1600	Felix Plater	"Perturbation of the spirit of the brain when mixed with and kindled by other matter can produce melancholia, or if more ardent, mania."
ca 1672	Thomas Willis	"[Manics and melancholics] are so much akin, that these Distempers often change, and pass from one into the other; for the Melancholick disposition growing worse, brings on Fury: and Fury or Madness [mania] growing less hot, oftentimes ends in a Melancholick disposition. These two, like smoke and flame, mutually receive and give place to one another."
ca 1735	Herman Boerhaave	"If Melancholy increases so far, that from the great Motion of the Liquid of the Brain, the Patient be thrown into a wild Fury, it is called Madness [mania]. Which differs only in Degree from the sorrowful kind of Melancholy, is its Offspring, produced from the same Causes, and cured almost by the same Remedies."

(continued)

Table 2.1 (continued)

Approx. date	Author	Quote
ca 1744	Robert James	"There is an absolute Necessity for reducing Melancholy and Madness [mania] to one Species of Disorder, and consequently of considering them in one joint View…We find that melancholic Patients, . . ., easily fall into Madness, which, when removed, the Melancholy again discovers itself, though the Madness [mania] afterwards returns at certain Periods."
ca 1751	Richard Mead	"Medical writers distinguish two kinds of Madness, and describe them both as a constant disorder of the mind without any considerable fever; but with this difference, that the one is attended with audaciousness and fury, the other with sadness and fear; and that they call mania, this melancholy. But these generally differ in degree only. For melancholy very frequently changes, sooner or later, into maniacal madness; and, when the fury is abated, the sadness generally returns heavier than before."
ca 1845	Jean-Etienne-Dominique Esquirol	"Several distinguished masters, Alexander de Tralles, and Boerhaave himself, were of the opinion, that melancholy… was only the first degree of mania. This is in some cases true. There are in fact, some persons who, before becoming maniacs, are sad, morose, uneasy, diffident and suspicious."
ca 1854	Jules Baillarger	"There exists a special type of insanity characterized by two regular periods, the one of depression and the other of excitement….This type of insanity presents itself in the form of isolated attacks; or, it recurs in an intermittent manner; or, the attacks might follow one another without interruption." He called it 'la folie à double forme,' emphasizing that the manic and depressive episodes were not two different attacks but rather two different stages of the same attack
ca 1854	J.P. Falret	"There is a certain category of patient who continually exhibits a nearly regular succession of mania and melancholia. This seemed sufficiently important to us to serve as a basis for a specific mental disorder, which we call circular insanity because these patients repeatedly undergo the same circle of sickness, incessantly and unavoidably, interrupted only by rather brief respites of reason." 'Described a circular disorder (la folie circulaire), which for the first time expressly defined an illness in which this succession of mania and melancholia manifests itself with continuity and in a manner almost regular.
ca 1867	W. Griesinger	"Provided rich clinical descriptions of melancholia and mania, although he described primarily chronic states with poor prognosis. As Aretaeus had centuries before, Griesinger conceived of mania as an end-stage of a gradually worsening melancholia and both as different stages of a single, unitary disease."
ca 1881	E. Mendel	"Was the first to define hypomania as that form of mania which typically shows itself only in the mild stages abortively, so to speak."
ca 1882	K. Kalhbaum	"Described circular disorders (cyclothymia), which were characterized by episodes of both depression and excitement but which did not end in dementia, as chronic mania or melancholia could."

(continued)

Table 2.1 (continued)

Approx. date	Author	Quote
ca 1899	Emil Kraepelin	"Used the term manic-depressive to encompass the circular psychoses and simple manias, and expressed doubt that melancholia and the circular psychoses were really separate illnesses."
ca 1905	G. Specht	He wrote a paper titled "Chronic Mania and Paranoia," in which he said that "all psychoses derive from an abnormal effect." (Doran et al. 1986) Specht associated mania with both chronicity and paranoia. He wrote that chronic mania was "not at all a rare occurrence."
ca 1911	Eugen Bleuler	Although he departed from Kraepelin by conceptualizing the relationship between manic-depressive (affective) illness and dementia praecox (Schizophrenia) as a continuum without a sharp line of demarcation, he so minimized mood disorders, subservient to Schizophrenia, that Schizophrenia comprised the vast majority of his continuum. Any hint of psychosis demanded the diagnosis of Schizophrenia regardless of a predominance of mood symptoms.
ca 1913	Emil Kraepelin	"Virtually all of melancholia was subsumed under manic-depressive illness." "Kraepelin placed special emphasis on the features of the illness that most clearly differentiated it from "dementia praecox: the periodic or episodic course, the more benign prognosis, and a family history of manic-depressive illness." [He essentially reversed himself in 1920, saying that differences between Schizophrenia and Bipolar were obscure.]
ca 1979	K. Leonhard	"It was the work of Angst and Perris that helped spread my theory that Unipolar and Bipolar Diseases…have different clinical pictures. The Bipolar form displays a considerably more colorful appearance; it varies not only between the two poles, but in each phase offers different pictures. The Unipolar forms…return, in a periodic course, with the same symptomatology."
ca 1960's	D Dunner	Distinguished Bipolar I from Bipolar II based on the severity of the manic symptoms, calling mild mania hypomania and Bipolar II

Adapted from Goodwin and Jamison 1990

Plato (427–347 BCE) considered two forms of mania: one of divine origin and one due to physical exertion. It was a substantial accomplishment that many early physicians recognized that depression and mania were two phases of a single disease given the striking differences in the symptoms of each (Table 3.6). As shown in Table 2.1, *Themison* (100 BCE), *Soranus of Ephesus* (around 100 Common Era [CE]), and Celsus (130 CE) more firmly linked melancholia to mania, although Soranus believed that the two were distinct diseases with common prodromal symptoms requiring the same treatments. Today's drug treatments are once again the same for mania and depression—the mood stabilizers (Sect. 6.2). Soranus accurately described the signs and symptoms of both mania and depression that are consistent with current observations and Diagnostic and Statistical Manual (DSM) diagnostic criteria (Tables 3.3 and 3.4).

Table 2.2 Historical treatments for Bipolar through the centuries

Magical charms	Cupping
Herbs	Leeches
Invocations	Scarification
Music	Baths
Songs	Psychotherapy (after 1800)
Dances	Purgation
Listening to dripping water	Torture
Passive exercises	Whipping
Rocking	Beating
Isolation	Chaining
Bright light	Ducking/waterboarding
Dim light	Blistering
Darkness	Exorcism
Shaving the head	Castration
Warm oil to the head	Darwin's chair
Diet	Straitjackets
Starvation	Execution
Hellebore as an emetic	Burning at the stake
Other drugs: datura, digitalis, prussic acid, opium, purgatives	Electroconvulsive therapy (ECT)
Alcohol	Antipsychotic medications, excessive
No wine	Frontal lobotomy
Bloodletting/bleeding	

Prescribed treatments for these diseases have included isolation, bright or dim light, darkness, warm oil applied to the head, bloodletting, shaving of the head, cupping, leeches, scarification, passive exercises such as rocking, a careful diet excluding wine, listening to dripping water, hellebore as an emetic, starvation, opium, alcohol, music, love, whipping, torture including chains, and sudden brutal ducking (waterboarding) (Table 2.2).

By *150 CE, Aretaeus of Cappadocia* also wrote that depression was "… part of the disorder called mania" since he observed that "some patients after being melancholic have fits of mania … so that mania is like a variety of being melancholic." Aretaeus stressed the *frequency of relapses* and that mania and depression were of *lifelong duration* and *frequently terminated in "Dementia"* (Chap. 1, Case 1.1). His observation that cycling Bipolar could turn into a chronic noncycling dysfunctional state was later ignored in the mid-nineteenth century when Morel and then Bleuler instead named a new disease, "Schizophrenia," to account for such severe, chronic Bipolar clients. Many tens of thousands of severe Bipolar clients have subsequently been misdiagnosed with "Schizophrenia" and mismanaged since 1911 (Sect. 3.9).

Aretaeus described mania as "… furor [its most serious form], excitement, and cheerfulness." He suggested that "… mania was an end-stage of melancholia..." probably because of the frequency of repeated episodes of depression before the onset of a manic state in many clients. Aretaeus accurately described the cycling of such clients between depression and mania saying, "… *the client who previously was gay, euphoric, and hyperactive suddenly has a tendency to melancholy*; he becomes, at the end of the [manic] attack, languid, sad, taciturn… he complains that he is worried about his future, he feels ashamed. *When the depressive phase is over, such clients go back to being gay, they laugh, they joke, they sing... sometimes they laugh and dance all day and all night... sometimes [the manic client] kills and slaughters the servants*" (Goodwin and Jamison 1990). This is an early and scary prediction of some current-day psychotic manic mass murderers (Sects. 4.5 and 4.6).

Aretaeus even observed that spring and autumn were the most common seasons for these disorders, suggestive of Seasonal Affective Disorder (SAD) (Sect. 2.5). In about *575 CE, Alexander of Tralles* wrote that "… *mania is nothing else but melancholia in a more intense form.*"

During the Middle Ages in what would become Europe, between circa 400 and 1400, mental health care "fell into the hands of exorcising priests and *clerical witch hunters*…For *over a thousand years the mentally ill were again regarded as possessed* by the devil or evil spirits or were considered to be witches or sorcerers who could produce the illness in others…*therapists and physicians were excluded* from the field of mental illness…which was taken over by the *Inquisitors*…many devils were exorcised…*witches executed…burned at the stake*…" (Ackerknecht 1959).

Dominicans H. Kraemer and J. Sprenger published the infamous ***Malleus Maleficarum*** in 1486, which regarded anyone "…who showed the slightest psychological deviation or peculiarity as a witch or sorcerer…All misfortunes of life (a poor harvest, death, a broken marriage) were attributed to the works of a devil…" This book alone may have been responsible for the horrible deaths of thousands, if not tens of thousands, of innocent victims, many with mental illnesses, all in the guise of science and doing the right thing.

Gaddesden (1300) returned to reason: "… *mania and melancholia are different forms of the same thing.*" In *1549, Pratensis* believed that "Most physicians associate mania and melancholia…as one disorder..." Another "enlightened physician," *Paracelsus,* published his 1567 book ***Diseases Which Lead to a Loss of Reason***, stating that mental illnesses are *not caused by the devil but are physical diseases*. He specifically addressed a condition indicative of mania as a disturbance of reason that exhibited "excited and unreasonable behavior, agitation, and irritability with a tendency for relapse..." His theory of causation disputed Hippocrates' four humors and focused on one substance, the "*humor vitae.*" "If the temperature was high, the humor vitae would burn…its finer particles would be separated off and would rise upward… coagulating in the head where it *might change into worms* or lead to the formation of ulcers…" His treatment of mania was to allow the vapors to escape by "opening those parts of the body to which mania rises (toes, fingers, head)." Paracelsus' main contribution was his introduction of "chemical concepts" for the treatment of mental illness. The *"worms in the head" theory* of causation for mental illness is an index of the level of scientific sophistication at that time. Recognize that these physicians were on the "cutting edge" of scientific knowledge and methodology. Hopefully, today we are very close to the real causes and curses of Bipolar.

Plater (1536–1614) from Switzerland *used the term "kindled" in 1600* to *describe the gradual onset and worsening of melancholia and mania.* Kindling is a term used today to describe the phenomenon of a progressive lowering of the threshold for the initiation of a spontaneous manic or depressive episode after a first externally stimulated episode (Post 2009). Each subsequent episode tends to be worse than the last, building into severe, full-blown episodes like building a bonfire starting with small sticks. In the seventeenth century, Plater revived the Greek model of the four humors in his book titled ***Medical Practice***. Although the insane were still being "diligently burned at the stake as witches, in 1680 a royal edict in France abolished the death penalty for them" (Ackerknecht 1959).

Willis in 1672 wrote, "These two [manias and melancholias], like smoke and flame, mutually receive and give place to one another." In *1744, James* said that "There is an absolute necessity for reducing melancholy and madness [mania] to one species of disorder…" In *1798, Haslam*, the superintendent at *Bethlam Hospital* (initially called "Bedlam"), London, supported the concept that there was "…common ground between mania and melancholia: 'I would be strongly opposed to them being considered opposite diseases…We see every day the most furious maniacs suddenly sink into a profound melancholy; and the most depressed and miserable objects become violent and raving'" (Healy 2008) (Table 3.6).

During the eighteenth century, psychology gained recognition as an independent science. Those with insanity or mental illness began to be treated a bit more humanely, with less use of chains and other tortures. *By the middle of the eighteenth century, psychotherapy was recommended* and concluded to be more effective than previous methods of purgation and bloodletting. Other treatments continued to be brutal. The *Darwin chair* was introduced. It was rotated until "blood oozed from mouth, ears, and nose with reports of great successes." *Castration, starvation,* and drugs such as datura, camphor, and digitalis were used in large quantities to treat cases of insanity. The adverse effects of these drugs were substantial, even life-threatening, while any benefit was negligible.

In *1801, Pinel* in France emphasized observation and statistical analysis. Pinel's classification of mental illness included mania, melancholia, Dementia, and idiocy. He blamed the *ganglia in the abdominal cavity* for mania. He recorded bizarre, jolly, and also sad behaviors in his clients. He said the course of mania is self-limiting and *recovery is often possible*, noting that *melancholia often leads to refusal of food and suicide but can also generate into mania.* Pinel rejected the use of chains, beatings, extensive bloodletting, and ducking and advocated against use of the straitjacket for long periods of time. He emphasized *physical exercise*, work, and the maintenance of a *consistent day-to-day routine.*

In *1812, Rush* in the United States published his book on hospitals for the insane. His recognition that heredity and social environment cause mental illness remains accurate.

A major medical breakthrough occurred in about 1816 when it was observed that a high fever could cure syphilis. This discovery promoted the naming of new diseases and hope for finding causes and treatments for mental illnesses as well.

Pinel's student *Esquirol (1772–1840) localized mania as a brain disease*, as had Hippocrates some 2,000 years before him. He rejected Pinel's theory that mania was a disease of the gastrointestinal tract. Esquirol led the *French School of Psychiatry* in the first half of the nineteenth century with achievements in public health, the use of statistics, and the design of the 1838 French legal code addressing the administration of mental health. Yet it was the English in the nineteenth century who *did away with restraints for the mentally ill.*

In 1830, the superintendent of *McLean Hospital, Boston, Rufus Wyman*, detailed one of his cases.

Case 2.1: Client of Rufus Wyman, MD

"Exultation, and depression of passion, are sometimes manifested alternately in the same individual…without disease of the intellectual powers. During the state of depression, he talks little…scarcely answers questions…goes to bed early…sleeps well…rises late…takes food regularly…is indifferent about his dress…refuses to walk, or ride, or to attend church…writes no letters…reads no newspapers… discovers no interest in any person or kind of business. He is not anxious, or distressed on any subject…he is perfectly quiet and inoffensive. After being *depressed for 2–5 weeks*, he gradually becomes more active, gay, is full of business. As a first change, he begins to smile, and answer questions; then to sit up later, sleep less and rise earlier…walks, and rides when requested. In a few days he begins to converse freely, read newspapers and play at chess. Next he calls for his best clothes…is anxious to attend church, visit everywhere, and see everybody…plans voyages…writes letters to all parts of the United States, to England, France, Holland, etc. … becomes gay…dances… sings…is irascible…offended when opposed…*passionate and violent*…tears his clothes…*breaks windows*, swears, strikes, kicks, bites, *dashes drinks in the faces of attendants*…The paroxysms of passion in various degrees are *repeated many times in a day*, from the most trifling causes, and *without malice*. In this case, *the changes from depression to exultation of passion are usually sudden, and sometimes instantaneous*. His letters are well written, his plans of voyages are judicious…When the transitions are gradual he appears, *during the intervals, quite well for several weeks, and is a kind-hearted, intelligent, agreeable man*" (Healy 2008).

This case is an example of substantial mood swings into mild to moderate depressions, full-blown manias, and periods of euthymia. The client's intellectual functions remained intact at both poles.

The French made major contributions to the concept of Bipolar in the 1830s and 1840s. In *1835, Esquirol* wrote, "One remarkable, and not uncommon transition of insanity, is from great dejection, and distress, to ease and cheerfulness and sometimes to an uncommon flow of spirits." In *1845, Falret and Baillarger* came to the same conclusions about mania and depression. Falret "...described *a circular disorder [la folie circulaire*], which expressly defines an illness in which this succession of mania and melancholia manifests itself with continuity and in a manner almost regular." In that same year, "...Baillarger formally and accurately characterized what we now know as classic Bipolar cycling when he said, 'There exists a special type of insanity characterized by two regular periods, the one of depression and the other of excitement' ... calling it '*la folie à double forme*', emphasizing that the manic and depressive episodes were not two different attacks but rather two different stages of the same attack'" (Goodwin and Jamison 1990).

At the annual meeting of the Académie de Médecine de Paris on January 30, 1854, Baillarger eloquently restated his conclusions. "There are no states which show more marked differences one from the other and more striking contrasts than melancholia and mania. The melancholic is weak and irresolute; his life is spent in inertia and mutism; his concepts are slow and confused. The manic, by contrast, is full of confidence, of energy and audacity; he deploys the greatest activity and his loquacity has no limits. It would therefore seem, in theory, that two states so opposed must be foreign to one another, and that a great distance must separate them. This is not however that which is demonstrated by observation. Indeed we see, in many cases, melancholia succeed mania and vice versa, as if a secret bond united these two diseases. These singular transformations have been often reported" (Healy 2008) (Table 3.6).

Crichton in Edinburgh, Scotland, in the mid-nineteenth century, also reported cases of melancholia, "...terminating, or at least alternating, with the state of furious delirium, having all the true character of mania."

It is curious that one of Falret's assistants, *Morel (1809–1873), in the mid-1800s* carved out from Bipolar a separate disease he called Dementia Praecox for the most severely psychotic, chronic, and dysfunctional Bipolar clients; it was renamed "Schizophrenia" in 1911. These clients resembled demented clients in dysfunctionality but retained orientation; they were younger than those with the usual Dementia of old age. Morel's decision has been a disaster for functionally psychotic clients who actually have Bipolar disorders. For details of the development of the concept of "Schizophrenia," see Sect. 3.9.

Griesinger contradicted Morel when he observed that manic-depressive/Bipolar clients could progress to chronic psychotic states with poor prognoses, simulating Dementia, meaning that no new diagnosis was needed. He helped reform and develop *German Psychiatry* to a level of international repute. *In 1842*, he *attributed mental illness to brain dysfunction* and also emphasized the client's *heredity and upbringing* as important to causation. At this time, a majority of the institutionalized mental health population suffered from general paresis (syphilis), Dementia, alcoholism, or other organic diseases of the brain that at the time were not clearly differentiated from nonorganic disease such as psychotic mania or depression. In the mid-nineteenth century, a better understanding of the differences between physical and mental disease was advanced.

For example, in *1867, Griesinger* characterized depression by *guilt, paranoia*, agitation, estrangement, and withdrawal, noting that some of his clients "*may be silent for years.*" He said *depression may change into mania or Dementia* and that suicide is a danger "even in children." He described mania as "*raving madness, recognizable by restless, impulsive behavior and incoherence of ideas…extravagant volitional states with hallucinations and ideas of grandeur…*" Griesinger's treatments included baths, opium, digitalis, prussic acid, and datura, as opposed to bleeding, blistering, purgatives, and emetics.

Morel's misconception that a new disease, Dementia Praecox, was needed to explain chronically psychotic clients won out with support later from Kraepelin (1856–1926) (only initially), Bleuler (1857–1939), Schneider (1887–1967), and many others.

Kraepelin in 1899 used the term "Manic-Depressive Insanity" (MDI), and following Morel, he initially distinguished MDI from Dementia Praecox by "… the periodic or episodic course, a more benign prognosis, and a family history of Manic-Depressive Illness" in the former disease. After 1911, *the Kraepelinian dichotomy—the concept of two severe mental illnesses*, Manic-Depressive Insanity (*Bipolar) and "Schizophrenia"*—was established by Bleuler (1911). It was not seriously challenged until the 1970s (Pope and Lipinski 1978; Craddock and Owen 2005, 2010a, b). Later in his career, Kraepelin did reverse his belief that there are differences between "Schizophrenia" and severe Manic-Depressive Insanity/Bipolar Disorder, but this reversal was too late to impact Academic Psychiatry and, therefore, psychologists, psychiatrists, and mental health workers around the world. Bleuler (1911/1950) and Schneider (1959) were heavily invested in "Schizophrenia" and the two-disease concept (Bipolar and "Schizophrenia"). They mistakenly emphasized the importance and prevalence of "Schizophrenia" over Bipolar to the detriment of many tens of thousands of clients who have been misdiagnosed with "Schizophrenia." The teachings of Bleuler, Kraepelin (his early idea), and Schneider have overwhelmingly influenced the fields of psychology and psychiatry for 100 years, teaching that "Schizophrenia" is a bona-fide diagnosis. It remains in the DSM-5-TR (2022).

Kasanin (1933) broke with Bleuler's ideas that "Schizophrenia" was the diagnosis in all cases of severe mental illness, when he associated "Schizophrenia" with Bipolar in psychotic clients with a full complement of Bipolar symptoms. He initiated the new diagnosis of "*Schizoaffective Disorder*" for these psychotic Bipolar clients. His paper (1933) was a brave step away from the dominant canon that the occurrence of psychosis demands the diagnosis of "Schizophrenia" regardless of Bipolar symptoms.

Bipolar began to be separated from Unipolar (UP) depression only by the mid-twentieth century. *Bipolar* was formally canonized in *1979 when Leonhard differentiated Unipolar from Bipolar Mood Disorders* (Tables 3.1 and 3.2). The DSM III reflected this refinement (APA 1980). Dunner (2017) *distinguished Bipolar I from Bipolar II* while at the NIMH. Bipolar II was finally recognized in the DSM IV in 1994 (APA 1994).

An important point to be taken from the history of Bipolar Disorder is the linkage of severe episodes of either mania or depression with some clients' psychosis, paranoia, chronicity, and deterioration to a Dementia-like state. Specht (1905), even before "Schizophrenia" was named, believed that chronic mania, leading to cognitive deterioration, was common. Documenting Griesinger's and Specht's early observations, NIMH studies with long-term follow-up of Bipolar clients show that initially classic cycling clients can deteriorate to a persistent psychotic depressive state without remission (Carlson and Goodwin 1973; Evans 2000; Goodwin and Jamison 1990, 2007; Post 1992). Others have also recorded chronic paranoid psychosis in Bipolar clients (Abrams et al. 1974; Swartz and Shorter 2007; Lake 2008a, b, c, d) (Table 3.8). See the case of Mr. S. T. (Sects. 1.3 and 3.9; Case 1.1).

Another important point to be taken from this 2,000-year history of manic and depressive cycling individuals is the consistency of the descriptions of symptoms. Such a consistency and uniqueness of signs and symptoms over such an extensive period of time described in detail by a wide variety of mental health workers from around the world strongly supports the scientific validity of Bipolar as a bona-fide disease (Sects. 3.2 and 3.9; Table 2.1).

The treatment for Bipolar clients through the centuries has at times been brutal. Torture and even execution were common in the Dark Ages when the mentally ill were considered to be witches or possessed by the devil. Multiple other brutal treatments such as frontal lobotomy were used to treat severe mental illness into the mid-twentieth century (Table 2.2).

2.2 Bipolar Is Common

> "As many as *one of every 20* people in the US will suffer an episode of mania or hypomania, recognized or not, in their lifetimes and thus have Bipolar. Many will seek therapy. Among psychotherapy clients, as many as one in 10 or more may have Bipolar." (Lake 2022)

Bipolar is *more common* than previously recognized. Recent 12-month prevalence figures of Bipolar from the National Institute of Mental Health (NIMH) and the Harvard National Comorbidity Survey-Replication (NCS-R 2017) are around 2.7% of adults living in the United States; *lifetime prevalence is 3.9–4.4%*. These figures contrast with quotations of 1% lifetime risk only a few years ago, but they are still likely to be low (Gold and Sylvia 2016).

The average Bipolar individual suffers with episodes of mania for 10 years before receiving an accurate diagnosis and proper management. Many Bipolars are unsure if they have it or, more likely, are sure that they do not and go uncounted. Also uncounted are homeless and incarcerated undiagnosed Bipolar individuals. According to Torrey et al. (2010), there are more than three times as many seriously mentally ill persons primarily with Bipolar in jails and prisons than in hospitals. For example, Kemp et al. (2008) find that *30% of men* in a Cleveland, OH, prison had previously undiagnosed and untreated Bipolar.

Among clients diagnosed with UP or MDD, as many as 50% will subsequently incur a manic episode. They will actually have had Bipolar depression and never MDD. If the hypomania is mild, their Bipolar may never be recognized (Fig. 3.1, Curve E).

More than 50% of Bipolars have one or more comorbid medical diagnoses that may mask the presence of Bipolar. Another source of unrecognized Bipolar comes from *childhood onset Bipolar,* which, in spite of considerable controversy earlier, is increasingly recognized (Post 2009) (Sect. 2.7). Despite this, many children and adolescents with Bipolar are still unrecognized, misdiagnosed, and uncounted (Sect. 2.7).

Considering the data above, a more accurate lifetime prevalence figure could *exceed 5% of the US population*, recently estimated at 330 million. This amounts to as many as *16 million individuals in the United States* with a *lifetime Bipolar Disorder*, diagnosed or not. As many as *one of every 20* people in the United States will suffer an episode of mania or hypomania in their lifetimes and thus have Bipolar. Many will seek therapy. Among psychotherapy clients as many as one in 10 or more may have Bipolar, some unrecognized. Recognition is improving as demonstrated by the four-fold increase in the lifetime prevalence figures from less than 10 years ago.

2.3 Bipolar Is Expensive

> "…assessing the current total and excess costs of Bipolar is particularly important to better understand the magnitude of the resources that are being spent on Bipolar from a societal perspective. The results show the need for more effective treatments and practices to reduce the economic and disease burdens on society." (Cloutier et al. 2018)

Bipolar, the *fourth leading cause of disability worldwide*, constitutes a major expense (Harrison et al. 2018). Bipolar clients have substantial *direct health care costs* that include emergency department (ED), inpatient and outpatient medical, psychotherapeutic, and pharmacological treatments. Estimates of medical costs of Bipolar include the high rate of attempted and successful suicides and increased comorbidities with multiple medical diseases. *Direct nonhealth care costs* take into account Substance Use Disorder–related expenditures, such as costs connected with motor vehicle accidents, and those associated with the criminal justice system, such as property and personal losses incurred by victims of violence and crimes perpetrated by intoxicated Bipolars. *Indirect costs* involve those related to productivity loss from unemployment, incarceration, reduced productivity when at work, productivity loss from premature mortality from all causes, and, especially, suicide-related deaths. Also caregiving costs for Bipolar clients are substantial.

Cloutier et al. (2018) estimate the economic burden of Bipolar for the year 2015 based on that year's Bipolar I and II *lifetime prevalence of 1%* of the US adult population. The 2,477,737 Bipolar individuals cost *an average of $81,555 each per year for a total of $202.1 billion*. The major contributors include unemployment (36%), caregiving (25%), and direct health care costs (23%). Subtracting the costs in the non-Bipolar population from those of Bipolars shows an annual *excess of $119.8 billion overall and $ 48,333 per individual Bipolar client.*

Eight years later, the cost of Bipolar continues to rise because of increases in both the US population overall and in the numbers of diagnoses of Bipolar. Undiagnosed and misdiagnosed Bipolar individuals add additional uncalculated costs (Sect. 2.2). A calculation using a 5% lifetime prevalence instead of 1%, and a US population of about 330 million shows that some *16 million individuals may now suffer with Bipolar.* These updated figures and Cloutier's calculations suggest a more realistic total annual cost for Bipolar in the United States is over a *trillion dollars*. Beyond fiscal costs, the emotional cost burden of Bipolar is enormous.

2.4 Bipolar Is a Genetic Disease of the Brain

> "Mental illnesses are brain diseases. Based on biomedical research, there is absolutely no justification for separating out mental disorders from other serious brain disorders. They are brain diseases just as a stroke or brain tumor is a brain disease." (Steven Hyman, past Director, NIMH, 1996–2000)

Now recognized as *dynamic*, the brain is the most complex organ in the body, encoding memories and regulating thoughts, emotions, cognition, judgement, mood, behavior, circadian rhythms, and Bipolar. "Maladaptive maturation of the brain underlies mental illness. Genes and external factors interact from conception on to instruct this maturation process toward more or less illness risk" (Erwin and Weinberger 2022). The translation of genetic studies of psychiatric disorders is needed for clinically actionable information to transform diagnostics and therapeutic interventions (Brennand 2022).

Bipolar brains differ structurally from the brains of non-Bipolar individuals; specific brain areas implicated for such differences include the *medial prefrontal cortex* and the *limbic system, which* contains the *hippocampus, amygdala, and anterior cingulate gyrus*. Neuronal activity in the *prefrontal cortex regulates judgement, decision-making*, logic, the distinction between *right and wrong,* and the understanding of *consequences* based on past experiences. The *limbic system* generates *emotion, motivation*, memory, fear, *reactivity, and impulsive behavior*. All are intimately involved in bipolarity. Progressing episodes of Bipolar and recurrent depressions are associated with reduction in gray matter volume, an index of neuronal loss, visible as *shrinkage of the prefrontal cortex* and the temporal lobes, while the limbic system in mania experiences an *excessive increase in neuronal activity*.

This suggests that there is a reduction in adaptability to new circumstances, judgement, the appreciation of consequences, and a loss of normal balancing of mood and behavior. Greater limbic function with decreased prefrontal activity results in increased emotions, reactivity, and impulsive behavior with less judgment and consideration of consequences based on diminished prefrontal cortex regulation. This causes impulsive decisions and behavior with more potential for negative outcome, compatible with mania.

In addition to structural differences, there are also differences in brain function between Bipolars and non-Bipolars that correlate with the structural abnormalities shown in brain imaging during subjects' responses to emotional facial expressions presented under standardized testing circumstances. Bipolar clients made over twice as many mistakes interpreting facial expressions as did subjects without a Mood Disorder, suggesting that Bipolar clients use their *medial prefrontal cortex* less effectively than non-Bipolar subjects when making decisions under time pressure. This brain area, known to *inhibit impulsive action, is reduced* in volume and underactive in Bipolar even during euthymia. These functional data confirm the structural abnormalities and lead to the conclusion that *Bipolar brains generate more emotion and regulate it less.*

Family, twin, and adoption studies documenting Bipolar as gene-regulated and, therefore, a physical disease show that Bipolar is among the *most heritable* of psychiatric diseases. There are estimates that between 60% and 85% of that heritability is due to genetic factors rather than environmental influences. Although genetic, Bipolar is not partial to sex, race, age, ethnic group, social class, or financial status. Bipolar cosegregates with intelligence, success, Substance Use Disorders, and other medical conditions.

Lifetime Bipolar incidence in the general population is about 5%, but if a first-degree relative has it, chances double to about 10%. Offspring of one biological parent with Bipolar have a 15–30% chance to develop either a Bipolar or a Unipolar illness. If both parents have Bipolar, the risk increases to 50% or more. When an *identical twin* has Bipolar, the co-twin has a *40–70% chance of developing Bipolar* (Fig. 2.1). Monozygotic concordance is not 100%; therefore, environmental factors, especially in early childhood, and client habits such as substance use are involved but not predominant.

CONCORDANCE OF MONO- AND DIZYGOTIC TWINS IN MOOD DISORDERS (Faraone and Tsuang, 1987)

	#STUDIES	#MZ PAIRS	%MZ CONCORDANCE	#DZ PAIRS	%DZ CONCORDANCE
UP PROBAND	4	50	42	53	13
BP PROBAND	8	117	69	263	23

Fig. 2.1 Concordance of mono- and dizygotic twins in Mood Disorders (Faraone and Tsuang 1987)

The concordance of 69% in monozygotic (MZ) twins confirms that Bipolar is genetically regulated and therefore a biological condition. That the concordance is not closer to 100% suggests some environmental input to the heritability of Bipolar.

Despite the fact that Bipolar aggregates in families, no specific genetic model has been identified. Bipolar does not fit a single-gene model; instead, hundreds of different genetic variants of small effect size contribute to susceptibility. Over 226 genes appear to be involved in this polygenic risk, with multiple different combinations of these genetic influences potentially causing overlapping phenotypes or symptoms of Bipolar from mild to psychotic. In contrast, a recently identified gene, AKAP 11, is the first found to have a large effect on Bipolar risk, raising the risk several-fold (Palmer et al. 2022).

The genetic code informs the structure, function, and timely expression of proteins, which are the basic building blocks of the cell machinery. Now under investigation are brain gene changes in Bipolar clients that are involved in the expression of proteins implicated in synaptic function that regulate mood, emotions, judgement, and behavior. Efforts to identify specific susceptibility genes that coordinate biological processes involve the study of how "silent" genetic loci influence the expression of other genes. The genetic candidates under consideration code for receptors, enzymes, transporters, neurotransmitters, and additional molecules.

The *Encyclopedia of DNA Elements (PsychENCODE) Consortium* was established in 2015 using some $50 million from the National Institute of Mental Health (NIMH) with the goal of linking genes, molecules, and their regulatory elements to human behavior. This multidisciplinary team of investigators involves scientists from multiple research institutes working to characterize the spectrum of genomic elements active within the human brain throughout the lifespan. The goal is to clarify the roles of such genomic elements in neuropsychiatric disorders, including Bipolar (PsychENCODE Consortium 2018).

Studies on more than *2,000 normal human tissue bank brains* focused on 16 brain regions. To trace healthy molecular brain development, *seven prenatal brains between five and 27 weeks after conception* along with brains from newborns to 64 years of age have been studied. Comparisons with *tissue bank brains from Bipolar clients* have revealed multiple sites of DNA differences.

Genetic changes in the brain that cause neuropsychiatric disorders can occur years to decades before symptoms appear. Mounting evidence shows that Bipolar Disorders begin early in life with risk emerging from both genetic and early-life environmental risk factors that may begin as early as *fetal life*. For example, Li et al. (2018) report that the greatest differences in cell types and gene expression activity that modulate neuropsychiatric disorders occur early in the womb, decrease late in pregnancy and early childhood, and begin to increase again in early adolescence. This is consistent with some of the clinical observations of Papolos and Papolos (2006) (Sect. 2.7).

Another productive strategy involves *cell culture studies*. *Human stem cells* have been "coaxed" to develop into brain organoids, which are collections of neural cell types that mimic the early stages of human brain development. In these studies, the activity of gene regulatory networks can be followed over time in fetal cortical development, which is a period that carries considerable genetic risk. Stress can challenge the plasticity of the brain and can alter the normal transcriptional profile of neurons and glia that are likely involved in the development of Bipolar.

2.5 Bipolar, Sleep, and the Seasons

> "For me, my love of winter has come with time. I…find relief in the lack of sunlight, in the coziness of a long Alaskan night…The calmness of our darkest season eases the extremes of my moods… By the end of February… my mind, aggravated and stimulated by those persistent sunbeams, will wander until mid-April when the rapid cycling and the mixed episodes will peak." (Meyer 2020)

Disturbances in sleep, the most recognized manifestation of the biological clock, and Bipolar are intimately linked. The core genetic causes of Bipolar are coupled to a dysregulation of the circadian rhythm system and the biological clock. Sleep disruption is present in all phases of Bipolar encompassing mania, depression, and euthymia. The onset of a change in sleep often predates and predicts a Bipolar episode. It is established that sleep is critically important in the complex multifactorial cause of interepisode dysfunction, adverse health outcomes, and relapse in Bipolar.

The circadian system is regulated by neurochemical processes that have a 24-hour cycle or rhythm. The *anterior hypothalamus*, specifically the *suprachiasmatic nucleus (SCN)*, contains the nerve cells that form the "*master clock*" that is responsible for regulating circadian rhythms. Lesions in the SCN in animals result in loss of the circadian rhythm. This clock is synchronized through environmental cues, primarily the number of hours of daylight. Neurons sense when it is morning and start the biological activities needed during the day. They know when it is night, turning off daytime rhythms and turning on nighttime functions such as the secretion of melatonin. The neurotransmitter *adenosine* is involved in this regulation of sleep-wake homeostasis as it increases during wakefulness. Levels differ in Bipolar clients. Secretions of melatonin and cortisol are circadian hormones that are abnormally released in Bipolar. There is ample evidence to support the conclusion that Bipolar is related to circadian rhythm disruptions.

The *CLOCK gene* is one of several known circadian genes. Animal models with an altered CLOCK gene show manic-like behaviors. Light therapy has an antidepressant effect in some depressed clients (Phelps 2014). *Sleep deprivation* has been used in treatment of Bipolar depression. A single night of sleep deprivation can sometimes bring short-lived relief. A switch rate into mania averages about 5%, which is comparable to some reports of the switch rate caused by antidepressant medications.

Additional data linking sleep and mood derive from studies of the *amygdala*, which, like the hypothalamus, is part of the limbic system in the brain associated with the regulation of emotion. In normals, activity in the amygdala increases when there is a decrease in sleep followed by increased emotionality, irritability, and easy frustration. In mania the baseline activity in the amygdala is already increased so less sleep further aggravates emotionality.

Sleep loss can initiate a manic episode, so situations such as travel across time zones, shift work, "all nighters" for exams, meeting deadlines, or partying do present risks that deserve consideration. Therapists can inform employers that their Bipolar employees on night shift risk manic episodes and that they need day shifts.

Such requests constitute reasonable accommodation under the Americans with Disabilities Act.

Because sleep apnea causes disturbed sleep and sleep loss, understanding more about it is important in treating Bipolar. Sleep apnea is characterized by breathing pauses, or periods of shallow breathing while sleeping. During these episodes there is closure of the trachea that causes a pattern of snoring that progresses from mild snoring to very loud and effortful—almost gasping—snoring, followed by a momentary wakening. Each pause or period can last for seconds to a few minutes and happens many times a night. These are usually not remembered; clients are unaware on their own. There may be a repositioning in bed and the pattern begins again (Phelps 2019). In addition to its link to Bipolar through sleep loss, those affected with sleep apnea usually experience sleepiness during the day. In children there may be difficulty in school or hyperactivity. Some Bipolar clients gain substantial improvement in their symptoms after treatment for their sleep apnea. Overweight Bipolar clients are encouraged to have themselves evaluated for this breathing disorder.

The changes in sleep during mania are most striking. *Sixty-nine to 99% of manic clients report a decreased need for sleep* and difficulties in falling and staying asleep. During mania, the decreased need for sleep coupled with paradoxically high energy and activities is unique among medical diseases. The degree of sleep disturbance affects the overall course of Bipolar, the effectiveness of its treatment, and the client's quality of life.

Bipolar depression is associated with high rates of increased sleep, time in bed, and at the same time, severe insomnia. During mixed Bipolar episodes a sleep disruption is present 100% of the time. Sleep disturbances in Bipolar persist despite mood state, including euthymia, when insomnia occurs 67% of the time. *Poor sleep associates with a worse course in Bipolar.*

Further evidence of the linkage of Bipolar to circadian rhythms derives from the association of Bipolar episodes with *changes in the seasons*, more specifically, *changes in hours of daylight. Seasonal Affective Disorder (SAD)* is a type of Mood Disorder in which depression usually occurs in late summer and fall and mania begins in late winter and spring. The regulating factor is the change in the number of daylight hours, with decreasing daylight associated with depression and increasing light, with mania. Such changes in daylight hours are exaggerated at extreme latitudes.

Case 2.2: Ms. Caren Meyer, Alaska

The case of Ms. Caren Meyer from Alaska is an example of late winter, spring, and early summer Bipolar SAD. "Every year the returning sunlight in February marks the coming of my most dangerous season, and so begins my preparation for another Bipolar spring… I have my very own Bipolar calendar…Every spring, like clockwork, the *sun returns to southern Alaska with an unnecessary force*, and with it come the *manic eruptions* that signal the end of the comforting darkness of winter... For me, my love of winter has come with time. I...find relief in the lack of sunlight, in the coziness of a long Alaskan night...The calmness of our darkest season eases the extremes of my moods... And so when February greets me with days that grow longer and longer, I begin to plan. Expectant and nervous...another spring is coming with its sharp rays of sunlight...By the end of February, I will not have much time...there will be a jolt with daylight savings in March...My mind, aggravated and stimulated by those persistent sunbeams, will wander until mid-April when the rapid cycling and the mixed episodes will peak. I will love my new-found energy for a short while, and then I will hate it, and then the loving and the hating will merge until I do not know anything but a confused, dream-like state...and so I prepare...I see my psychiatrist and my therapist and I set up appointments for regular, frequent visits...we bolster my medication...My husband tacks a heavy quilt over the curtains on our bedroom window...I set a strict sleeping schedule and commit to being indoors by the early evening... I get out my darkest sunglasses and a baseball cap...I commit to avoiding spring's evening barbecues and many outdoor activities that will extend later and later into the sunlit Alaskan night...Nearly two decades ago, when I was first diagnosed, April brought so many weeks of extreme agitation that...I could no longer separate day from night...*I became paranoid...thought I was a messiah*" (Meyer 2020). This last statement documents manic paranoia and grandiosity that has reached psychotic proportions (Sect. 3.9).

Poor sleep affects Bipolar women more than men. Women are more susceptible to relapse following sleep loss, are more likely to have insomnia, and are likely to experience more emotional dysregulation following sleep deprivation than men, possibly due to greater variability in reproductive hormones that affect circadian rhythms (Lewis et al. 2017). Poor sleep in women predicts increased severity, variability, and frequency of mania and depression (Saunders et al. 2015). *Attention to sleep quality* is important in the treatment of Bipolar, especially in women.

For this reason, *clients must chart their mood and sleep-wake schedules* daily and bring their records to every session for review and discussion. There are numerous options, from forms to be marked to apps that allow digital records. Clients will need consistent reminders (Sect. 6.4).

Normal sleep time is between 6.5 and 8.5 hours per night; short sleep time, less than 6 hours and long sleep, over 9 hours per night. Reduced sleep duration predicts mania in Bipolar clients, so in Bipolar depressed clients who begin to experience decreasing sleep duration, immediate, intensive treatment is warranted in an attempt to avoid a full-blown manic episode.

Life events and disruptions in social routine can impact circadian rhythms. A *social rhythm disruption* is a disturbance in daily routine that can involve emotions, mood, sleeping, eating, exercising, and social interactions that change patterns of brain activity tied to mood regulation. Sixty-five percent of Bipolar clients have at least one social rhythm disruption in the eight weeks before the onset of a manic episode. Circadian disruptions, especially sleep, have clear roles in the cause and maintenance of Bipolar episodes often triggering an episode. Social rhythm disruptions predict mood episode recurrence and a worse prognosis overall. They seem to lead into manic episodes more often than depressive ones. Like Bipolar, sleep disturbances also associate with Cardiovascular Disease (CVD), Diabetes Mellitus (DM), weight gain, decreased cognitive function, low work performance, and suicide.

Recognition and treatment of sleep disturbances help stabilize Bipolar. Section 6.4 discusses the importance of identifying triggers and subtle early symptoms that herald an episode. Again, sleep changes are a common trigger and sign of an oncoming episode.

2.6 Women and Bipolar

> "An episode of PPD can be an initiator of a lifetime course of Bipolar with subsequent non-delivery related MDEs and manic episodes." (Goodwin and Jamison 2007)

Bipolar affects men and women equally, but women are more subject to depression and MDD. Two types of depression specific to women are Premenstrual Dysphoric Disorder (PMDD) and Postpartum Depression (PPD). For a diagnosis of PMDD, at least five symptoms of depression must occur in the *final week before the onset of menses* and symptoms must start to improve after the onset and become minimal or absent in the week after menses. This diagnosis requires a marked change from baseline mood to include depressed mood, hopelessness, and self-deprecating thoughts accompanied by increased anxiety. In PMDD, there can be notable affective lability, sudden mood swings, and increased sensitivity to rejection. There are usually increased irritability, anger, and more interpersonal conflict. Also typical are a decreased interest in usually enjoyable activities, reduced ability to concentrate, decreased energy, changes in appetite, hypersomnia or insomnia, and bloating or weight gain. For the PMDD diagnosis, these symptoms must cause "significant distress, interference with work, school, social activities, or relationships." Therapists can make this diagnosis and successfully treat these clients with psychotherapy.

Postpartum Depression (PPD) is also unique to women. Over their reproductive lifetime, women may be most susceptible to depression after delivery. According to the Cleveland Clinic, 50–75% of new mothers experience some depression after delivery, sometimes referred to as the "baby blues." As many as 15% of first deliveries are accompanied with a much more severe Major Depressive Episode (MDE) that lasts weeks to months, warrants medication and intensive psychotherapy, and has been referred to as PPD. If a woman has had depression after her first delivery, she has a 30–50% chance of having PPD after subsequent deliveries. About 0.1% of women suffer Psychotic Depression after delivery, endangering both mother and child (Sect. 4.6). The presence of MDD or PMDD increases the risk for PPD, which associates with Bipolar. An episode of PPD can be an initiator of a lifetime course of Bipolar with subsequent nondelivery-related MDEs and manic episodes. Note that certain nonmanic Bipolar factors suggest that a PPD is part of Bipolar rather than MDD (Sect. 3.5; Table 3.11).

2.7 Children and Bipolar

> "Diagnosed early, and treated appropriately, these Bipolar children and their families can live infinitely more stable lives. The first step, then, is the [rapid and accurate] diagnosis of the [Bipolar] disorder ..." (Papolos and Papolos 2006)

> "Their explosive behavior and mood changes render family life difficult and social relationships with other children virtually nonexistent." (Post 2009)

> "There is a group of children whose entire clinical picture of Conduct Disorder [ADHD, IED, ODD] may evaporate if you treat the manic symptoms." (Biederman et al. 1996)

Of special interest to psychotherapists who treat children and adolescents, *Bipolar is best understood as a pediatric-onset illness* that can go unrecognized for years to decades. Some 30% of adult Bipolars remember the onset of their Bipolar symptoms before age 14. Mounting evidence indicates that a sizeable number of children experience first symptoms of their Bipolar Disorder in the earliest years of life, if not in utero (Papolos and Papolos 2006; Post 2009; Post et al. 2017). The existence of early childhood-onset Bipolar is no longer questioned, and its recognition and prevalence continue to increase (Goldstein et al. 2017).

Investigation is ongoing in pursuit of understanding the very early genetically regulated onset of Bipolar (Sect. 2.4). Molecular genetic studies from fetal brains and in-vitro stem cell cultures suggest that the genetically misguided dysfunction in neuronal signaling responsible for *Bipolar may occur before birth.* The clinical observations of Papolos and Papolos (2006) support this idea. They write, "Many of the mothers [of subsequently diagnosed Bipolar children] we interviewed remembered their [Bipolar] babies' excessive activity even in utero…'While my daughter was *in the womb, she kicked so hard* and so often that I had very little rest….much of the time it felt like she was in a fight…rolling and tumbling around inside of me and then, when she was born… she kept all the other babies up all night with her screaming…' [A second mother said] 'Uh oh, the baby is angry again. His kicks would last for an hour as I doubled over in pain toward the end of pregnancy…'" These pregnancies were different from these mothers' other pregnancies with non-Bipolar babies. These hyperactive children developed symptoms of Bipolar very early in their lives, if such symptoms were not present before birth.

Other examples of Bipolar behavior in the first years of life are described by Papolos and Papolos (2006). "These children [eventually diagnosed with Bipolar] seem to burst into life and are on a different time schedule from the rest of the world right from the beginning. Many are *extremely precocious and bright*…doing everything early and with gusto. They seem like *magical children*, their creativity can be astounding and the parents speak about them with real respect, and sometimes even awe: 'She started talking at eight months, walked at nine months…was speaking in complete sentences by a year…was writing small novels in second grade…acted and danced and sang way beyond her years'…[Another mother writes that her son] '…has never been a child; he always thought like an adult.'" Other more troubling characteristics of very early-onset Bipolar children are recorded: "…a child is typically triggered by a simple parental 'no'; the child goes into…a tantrum where *he kicks, hits, bites, punches, breaks things, and screams foul language*. This can go on for *three hours at a time*, several times a day, and can persist through adolescence if the child is not treated." A young Bipolar woman describes her own childhood rage: "It comes out so quickly; faster than a knee-jerk reaction. It's like electricity shoots through me…or being struck with lightning…I would throw things, smash a couple of frogs between rocks. *I was raging all the time, every day*, multiple times a day, verbally abusive, nasty, negative…" Another parent described, "the look…the pupils of the eyes dilate and the eyes become wild looking…it's feral. He looks feral when he rages…he just exudes this primal rage." Some parents are noted to have avoided buying furniture for years because it all gets broken during a manic rage "*…it's like living in a war zone*." A seven-year-old's major raging cycle is described as "…going on for several weeks, raging violently, throwing things, attacking me, throwing a chair out the window, going through a *knife drawer saying he was going to kill me*."

Detrimental to these early childhood onset Bipolars, an unacceptable percentage of cases go unrecognized or, worse, misdiagnosed because Bipolar in childhood rarely fits the DSM clinical course for adult Bipolar and because the symptoms overlap substantially with historically more commonly diagnosed childhood disorders. Differing significantly from most adult cases and thus obscuring diagnosis, Bipolar children often have more irritability, explosive rage episodes, and persistent ultra-rapid cycling that *appears chronic*. Most cycle monthly; many, called ultra-rapid cyclers, do so weekly or daily; and some, called ultradian, *cycle several times per day*. Papolos and Papolos (2006) describe their experiences: "…almost all Bipolar children tend to be *hyperactive, inflexible and oppositional, very irritable*, exhibit episodes of *explosive rage*, sometimes for hours when *…holes get kicked in walls and parents, siblings, and pets are threatened or hurt*." Some *75% of children with Bipolar* between the ages of six and 16 suffer with *intense irritability, mixed states, psychosis, suicidality, or homicidality*. "Their explosive behavior and mood changes render family life difficult and social relationships with other children virtually nonexistent" (Post 2009). These clients may be misdiagnosed. Additional symptoms common to childhood Bipolar include excessive and intense separation anxiety; super sensitivity to stimuli of all sorts; negative hyperactivity; racing thoughts; pressured speech; distractibility; impulsivity; restlessness; risk taking; interpersonal conflicts; periods of extremely "silly, giddy, or goofy behavior"; obsessive-compulsive symptoms; initial insomnia; grandiosity; hypersexuality; manipulative and bossy behavior; night terrors; vivid nightmares; fascination with gore, blood, and morbid topics; anger and violence; destruction of property; conflicts with law enforcement; Substance Use Disorders; paranoia; psychosis; and when depressed, low energy; withdrawal; low self-esteem; carbohydrate cravings; feelings of shame; neurocognitive deficits; lack of organization; absence of peer friendships; self-mutilating behavior, and suicidal thoughts (Mendez et al. 2019; Goldstein et al. 2017) (Table 2.3).

For depressed children without an obvious manic episode, a new DSM diagnosis among the depressive disorders that is limited to six- to 18-year-olds is *Disruptive Mood Dysregulation Disorder (DMDD)* (Table 2.4). According to the DSM, this diagnosis cannot coexist with Oppositional Defiant Disorder (ODD), Intermittent Explosive Disorder (IED), or any Bipolar Disorder because of substantial overlap of symptoms and behaviors among DMDD, ODD, IED, and mixed Bipolar depression especially in children with irritable depression. Like DMDD, ODD and IED diagnoses are specific for individuals under 18.

Table 2.3 Common symptoms in Bipolar children

Rapid to ultradian cycling, frequent mixed states
Hyperactivity
Inflexibility
Oppositional Behavior
High irritability, anger, explosive rage, and violence
Impulsivity
Distractibility
Racing thoughts, pressured speech
Restlessness
Risk taking
Hypersexuality
Silly, giddy behavior
Night terrors and vivid nightmares
Fascination with gore, blood, and morbid topics
Destruction of property with conflicts with law enforcement
Paranoia to psychosis
When depressed, self-mutilating behavior and suicidal thoughts

Table 2.4 DSM-5-TR diagnostic criteria for Disruptive Mood Dysregulation Disorder (DMDD)

A. Severe recurrent, verbal or physical temper outbursts which are commonly out of proportion to the situation or provocation
B. The outbursts are inconsistent with developmental level
C. The outbursts average three or more times a week
D. In between outbursts, the mood is persistently irritable or angry almost 24/7
E. The criteria above (a-d) have been present for 12 months or more without a three-month period of no symptoms
F. Criteria a and d present in two of three settings and are severe in at least one
G. Must be diagnosed initially between six and 18 years of age
H. By history, the age of onset of criteria a-e is before 10
I. No manic or hypomanic episodes for more than one day
J. The behaviors do not exclusively occur during an episode of major depression nor are explained by any other psychiatric condition
K. Symptoms are not caused by a substance or another medical condition

Modified for brevity

A diagnosis of DMDD addresses the need for a Mood Disorder diagnosis in children and adolescents without mania who present with persistent irritability and depression coupled with recurrent temper tantrums. DMDD allows for a change from the more popular diagnoses of ODD or IED to a Mood Disorder, enabling treatment with mood-stabilizing medications rather than second-generation anti-psychotic drugs (SGAs) used in ODD and IED. The SGAs have substantial adverse effects (AEs), especially in children (Sect. 6.3). The Bipolar spectrum concept applies to DMDD in children, so in cases with depressive presentations, assessing the nonmanic Bipolar markers is necessary (Sect. 3.5; Table 3.11). Psychotherapy is the treatment of choice and *lithium, valproic acid (Depakene, Depakote), and lamotrigine (Lamictal)* also have potent antidepressant properties. Sedation can be a useful side effect in such children.

Papolos and Papolos (2006) have written further discussions about the difficulty of an accurate diagnosis in Bipolar children. They address "…very disturbing findings about the misdiagnosis and treatment of early-onset Bipolar Disorder. Because of the mixed-symptom picture of these children…many appear hyperactive and are oppositional and defiant or have comorbid Obsessive-Compulsive (OCD), Anxiety [or Depressive] Disorders …most are being shunted off into these diagnostic groups without the possibility of a Bipolar Disorder diagnosis even being considered." Over 50% with Bipolar also have an Anxiety Disorder; almost 70% of children with Obsessive-Compulsive Disorder (OCD) have a Mood Disorder. The comorbidity of severe Bipolar in children approaches 70% for ODD and IED diagnoses because their symptoms overlap with those of Bipolar.

The symptoms of *Oppositional Defiant Disorder (ODD)* duplicate the symptoms of mania and *Disruptive Mood Dysregulation Disorder (DMDD)*. For example, the DSM diagnostic symptoms of ODD include "…A pattern of angry/*irritable mood*, argumentative/*defiant behavior*…often *loses temper*…easily *annoyed*…often *argues* with authority figures…" Bipolar, especially in children, and DMDD are 100% consistent with these ODD symptoms and are characterized by irritability, anger, defiance, and a low threshold for frustration.

Similar to ODD, the DSM diagnostic criteria for *Intermittent Explosive Disorder (IED)* also match up with mania and DMDD. Diagnostic symptoms of IED include "Recurrent behavioral *outbursts*…a failure to control *aggressive impulses*… *temper tantrums*, tirades…fights…physical *aggression*…not premeditated…associated with financial and legal consequences."

The diagnostic criteria of the traditional childhood Conduct Disorders are based on disease nonspecific symptoms common to more than one diagnosis. Conversely, Bipolar has shown itself to be an established neurogenetic disease of the brain (Sects. 2.1 and 2.4). Diagnosticians must exercise care in diagnosing any of the several more traditional childhood disorders that have such symptoms corresponding to Bipolar.

ADHD has been the go-to diagnosis among child and adolescent psychotherapists and psychiatrists for many decades; an ADHD diagnosis is often pushed for disruptive school children by their grammar school teachers. Data suggest that "More than half [of ADHD children] are first diagnosed by their teachers with some physicians asked to 'rubber stamp' the finding and put the student on [stimulant] medication" (Sax et al. 2003). Isaac (2001) emphasizes the symptom redundancy between children and adults with Bipolar and ADHD in his book *Bipolar Not ADHD: Unrecognized Epidemic of Manic-Depressive Illness in Children* and says "...there is a *dangerous tendency to refuse to let go of a diagnosis of ADHD*..." Geller et al. (2008) also believe that ADHD is overdiagnosed and misdiagnosed for mania and Bipolar. The rate of ADHD diagnosis jumped by more than 50% in two- to five-year-olds between 2007 and 2011, and the Centers for Disease Control (CDC) reports that 9.4% of children between two and 17 years old are diagnosed with ADHD. Some, if not many, of these children likely have Bipolar instead. Joining Isaac (2001), Geller et al. (2008), and Papolos and Papolos (2006) go further by implying that *ADHD is a misdiagnosis of Bipolar*. They report that 93% of their Bipolar children meet DSM criteria for ADHD; "...ADHD may be, for many, an early stage on a developmental path that culminates in a full-blown Bipolar Disorder." Diagnosticians must exercise care in diagnosing any of the traditional childhood disorders that have such symptoms overlapping with Bipolar (Table 2.5).

Papolos and Papolos (2006) quote Biederman to say, "There is a group of children whose entire clinical picture of Conduct Disorder (CD) [ODD, IED, ADHD] may evaporate if you treat the manic symptoms." Table 2.5 summarizes pediatric Bipolar comorbidities. As emphasized by Papolos and Papolos (2006), "...Bipolar Disorder should be ruled out before any of the stimulant or antidepressant drugs are prescribed. Instead, *mood-stabilizing drugs must be considered as a first line of treatment*..." Therapists must have a role in this process by communicating their management judgements to the client and their prescribers.

Table 2.5 Potential misdiagnoses in Bipolar children

Attention Deficit Hyperactivity Disorder (ADHD)
Major Depressive Disorder (MDD)
"Schizophrenia" (SZ)
"Schizoaffective Disorder" (SAD)
Oppositional Defiant Disorder (ODD)
Intermittent Explosive Disorder (IED)
Conduct Disorder (CD)
Antisocial Personality Disorder (APD)
Borderline Personality Disorder (BPD)
Disruptive Mood Dysregulation Disorder (DMDD)
Anxiety Disorder (AD)

Still, Charlie Popper records some subjective differences between the two: According to Popper (1996), ADHD children break things carelessly, while Bipolars do so purposefully during anger and rage. ADHD children usually calm down within 30 minutes, while Bipolar children may rage for hours. ADHD children are triggered by sensory and emotional overstimulation, whereas Bipolar children can explode when limits such as a simple "no" are set. Bipolar children report more severe sleep disturbances that include nightmares and night terrors with themes of gore and bodily mutilation. Bipolars can demonstrate giftedness in verbal and artistic skills. They have strong early sexual interest and behavior compared to ADHD children. Bipolar children can have psychotic features in contrast to ADHD children who do not. Lithium improves Bipolar but not ADHD.

A trial of lithium may be diagnostic with therapists' close follow-up after lithium is started; compliance must be monitored. These subjective differences presented by Popper could identify some ADHD children but also represent a spectrum of Bipolar severity and variability.

Rengasamy and Birmaher (2019) differentiate Bipolar from ADHD, ODD, and IED by contrasting the episodic nature of Bipolar with the persistence of the other diagnoses. Rapid-cycling children with persistent irritability appear chronic; this is less the case for adult Bipolars. Papolos and Papolos (2006) emphasize the appearance of a chronic, persistent nature to many *childhood Bipolar* cases because of their ultra-rapid cycles.

To accommodate the approximately 50% of Bipolar children and adults who do not meet strict DSM diagnostic criteria, a diagnosis of *Bipolar Disorder-Not Otherwise Specified (BP-NOS)*, has been used. More recently, the DSM-5 (2013) and the DSM-5-TR (2022) have dropped this diagnosis and refer to these clients as having *Other Specified (OSBD)* or *Unspecified Bipolar Disorder (USBD)*, further complicating the diagnostic schema. Some therapists still use BP-NOS because years of research have used this terminology.

BP-NOS/OSBD/USBD in children can be severe. Such clients are highly impaired, certainly as severely ill as those with Bipolar I and Bipolar II. They take longer to achieve stabilization and show similar rates of dysfunctionality, psychosocial impairment, and suicide attempts and have rates of positive family histories for Bipolar similar to those with Bipolar I or Bipolar II (Birmaher et al. 2009a, b). Further reiterating the severity of BP-NOS/OSBD/USBD is that as many as 40% convert to Bipolar I or Bipolar II by adolescence and early adulthood. Like adults, approximately 25% of youth with Bipolar II will convert to Bipolar I and incur more severe and more frequent manic episodes. The conversion rate is higher in those with a family history positive for Bipolar. Psychotherapists can institute mood charting and other life changes to modify episodes such as increasing the number of therapy sessions and recommending certain life and medication changes in collaboration with the client and the psychiatrist (Sects. 6.2 and 6.4).

When psychotic symptoms occur in childhood Bipolar Disorder, once street drug use, medication, and medical/surgical causes are eliminated, the therapist can conclude that the psychotic symptoms are due to a severe Mood Disorder, either psychotic mania or depression. In this author's opinion, there is no consideration of

"Schizophrenia" or "Schizoaffective Disorder" because these are misdiagnoses of a severe, psychotic Mood Disorder (Lake 2012; Sects. 3.7 and 3.9).

When a new client presents with a diagnosis of "Schizophrenia" or "Schizoaffective Disorder," gently explore these diagnoses only after establishing a therapeutic relationship. Such clients and their parents or guardians can be reluctant to give up these diagnoses because of disability status.

Another obstacle to a Bipolar diagnosis is the resistance to give up a diagnosis of ADHD for Bipolar because the stimulants, often sought for their stimulant effects, will be discontinued. Also the successful function in some hypomanic Bipolar II children obscures the benefits of treatment and can cause families to avoid seeking help. Other factors that contribute to this delay in recognition of Bipolar in children include the following: The early child literature discounted the existence of Bipolar in children. More popular disorders are diagnosed, such as ADHD, ODD, and IED. Comorbid diagnoses, both medical and psychological, can confuse the differential diagnosis. Some of the medical comorbidities that can present with symptoms of mania or depression include Hypo- or Hyperthyroidism, Substance Use Disorders and others discussed in Sects. 3.6 and 3.7 (Table 2.5).

These diagnostic challenges result in an average time of about 10 years between actual onset of Bipolar symptoms and their ultimate accurate diagnosis and treatment in both children and adults. Moreover, for each year of untreated Bipolar, children have a 10% lower likelihood of full recovery (Lish et al. 1994). Many of these clients with undiagnosed Bipolar will have been mismedicated with stimulants for ADHD or antidepressants for depression or antipsychotics for ODD and IED in the interim. Based on Post's research at the NIMH that stimulants and antidepressants cause kindling or sensitization of the brain and promote Bipolar recurrences, this is a tragic oversight. Reducing the severity of the course of Bipolar depends upon early recognition and treatment to inhibit kindling (Post 2009).

Most Bipolar children, especially Bipolar II, first present with major depression and risk being misdiagnosed with MDD or DMDD and mismanaged. As in adults with MDD, about 50% of depressed children diagnosed with MDD will eventually be rediagnosed with a Bipolar Disorder. Bipolar children misdiagnosed with ADHD or MDD are treated with stimulants and antidepressants that switch about 5% of such children into mania, some to a manic psychosis with paranoia and violence that increase the risk of hospitalization, the rate of cycling, and suicide. Faedda et al. (2004) find that *58%* of initially misdiagnosed Bipolar children and adolescents switched to mania after stimulant or antidepressant therapy.

Aids in diagnosing Bipolar in youth are symptom rating instruments that include the Kiddie Schedule for Affective Disorders and Schizophrenia for School-Age Children, the Child Mania Rating Scale, and the General Behavior Inventory (Sect. 5.4). In addition to use of such instruments and the initial assessment, accurate clinical diagnosis involves collaboration with parents, teachers, and peers when possible in addition to the children themselves. Especially difficult is the assessment for subtle past episodes of hypomania in cases presenting with depression, making parents' input critical.

Further understanding of childhood Bipolar presentations is helped by the estimate that about 40% of the average pediatric Bipolar client's time is spent in euthymia, 35% in depression, and about 25% in mania, with a possibility of frequent cycling among these three states. For example, the *two-year relapse rate* after recovery from a Bipolar episode is *65–85%*. For Bipolar youth in general, a recurrence typically comes 20 to 45 weeks after the end of the last episode (Miklowitz et al. 2014; Birmaher et al. 2009a, b). Mendez et al. (2019) have developed a "risk calculator" to predict recurrences in Bipolar youth. Relapses can be predicted within six months with an accuracy of 72% and an 82% accuracy within five years. Over half of the recurrences are depressive episodes, and about 25% are manic, hypomanic, or mixed episodes.

2.8 A Defective Brain Selective-Attention Filter in Bipolar

The concept of a brain selective-attention filter defect in Bipolar can help with understanding the source for the broad spectrum of Bipolar symptom severity, especially thoughts and speech (Sect. 3.3). Experimental models, including Broadbent's filter theory and various cognitive neuroscience techniques in mentally ill clients, have focused on selective attention and its malfunction (Driver 2001; Politis et al. 2004; Olincy and Martin 2005).

The human brain possesses the ability to selectively process incoming information. Attention is part of this processing and is a multidimensional construct. Selective attention refers to those mechanisms which lead consciousness to be dominated by one thing rather than another (Driver 2001). Stimuli come from all five senses and myriad internally generated thoughts and ideas. Partly under voluntary control, partly subconsciously, and partly dependent on the predetermined stimulus salience for each individual, most stimuli are blocked while others are prioritized and processed more thoroughly.

Selective attention appears to govern an initial filtration process that is linked with a prioritization mechanism before stimuli reach consciousness. Those stimuli that reach consciousness are the basis of thoughts, verbalizations, emotions, and actions. The filter/prioritizer enables one to screen out and avoid attending to extraneous distractions during a conversation or other focused activity, such as an initial diagnostic interview. Although there is individual variability in what is likely to attract or distract one's attention, stimuli indicating an emergency or a life-threatening situation are universally given priority in euthymic individuals. For example, the sudden smell of smoke appropriately overrides most conversations (Fig. 2.2). By contrast, at a ball game, depending on their individual interests, a home run or touchdown might appropriately distract some from a serious discussion while others are appropriately oblivious to a score and continue their conversation, all depending on each individual's unique selective attention settings.

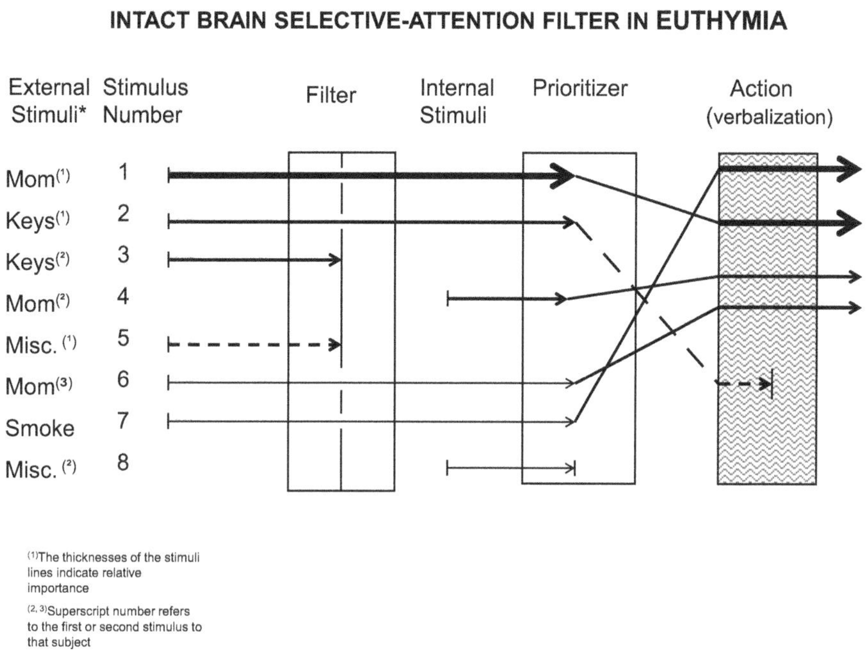

Fig. 2.2 Intact brain selective-attention filter in euthymia
Three areas of CNS data processing are denoted by three boxes representing the state of euthymia. The examples of the stimuli used in the figure are hypothesized and extended from an actual interview of a client during a student case conference (see Sect. 2.8). External stimuli appear to meet a filter that eliminates trivial data (first box) in euthymia while most or all stimuli pass through the filter in mania (Fig. 2.3). More stimuli may be stopped at the filter in depression. Internal stimuli are shown but their filtration is not indicated in the figure.
A second data processing mechanism is represented by the second box and is likely a prioritizing function that can rearrange the importance of stimuli, diminishing or exaggerating attention to incoming data. The time elapsed during processing of the interview material differs between mood states. In euthymia, the eight stimuli take about 10 minutes; the 10 stimuli in mania, two minutes, and the five steps in depression, 10 minutes.
In euthymia, the psychologist's questions about "Mom" are prioritized and are not overridden by the "Keys" (neither "Keys" stimulus 1 or 2) or by miscellaneous stimulus 1 or 2. The first "Keys (1)" stimulus is impactful enough to pass the filter but is shown as downgraded by the prioritizer function and there is no action or verbalization. A second "Keys (2)" stimulus when the professor picked up his keys does not pass filtration. Internal stimulus 4 ("Mom 2") and external stimulus 6 ("Mom 3" as in the form of another question from the interviewer) are appropriately prioritized and verbalized in continuing with the interview. The dialogue about the topic of "Mom" may last 10 minutes and is only overridden by a hypothetical stimulus, "Smoke." The sight or smell of smoke (stimulus 7) readily passes the filter and is highly prioritized. Note increase in line thickness and elevation to the top of the "action" box, receiving immediate attention above the "Mom" topic.

Bipolar is a disorder of thinking, as demonstrated by its manic symptoms of distractibility and disorganized thoughts, speech, and behavior. In worsening mania, the selective-attention filter/prioritizer function appears to become more porous forcing attention to inappropriate and unrelated stimuli that steal focus away from important data which are lost in a flood of irrelevant data (Fig. 2.3). This defect is described by Bipolar clients as racing thoughts and a flight of ideas. As the porous manic filter allows more and more extraneous stimuli through to consciousness, the manic brain cannot prioritize them but seems to attempt to attend to each idea and say them all, jumping from one to another seemingly unrelated idea.

The rate and degree of impairment of manic thoughts and speech is an index of the severity of the breakdown in selective attention, information processing, and the intensity of the mania. A mild increase in filter porosity associates with a mild increase in the rate of speech and the possibility of fame and success. A client, Ms. H. L., said her best friend whom she talked to weekly has repeatedly been the first to recognize her increased rate of speech that heralded a manic episode. She did not experience any change herself (Sects. 4.2 and 4.4; Case 4.6).

In mild mania, the defect in the filter/prioritizer system is minimal, promoting acceptance of new-edge ideas that might normally have been blocked but hold promise for breakthrough ideas and success. Hypomanic clients typically become more productive in their areas of endeavor as well as in additional ventures. History demonstrates that some of the most famous, productive, accomplished, and successful writers, composers, musicians, artists, designers, media personalities, generals, religious leaders, scientists, and politicians have both suffered and benefited from Bipolar Disorders (Table 1.1).

When the filter/prioritizer mechanism becomes less discriminating and more porous, the manic brain struggles to deal with the overwhelming overload of unprioritized stimuli. Speech becomes more rapid, nonstop, intrusive, and dominating, overriding input from anyone else. The distractibility becomes disruptive, judgement fails, and the quality of productivity dccrcascs. Kanyc Wcst's rccordcd spccch at his visit to the White House suggests a filter porosity that is characteristic of moderate to severe mania in Bipolar Type I. He had many bizarre ideas but in the past some of them have become major successes (Sects. 4.3 and 4.4; Case 4.19).

In moderately severe mania, multiple ventures may be undertaken with initial enthusiasm, but none completed due to an inappropriate mania-driven distractibility leading to a shift of attention to the next new activity felt to be more important. With increasing porosity, stimuli reach consciousness and demand attention even though they are tangential or seemingly unrelated to the subject of a conversation or current task. For example, during an initial diagnostic interview, a client with moderate mania may be unable to maintain focus on the interviewer's questions but instead turn his/her attention to irrelevant stimuli such as pictures on the wall, a clock, noises outside, the interviewer's keys, tie, jewelry, or hair and other inappropriate distractions that are normally blocked from consciousness in non-manic individuals. The interviewer's questions that govern the client's disposition are ignored. Redirection of the client may become difficult due to increasing distractibility and irritability.

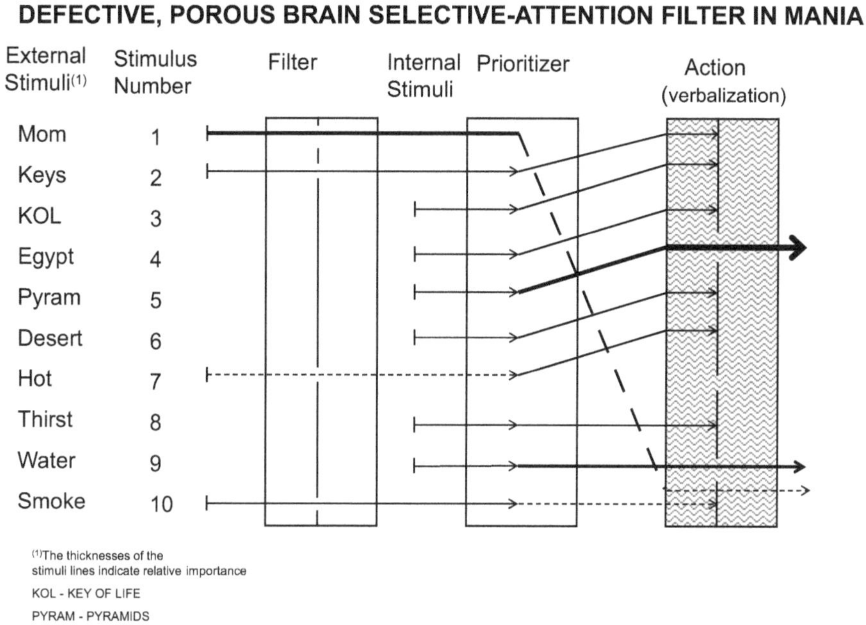

Fig. 2.3 Defective, porous brain selective-attention filter in mania
Three areas of CNS data processing are denoted by three boxes representing the state of mania. The examples of the stimuli used in the figure derive from an actual interview of a client during a student case conference (see Case 2.3). External stimuli appear to meet a filter that eliminates trivial data in euthymia while most or all stimuli pass through the defectively porous filter in mania. More stimuli may be stopped at the filter in depression.
A second data processing mechanism is represented by the second box and is likely a prioritizing function that can rearrange the importance of stimuli, diminishing or exaggerating attention to incoming data. This mechanism seems to be most defective in mania.
Internal stimuli are shown that inappropriately are all prioritized. The time elapsed during processing of the interview material differs between mood states. In euthymia, the eight stimuli take about 10 minutes; the 10 stimuli in mania, two minutes.
In mania the subject of "Mom" is inappropriately lost when stimulus 2, the "Keys", is passed through the filter and prioritized, possibly due to its being the most recent stimulus. The "Keys" idea is not verbalized because of a flurry of subsequent internal stimuli based initially on "Keys" and then on subsequent internal stimuli generated by the keys (see Case 2.3). This series of internal stimuli includes numbers 3 9. Stimulus 7 is shown as a dashed line of external input as the room may have been warm. Only 5 and 9 are verbalized. Although there are connections to each thought based on the client's report, the failure to filter and prioritize causes stimuli to come so fast and demand attention (apparently based on most recent order) that there is not enough time to verbalize all of them. An observer hears only "mom," "pyramids" and wanting water, concluding there has been a "blockage of thought." The present explanation is predicated on the core manic symptoms of distractibility, flight of ideas, and racing thoughts. Manic thought is indeed disordered.
A hypothetical but potentially critical external stimulus of "Smoke" (number 10) may pass the filter but may not be adequately prioritized in mania to receive action. "Smoke" may be quickly overridden by the next stimulus, such as "cigarettes are expensive" or "Smokey the Bear is cute." The first nine stimuli are actual thoughts of the client as discussed in the text; stimulus 10 is hypothesized. This exchange and series of thoughts might occur in as little as two minutes.

In severe mania, the brain's filter/prioritizer is very porous to inappropriate distractions. The ability to distinguish and thus to block out trivial sensory input is lost and the manic brain seems to attempt to process and vocalize myriad stimuli (Fig. 2.3). Words used to describe such thought and speech defects include extreme flight of ideas, pressed speech, tangentiality, loose associations, derailment, blocking, echolalia, clanging, punning, rhyming, word salad, speaking in tongues, and incoherence (Sect. 2.8; Cases 2.3, 2.4, 2.5). New ideas and thoughts come so fast that even speaking as rapidly as possible, a manic client may be able to verbally express only a small percentage of them. Conversely, critical stimuli may be overlooked. Rational conversation becomes impossible because what such clients verbalize is unintelligible. The clients themselves may feel in control and logical despite experiencing sensory and thought overload and seem to try to express it all as demonstrated by the cases below.

Case 2.3: Mr. D. M.

The case of Mr. D. M., a 56-year-old married male, recently readmitted to the acute inpatient unit in a psychotic state, was presented in a weekly student conference. He had carried the diagnosis of "Schizophrenia" for decades. The student reported his presenting symptoms of derailment, loose associations, blocking, delusions, functional deterioration, and gross disorganization of thoughts, speech, and behavior for over six months. The client fulfilled DSM criteria for "Schizophrenia" and demonstrated additional signs and symptoms associated with his diagnosis. After the student's presentation, the client was invited into the conference room for an interview with the attending professor. About two minutes into the interview, as the client answered a question about his mother, with a normal rhythm but a modest pressure, the professor "accidentally" knocked his heavy key chain off the table onto the floor. The client stopped talking, remained silent for about 10 seconds, and then said, with appropriate emotion, "*The pyramids are magnificent structures*." After another unusual pause, the client said, "*May I have a glass of water*?"

These appear to be textbook examples of "Schizophrenic thought blocking," described by Bleuler in 1911 as the sudden obstruction or loss of a thought during a flow of thoughts, and observed as an unusual silence followed by the emergence of a totally unrelated subject. There is no obvious association between "mother," "pyramids," and wanting water. This presentation appeared to meet all the DSM criteria for "Schizophrenia," but mania, as a psychotic Mood Disorder, had been overlooked in this client for decades.

The attending professor asked the client to try hard to concentrate his attention and explain how his thoughts had jumped from discussing his mother to pyramids to wanting water. With considerable redirection, the client was able to maintain focus enough to say that the professor's key chain hitting the floor stimulated the thought of "the key of life," leading to the idea that life began in Egypt's Nile River valley. "Egypt" brought him to pyramids and how "magnificent" they must be. His racing thoughts were going so fast that he only had time to make his "pyramids" statement but not his other thoughts leading to "pyramids." He then said that Egypt also stimulated the thought of a desert, of feeling hot and then thirsty, so he asked for a glass of water. This sequence of thoughts occurred in a matter of seconds. In his mind, his thoughts were linked and logical, but for observers, there were distractibility, racing thoughts, flight of ideas, apparent derailment, and disorganization of thoughts. This sequence may be explained by a substantial defect in the selective-attention function considered typical to mania. The client's filter/prioritizer failed to prevent his inappropriate distraction to and his processing of "keys" (Fig. 2.3). His consciousness inappropriately took up the keys so he was unable to maintain focus on the interviewer's questions about his mom and this theme was lost. The client's mind was racing to such an extent that he only had time to verbalize "pyramids are magnificent" and wanting water. Such a selective filter/prioritizer breakdown apparently allows so many thoughts to reach consciousness that there is not enough time to say them all. By the client's report, there were connections to all his thoughts, but an observer is oblivious to the connections because only about 20% of his thoughts are verbalized, and none have any relationship to the subject of "mom."

During euthymia, distraction to the keys falling to the floor would usually be blocked at the filter or given such low priority that the interview subject of "mom" would continue to hold focus appropriately uninterrupted (Fig. 2.2). In depression, exclusion of stimuli may be increased.

Some clinicians would diagnose "Schizophrenia," but in this case, upon additional inquiry, the client under discussion endorsed the DSM disease-specific symptoms diagnostic of a manic episode. The client's mom confirmed his manic symptoms. Mood-stabilizing medications were added.

Case 2.4: Mr. L. M.

An example of such manic incoherence comes from Mr. L. M., a euthymic 25-year-old Bipolar client who said that, when manic, his mind raced so fast that he was able to focus on the first letter of each word spoken by others and to "make entire [de novo] sentences beginning with each of those letters." His speech had been incoherent (word salad) and his behavior, disorganized, delusional, and psychotic, yet he said he had felt organized. He met disease-specific DSM criteria for Bipolar I, Manic, Severe with Psychotic Features.

Case 2.5: Mr. M. E.
Another extremely disorganized and incoherent 45-year-old married male, Mr. M. E., was brought to the Emergency Department (ED) by the police accompanied by his wife. He had been apprehended from the middle of a busy intersection gesturing frantically and speaking rapidly, nonstop, in a *"foreign language" or "in tongues"* to any one or no one. In the ED, he continued to speak rapidly without pause but with a rhythm, emotion, and body and hand gestures that indicated he was desperately trying to tell us something important. No English words were discernible. His affect was of extreme excitement and agitation, like he was *preaching for his life*. His wife denied that he spoke a foreign language and said he had never traveled beyond the county limits. She said that he had been in this mental state for *two days without sleep or food*. In retrospect, his initial diagnosis of "Disorganized Schizophrenia" was incorrect because he suffered from excited Bipolar I, Manic, Severe with Psychotic Features. Such a presentation can be understood as a severe disintegration in the manic filter/prioritizer function. A productive strategy in this case in the ED would have been to interview the client's wife asking the questions given in Tables 5.1 and 5.2 relevant to the diagnosis of mania. This case emphasizes the importance of considering a diagnosis of mania in disorganized, incoherent individuals observed to be "speaking in tongues" and inappropriately "preaching" on street corners.

The description of other clients' speech and behavior demonstrating even more porous filters and more severe disorganization and incoherence are detailed below. In severe psychotic mania with even more extensive damage to the filter/prioritizer mechanism, clients may only focus on words or sounds that rhyme or may only be able to say words or make sounds with no apparent relationship to one another. These disorganized and incoherent patterns of speech, called rhyming, punning, clanging, echolalia, and word salad, are traditionally associated with "Schizophrenia" and not mania, but they are classic symptoms of manic thought and speech.

In depression, all cognitive processes appear to be slowed. In an initial interview a depressed client may have difficulty maintaining focus on "mom" not because of subsequent interrupting stimuli but because of a defect in concentration and focus associated with depression. Other stimuli may be passively and inappropriately overlooked or receiving an unwarranted reduction in prioritization.

References

Abrams R, Taylor MA, Gaztanaga P. Manic-depressive illness and paranoid schizophrenia. Arch Gen Psychiatry. 1974;31:640–2.

Ackerknecht E. A Short History of Psychiatry. London: Hafner Publishing Co. Ltd.; 1959.

American Psychiatric Association (APA). Diagnostic and statistical manual of mental disorders. Washington, D.C.; 1994.

American Psychiatric Association (APA). Diagnostic and statistical manual of mental disorders (3rd Edition) (DSM-III). Washington, D.C.; 1980.

Biederman J, Faraone S, et al. Attention-deficit hyperactivity disorder and juvenile mania: an overlooked comorbidity? J Am Acad Child Adolesc Psychiatry. 1996;35:997–1008.

Birmaher B, Axelson D, Goldstein B, Strober M, Gill MK, Hunt J, Houck P, et al. Four-year longitudinal course of children and adolescents with bipolar spectrum disorders: the course and outcome of bipolar youth (COBY) Study. Am J Psychiatry. 2009a;166(7):795–804.

Birmaher B, Axelson D, Monk K, Kalas C, Goldstein B, Hickey MB, Obreja M, Ehmann M, et al. Longtime psychiatric disorders in school-aged offspring of parents with bipolar disorder. Arch Gen Psychiatry. 2009b;66(3):287–96.

Bleuler E. Dementia praecox or the group of schizophrenias. New York: International Universities Press; 1911/1950.

Brennand KJ. Using stem cell models to explore the genetics underlying psychiatric disorders: linking risk variants, genes, and biology in brain disease. Am J Psychiatry. 2022;179:322–8.

Carlson GA, Goodwin FK. The stages of mania: a longitudinal analysis of the manic episode. Arch Gen Psychiatry. 1973;28:221–8.

Cloutier M, Greene M, Guerin A, Touya M, Wu E. The economic burden of bipolar I disorder in the United States in 2015. J Affect Disord. 2018;226:45–51.

Craddock N, Owen MJ. The beginning of the end for the Kraepelinian dichotomy. Br J Psychiatry. 2005;184:384–6.

Craddock N, Owen MJ. Molecular genetics and the Kraepelinian dichotomy: one disorder, two disorders, or do we need to start thinking afresh? Psychiatr Ann. 2010a;40:88–91.

Craddock N, Owen MJ. The Kraepelinian dichotomy-going, going … but still not gone. Br J Psychiatry. 2010b;196:92–5.

Diagnostic and Statistical Manual (DSM-5-TR). American Psychological Association, 2022.

Doran AR, Breier A, Roy A et al. Differential diagnosis and diagnostic systems in schizophrenia. Psychiatr Clin N Am. 1986;9:17–33.

Driver J. A selective review of selective attention research from the past century. Br J Psychiatry. 2001;92:53–78.

Dunner D. Editorial bipolar II disorder. Bipolar Disord. 2017;19(7):520–1.

Erwin J, Weinberger Daniel R. To model developmental risk in a dish. Am J Psychiatry. 2022;179:319–21.

Evans DL. Bipolar disorder: diagnostic challenges and treatment considerations. J Clin Psychiatry. 2000;61:26–31.

Faedda GL, Baldessarini RJ, Glovinsky ID, et al. Treatment-emergent mania in pediatric bipolar disorder: a retrospective case review. J Affect Disord. 2004;82(1):149–58.

Faraone SV, Tsuang MT, Gutierrez JM. Longterm outcome and family psychiatric illness in munipolar and bipolar disorders. Psycopharm Bull. 1987;23:465–7.

Geller B, Tillman R, Bolhofner K, Zimmerman B. Child bipolar I disorder. Arch Gen Psychiatry. 2008;6(5):1125–33.

Gold AK, Sylvia LG. The role of sleep in bipolar disorder. Nat Sci Sleep. 2016;8:207–14.

Goldstein B, Birmaher B, Gabrielle A, Carlson G, Melissa P, Delbello M, Findling R, et al. Task Force Papers: the international society for bipolar disorders task force report on pediatric bipolar disorder: knowledge to date and directions for future research. In: Bipolar disorders. Hoboken: Wiley; 2017.

Goodwin FK, Jamison KR. Manic-depressive illness: bipolar disorders and recurrent depression. 1st ed. Oxford: Oxford U Press; 1990.

Goodwin FK, Jamison KR. Manic-depressive illness: bipolar disorders and recurrent depression. 2nd ed. Oxford: Oxford U Press; 2007.

Harrison PJ, Geddes JR, Tunbridge EM. The emerging neurobiology of bipolar disorder. Trends Neurosci. 2018;41(1):18–30.

Healy D. Mania: a short history of bipolar disorder. Baltimore: Johns Hopkins University Press; 2008.

Hyman S. 1996–2000 Past Director, NIMH.

Isaac G. Bipolar not ADHD: unrecognized epidemic of manic-depressive illness in children. San Jose: Writers Club Press; 2001.

Kasanin J. The acute schizoaffective psychoses. Am J Psychiatry. 1933;13:97–126.

Kemp D, et al. Screening for bipolar disorder in a county jail at the time of criminal arrest. J Psychiatr Res. 2008;42(9):778–86.

Lake CR. Hypothesis: grandiosity and guilt cause paranoia; paranoid schizophrenia is a psychotic mood disorder; a review. Schizophr Bull. 2008a;34:1151–62.

Lake CR. Disorders of thought are severe mood disorders: the selective attention defect in mania challenges the Kraepelinian dichotomy – a review. Schizophr Bull. 2008b;34:109–17.

Lake CR. How academic psychiatry can better prepare our students for their future patients: part I: the failure to recognize depression and risk for suicide in primary care; problem identification, responsibility and solutions. Behav Med. 2008c;34:95–100.

Lake CR. How academic psychiatry can better prepare our students for their future patients: part II: a course in ultra-brief initial diagnostic screening suitable for future primary care physicians. Behav Med. 2008d;34:101–16.

Lake CR. Schizophrenia is a misdiagnosis: implications for the DSM-5 and the ICD-11. New York: Springer; 2012.

Lake CR. Bipolar. London: Elsevier Academic Press; 2022.

Lewis KS, et al. Sleep loss as a trigger of mood episodes in bipolar disorder: individual differences based on diagnostic subtype and gender. Br J Psychiatry. 2017;211(3):169–74.

Li M, et al. Integrative functional genomic analysis of human brain development and neuropsychiatric risks. Science. 2018;362:6420.

Lish JD, Dime-Meenan S, Whybrow PC, Price RA, Hirschfield RM. The national depressive and manic-depressive association (DMDA) survey of bipolar members. J Affect Disord. 1994;31:281–94.

Mendez I, Axelson D, Castro-Fornieles J, Hafeman D, Goldstein B, Diler R, Borras R, et al. Psychotic-like experiences in offspring of parents with bipolar disorder and community controls: a longitudinal study. J Am Acad Child Adolesc Psychiatry. 2019;58(5):534–43. On line 2018.

Meyer C. Setting the rules for your 'bipolar calendar' as the seasons change. Bipolar mania. bpHope Blog: Dedicated to Living Well with Bipolar Disorder posted February 23, 2018; updated 2020. Captured 3/12/2018 and 2/27/20.

Miklowitz DJ, Schneck CD, George EL, et al. Pharmacotherapy and family focused treatment for adolescents with bipolar I and II disorders: a 2-year randomized trial. Am J Psychiatry. 2014;171(6):658–67.

NCS-R National Comorbidity Survey Replication 2017 available at http://www.icpsr.umich.edu/icpsrweb/ICPSR/studies/20240

Olincy A, Martin L. Diminished suppression of the P50 auditory evoked potential in bipolar disorder subjects with a history of psychosis. Am J Psychiatry. 2005;162:43–9.

Palmer D, et al. Exome sequencing in bipolar disorder identifies *AKAP11* as a risk gene shared with schizophrenia. Nat Genet. 2022;54:541–7.

Papolos D, Papolos J. The bipolar child. 3rd ed. New York: Broadway Books; 2006.

Phelps J. Light therapies for depression: circadian rhythms, natural therapies. Psych Ed. 17 September 2014. On line.

Phelps J. The biological basis of bipolar: Chapter 3 Central role of biological clock. PsychEducation.org. Captured 3/26/2019.

Politis A, Lykouras L, Mourtzouchou P, Christodoulou GN. Attentional disturbances in patients with unipolar psychotic depression: a selective and sustained attention study. Compr Psychiatry. 2004;45:452–9.

Pope HG, Lipinski J. Diagnosis in schizophrenia and manic-depressive illness: a reassessment of the specificity of 'schizophrenic' symptoms in the light of current research. Arch Gen Psychiatry. 1978;35:811–28.

Popper CW. Diagnosing bipolar vs ADHD, a pharmacologic point of view. Link 13. 1996.

Post RM. Transduction of psychosocial stress into the neurobiology of recurrent affective disorder. Am J Psychiatry. 1992;149:999–1010.

Post RM. Etiology. In: Kowatch RA, Fristad MA, Findling RL, Post RM, editors. Clinical manual for management of bipolar disorder in children and adolescents. Arlington: Am Psychiatric Publ; 2009. p. 71–131.

Post RM, Altschuler L, Kupka R, McElroy S, Frye M, Rowe M, Grunze H, et al. More childhood onset bipolar disorder in the United States than Canada or Europe: implications for treatment and prevention. Neurosci Biobehav Rev. 2017;74:204–13.

PsychENCODE Consortium. Revealing the brain's molecular architecture. Science. 2018;2018(362):1262–3.

Rengasamy M, Birmaher B. Chapter 11: Bipolar II disorder in childhood and adolescence. In: Swartz HA, Suppes T, editors. Bipolar II Disorder. Washington, DC: APA; 2019. p. 241–62.

Saunders EFH, et al. Corrigendum: The effect of poor sleep quality on mood outcome differs between men and women: a longitudinal study of bipolar disorder. J Affect Disorder. 2015;185:246.

Sax L, et al. Who first suggests the diagnosis of attention-deficit hyperactivity disorder? Ann Fam Med. 2003;3:171–17.

Schneider K. Clinical psychopathology. New York: Grune & Stratton, Inc.; 1959.

Specht G. Chronische manie and paranoia. Centralbl Nervenheilk Psychiatr. 1905;28:590–7.

Swartz CM, Shorter E. Psychotic depression. New York: Cambridge University Press; 2007.

Torrey EF, Kennard A, Eslinger D, Lamb R, Pavie J. More mentally ill persons are in jails and prisons than hospitals: a survey of the states. Treatment Advocacy Center; 2010; On line.

Chapter 3
How Do You Know It's Bipolar?

> "The diagnosis you receive affects everything from the medication you'll need to how long the therapy will take, and you shouldn't tolerate mental health care that doesn't aim for a clear diagnosis …" (Barth 2014)

> "Advances in brain neuroscience will lead to diagnostic systems … that map much more clearly onto the functions and dysfunctions of the brain." (Craddock and Mynors-Wallis 2014)

> "In all of medicine the Bipolar Disorders are unique because despite being life-long, severe mental illnesses, they associate with intelligence, success, fortune, and fame, but also with life chaos and suffering, all in the same individuals." (Goodwin and Jamison 1990)

3.1 Why Diagnose?

The value of diagnosing clients with mental health issues is again scrutinized because of the recent publication in the USA of the *DSM-5-TR* (2022). Diagnoses contribute to health care but only if accurate. Complicating accurate diagnoses among mental illnesses is the fact that as yet, the causes and pathogenesis remain uncertain, leading to diagnoses based on subjective and descriptive data elicited during an initial interview and from clinical observation rather than on objective physical findings and laboratory results. This leads to skepticism of diagnoses in mental health. Misdiagnoses are more likely in psychological than in physical diseases.

A further challenge to diagnostic accuracy is that some psychological/psychiatric diagnoses listed in the DSM-5-TR (2022) and the ICD, 11th Revision, are based on criteria that are disease non-specific, i.e., their symptoms are common to more than one disease. Some of these DSM diagnoses were initiated in the first quarter of the twentieth century when links between symptoms and diagnoses were inconsistent. With such overlaps in symptoms across different disorders, the choice of a diagnosis may depend on the personal bias of the therapist.

An exception is classic Bipolar Type I, defined by an episode of mania. The diagnostic criteria are disease-specific, including unique cycles between two extremes in

C. R. Lake, *Bipolar for Psychotherapists and Their Clients*,
https://doi.org/10.1007/978-3-031-38750-0_3

mood. Historical descriptions of such cycling have been consistent through 2,000 years (Sect. 2.1; Table 2.1). Bipolar is a scientifically established neurological disease of the brain (Sect. 2.4). An issue here is that many Bipolar clients do not present with classic symptoms so that an accurate diagnosis requires knowledge of the disorder at the extremes of its symptoms (Sect. 3.3).

Some have proposed alternatives to diagnoses (Sartorius 2015). One example is the use of symptoms or categories of mental illness described by the level of impairment or degree of disability. Craddock and Mynors-Wallis (2014) and Love (2018) outline criticisms and benefits of diagnosing clients. Criticisms include labeling, stigma, overmedicalization of sometimes normal experiences, and underappreciation of life experiences. The potential for misdiagnoses holds substantial risk for negative outcomes.

The British Psychological Society has recommended the adoption in the UK of an alternative to psychological diagnoses referred to as "psychological formulation." This is described as a joint effort between the client and the psychologist to summarize difficulties, to make sense of them, and to explain why they may be happening. Past difficulties and experiences are considered, as are the client's strengths and resources.

Supporting the use of diagnoses, an accurate one contributes to treatment decisions and allows productive communication among mental health professionals, and between such professionals and their clients. A diagnosis can also reduce stigma for clients because it provides recognition that their aberrant thoughts and behaviors are not unique, mysterious, or unexplainable, and are not due to being bad, odd, lazy, intoxicated, or having a character flaw. By recognizing that a diagnosis is common to others as well, inappropriate feelings of blame and shame are reduced.

There will be a body of knowledge and appropriate self-help material for each diagnosis that can contribute to understanding the condition. A correct diagnosis will assist clients in making best decisions about their care, informing client and therapist as to thc most useful therapeutic approach and proper medications if appropriate. Finally, a diagnosis explains and helps clients understand why they are having certain symptoms and it is a common tool which puts client and therapist on the same page with clients more likely to endorse the treatment plan.

According to Barth (2014), "The diagnosis you receive affects everything from the medication you'll need to how long the therapy will take, and you shouldn't tolerate mental health care that doesn't aim for a clear diagnosis…your diagnosis should direct the course of treatment…You'll get better more quickly and experience fewer treatment-induced side effects if you get the right diagnosis early in the treatment process…" For example, Barth (2014) notes that Bipolar clients misdiagnosed with MDD and prescribed antidepressants are subject to manic episodes brought on by these medications.

There are limitations of making diagnoses, even accurate ones. Issues of causation, the severity and pattern of symptoms, and the degree of impairment in functioning must also be considered. For Bipolar Disorder, for example, the clinician must be aware of the initial and lifetime pattern of manic and depressive episodes; the presence and history of suicidal ideations; the presence and history of psychotic features; interepisode functioning; co-occurrence of Substance Use Disorders; identification of triggering issues, including that by antidepressants; and social, cultural, and spiritual aspects of the client's life experience. The client's unique life circumstances, relationships, and personality are also considered along with the diagnosis.

Precise diagnosis in the mental health field awaits the identification of objective biomarkers that will delineate specific mental health conditions. Advances in brain neuroscience will lead to "diagnostic systems…that map much more clearly onto the functions and dysfunctions of the brain" (Craddock and Mynors-Wallis 2014).

In formulating diagnoses, clinicians use a diagnostic system that is widely accepted such as the DSM-5-TR or the IDC 11th Revision. The diagnosis may be most effectively offered tentatively and explored in collaboration with the client. When hope is offered for the diagnosis, it is more likely to be experienced more positively.

3.2 Subtypes of Bipolar: Distinguishing Bipolar I, Bipolar II, Bipolar III, Seasonal Affective Disorder, and Cyclothymia

The Mood Disorders are a most important group among mental illnesses because they are biologically grounded, common, costly, have a high morbidity and mortality, and are usually lifelong (Tables 3.1 and 3.2). In all of medicine, the Bipolar Disorders are unique because despite being life-long, severe mental illnesses, they associate with intelligence, success, fortune, and fame, but also with life chaos and suffering, all in the same individuals (Goodwin and Jamison 1990) (Table 2.1).

Mood Disorders divide into Bipolar and Unipolar; Unipolar depression is the same as a Major Depressive Disorder (MDD) (Table 3.2). MDD has only depressions and becomes Bipolar with an episode of mania. Previously Bipolar and Unipolar Disorders were considered separate but now they are thought to form a spectrum (Sect. 3.5) (Table 3.11).

Appreciating these subtypes of Bipolar helps with recognition and understanding as well as promoting productive dialogue with clients and informing treatment. There are several subtypes of Bipolar Disorders, the criteria for which are listed in the DSM and the ICD as well as in this book (Table 3.2).

Table 3.1 Mood Disorders and other mental illnesses

Mood Disorders
"Schizophrenia" Spectrum Disorders
Neurodevelopmental Disorders
Anxiety Disorders
Obsessive-compulsive and related disorders
Trauma and stressor-related disorders
Dissociative Disorders
Somatic symptom and related disorders
Feeding and eating disorders
Sleep-wake disorders
Sexual dysfunctions
Gender dysphoria
Disruptive, Impulse-control, and Conduct Disorders
Substance-related and Addictive disorders
Neurocognitive Disorders
Personality Disorders

Table 3.2 Bipolar Mood Disorders

Bipolar disorders
Bipolar – I[a,b]
Bipolar – II[b]
Bipolar – III[c]
Cyclothymia[d]
Substance/medication-induced Bipolar Disorder[a,b]
Bipolar Disorder due to another medical/surgical condition[a,b]
Other Specified Bipolar and related disorders[a,b]
Unspecified Bipolar and related disorders[a,b]
[Bipolar Disorder Not Otherwise Specified (BP-NOS; not in DSM; can account for two entries above)][a,b]

[a]Manic episodes can be associated with psychosis, i.e., hallucinations, delusions, disorganization, catatonia, paranoia

[b]Depressive episodes can be associated with psychosis, i.e., hallucinations, delusions, disorganization, catatonia, paranoia

[c]Manic and/or hypomanic episodes initially occur only after use of antidepressant or stimulant medications

[d]Cycles of mild hypomania and mild depression lasting days to weeks occurring continually for two years or more

Bipolar has been defined strictly by a lifetime experience of at least one manic or hypomanic episode but more recently less strict criteria are accepted for mania and Bipolar. There are rare cases when a Bipolar individual has only manic episodes without depression; the diagnosis is still Bipolar. In contrast, the average client with Bipolar suffers considerably more time in depression than in mania. Typically, both Bipolar and Unipolar cases cycle back and forth through episodes of baseline mood called *euthymia*. In Bipolar, the cycling is among depression, euthymia, and mania, in any order. There can be several cycles in a row of depression or mania alternating with euthymia. Both depression and mania can switch directly from one to the other without euthymia (Fig. 3.1).

A very general estimate of the percentage of time an average Bipolar I client spends in mania, euthymia, and depression is 20% mania, 40% euthymia, and 40% depression. In some severe cases, even the euthymic time can be unstable, brief, and disruptive (Fig. 3.1).

Subtypes of Bipolar include Bipolar Type I with full mania, Bipolar Type II with only hypomania plus at least one MDE, Cyclothymia with only mild cycles, Seasonal Affective Disorder (SAD) when episodes are related to the seasons, Bipolar Type III with mania triggered by medication (usually a stimulant or an SSRI), and, for cases with manic symptoms that fall short of meeting full criteria, Bipolar Not Otherwise Specified (BP-NOS). The DSM-5 and DSM-5-TR have dropped BP-NOS in favor of Other Specified (OSBD) or Unspecified (USBD) Bipolar Disorder. BP-NOS was especially used in ultra-rapid cycling children and adolescents.

In each of these subtypes of Bipolar Disorders, the swings in mood, ups and downs, must be clearly greater than those cycles seen in the non-Bipolar population (Fig. 3.1). The core characteristics of elevated or manic mood are similar across all of the Bipolar subtypes but they are distinguished from one another by the *severity of the symptoms* of mania, the *length of time* the manic or hypomanic episode lasts, and especially the *degree of life disruption* (Sect. 3.3). For example, in *Bipolar I*, the manic symptoms must persist for *at least a week*, be present 24/7, and be severe enough to cause *a marked impairment* in social and occupational function or warrant hospitalization. *Three (four if the mood is only irritable)* of the following seven symptoms are present to a significant degree and are obvious changes from usual behavior (Table 3.3).

When severe, these symptoms dictate mania and Bipolar I (Fig. 3.1, Curves F, G); when less severe, hypomania and Bipolar II (Fig. 3.1, Curves D, E); when even less severe and accompanied with *mild* chronic cycles of depression, Cyclothymia; when episodes are governed by the number of daylight hours, SAD.

An episode of *decreased need or time for sleep coupled with an increase in activities and energy* is suggestive of mania or hypomania and therefore Bipolar. Grandiosity, euphoria, or even exaggerated self-confidence beyond one's baseline are also indicators but can be overlooked because of successes and client rationalization. Mania and, to a lesser degree, the hypomania of Bipolar II involve obvious if not extreme changes from the individual's normal thoughts and behavior. The differences are discussed in more detail below.

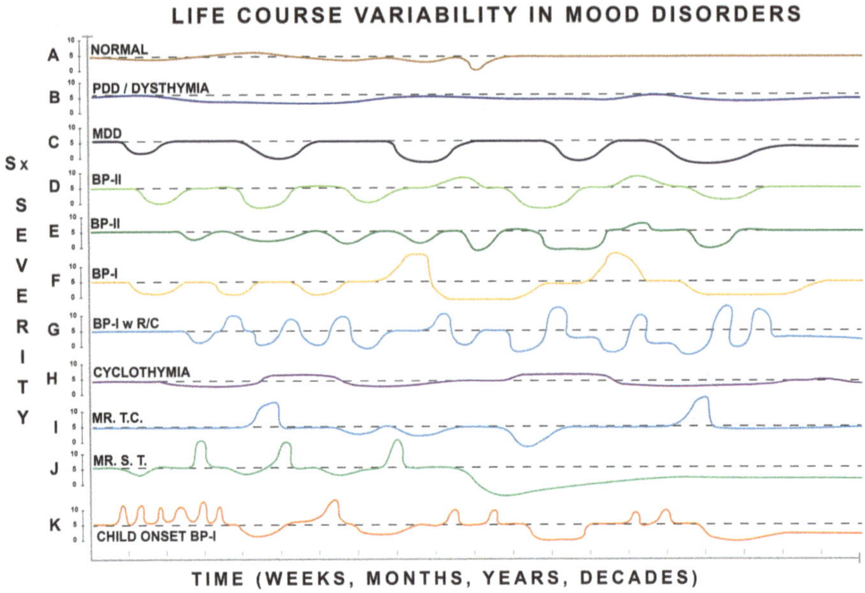

Fig. 3.1 Life course variability in Mood Disorders

The vertical axis depicts severity of symptoms. Each curve extends from 0 (most depressed) to 10 (most manic). The dashed line placed at five represents euthymia or normal mood.

The horizontal axis represents time across the life span. Each time interval represents approximately five years so that most of the cases found here begin by 15–20 years of age except "K," who has the onset of mania around five years of age.

Each curve describes a generalized case of a Mood Disorder. The curves represent mood swings into depression and/or mania throughout one's lifetime in average cases. Exceptions are the specific cases in curves "I" and "J;" "I" is the curve of Mr. T. C. (Case 3.2) and "J" is the curve of Mr. S. T. (Case 1.1).

Curve "A" represents that of a *normal* individual without Bipolar but with some minor mood swings and one moderate depression that was short lived.

Curve "B" represents *Persistent Depressive Disorder (PDD) or Dysthymia* (Table 3.10) where mood is slightly depressed for most of one's lifetime with a few returns, limited in time, to euthymia or normal mood.

Curve "C" represents Major Depressive Disorder (MDD) (Table 3.9). Throughout one's life there are multiple episodes of moderate to severe depression lasting an average of four to six months. There are returns to normal mood but never are there episodes of mood that rise above euthymia.

Curve "D" represents a variation of Bipolar Type II Disorder (Table 3.4) with more frequent and potentially severe depressive episodes accompanied by periods of euthymia and at least one mild, hypomanic episode at some point in one's life. The depressive episodes usually greatly outnumber the hypomanic episodes risking a misdiagnosis as MDD. Note the similarity of curves "C," "D," and "E" with the exceptions of the hypomanic episodes in later life in "D" and "E."

Curve "E" represents an even more subtle case of *Bipolar Type II Disorder* (Table 3.4) with only one minor hypomanic episode later in life after six moderate to severe depressive episodes.

Curve "F" represents a *Bipolar Type I* (Table 3.3). Three depressive episodes are seen beginning in childhood and recurring every four to five years until a psychotic manic episode at about 40 years old followed by a severe depression, brief euthymia, and another major manic episode.

Curve "G" represents a rapid cycling (R/C) adult case of *Bipolar Type I* (Table 3.3). Eight manic episodes and ten depressive episodes are depicted. Note: for Curve "G," the time scale is abbreviated with each time interval representing about six months so that there are four mood episodes in a year.

Table 3.3 DSM-5-TR diagnostic criteria for mania, Bipolar I Disorder

A. Distinct period for at least *one week* (or inpatient hospitalization) of abnormal and persistently elevated, expansive, or irritable mood accompanied by increased goal-directed activity, energy, and a marked decrease in need or time for sleep 24/7
B. In this period, three symptoms (four if mood is only irritable) persist to a significant degree:
1. Inflated self-esteem to grandiosity
2. Marked decreased need or time for sleep
3. More talkative than usual with pressure to keep talking
4. Flight of ideas and/or racing thoughts
5. Distractibility, tangentiality
6. Increased and excessive goal-directed activities with excessive involvement in pleasurable activities that have a high potential for negative outcomes and painful consequences such as gambling, midnight phoning, spontaneous travel, buying sprees, foolish business investments, multiple relationships, unsafe sex, excessive use of drugs and alcohol
C. Symptoms cause *marked impairment in functioning* (job, social, family) or *hospitalization* because of severity of the symptoms and dysfunctionality. These changes are very obvious to anyone knowing the client
D. Symptoms are not due to a substance or general medical condition

Modified for Brevity
Note: An episode meeting the above criteria constitutes a full manic episode and a lifetime diagnosis of Bipolar I Disorder

A differentiating factor between mania and Bipolar I versus hypomania and Bipolar II is the level of risk for harm that the client's behavior incurs. The *degree of deterioration of judgment* is important in determining the level of severity. Examples of areas of behaviors that reflect judgment from inappropriate to dangerous in Bipolar involve the excessive use of alcohol and substances, angry acting out, risky sex, reckless driving, and inordinate spending.

Changes in sexual desire are characteristic and potentially diagnostic in both poles of Bipolar. *Hypersexuality* is reported in 57% of manic clients (Goodwin and Jamison 2007). During mania or hypomania, there are increases in self-confidence with inflated self-esteem, energy, poor judgment, and intrusiveness that when coupled with hypersexuality have a potential for dangerous decisions involving

Fig. 3.1 (continued) Curve "H" represents *Cyclothymia* (Table 3.5). Here the mood cycles between very mild hypomania for months, shifting to euthymia for weeks and then into mild depression usually for months and back to hypomania when the cycle repeats usually for life.
Curve "I" represents the case of *Mr. T. C.* (Case 3.2). Mr. T. C. suffered a psychotic manic episode in college, three or four mild to moderate depressive episodes that occurred over 40 or more years, and then another psychotic manic episode at 64. Without his wife's history, he may not have been accurately diagnosed. His case represents the unusual range of occurrence of mania.
Curve "J" represents *Mr. S. T.* (Case 1.1). This is a tragic case of an intelligent successful individual who cycled in a classic manner before his cycling stopped and he deteriorated into a chronic persistent dysfunctional mildly psychotic state. His psychotic statement, "I'm doing just fine" prevented treatment. He may have died on the streets.
Curve "K" represents *child onset ultra-rapid cycling Bipolar Type I Disorder.* Note: the time interval is greatly reduced here as there are multiple episodes per day.
Abbreviations: *Sx* Symptoms, *PDD* Persistent Depressive Disorder/Dysthymia, *MDD* Major Depressive Disorder, *BP* Bipolar, *w R/C* with Rapid Cycling.

excessive and risky sexual behavior. Such behavior that increases the risk for one's life is consistent with Bipolar Type I. These hypersexual manic clients may rush into sex without considering consequences. They are more willing to experiment; to have unprotected sex multiple times per day with multiple partners; and to engage in extramarital affairs, excessive use of pornography, or masturbation. Negative consequences include STDs, broken marriages, broken hearts, jobs lost, and hours lost to masturbation or searching for a sexual partner. The following is an example of substantial risk-taking by a successful professional and mother with a Bipolar I diagnosis.

Case 3.1: Ms. C.S., RN and Mother of Six

Ms. C. S., a successful 45-year-old, college-educated RN and mother of six, became hypersexual during her manic episodes. She described putting her kids to bed, putting on ultra-tight short shorts without underpants, a t-shirt with no bra, and driving to the interstate after dark. She related that when there, she would find an 18-wheeler, pull alongside the cab, turn on her dome light, pull up her t-shirt exposing her breasts and signal to the driver to exit. She said that she was rarely rejected and would follow the 18-wheeler off the exit, get out of her car, get into the cab of the truck, and have sex. On other occasions she would dress the same and drive to a strip club where she would make it clear that she wanted sex. When asked about the risk to her life, she said she hoped to be killed. This is mixed mania, Bipolar Type I, Severe.

Table 3.4 DSM-5-TR diagnostic criteria for hypomania, Bipolar II Disorder

A. Distinct period of at least *four consecutive days* of abnormal and persistently elevated, expansive, or irritable mood accompanied by increased goal-directed activity, energy, and a decreased need or time for sleep 24/7
B. In this period, three symptoms (four if mood is only irritable) persist to a significant degree:
1. Inflated self-esteem to grandiosity
2. Marked decreased need or time for sleep
3. More talkative than usual with pressure to keep talking
4. Flight of ideas and/or racing thoughts
5. Distractibility and tangeniality
6. Increased and excessive goal-directed activities with excessive involvement in pleasurable activities that have a high potential for negative outcomes and painful consequences such as gambling, midnight phoning, spontaneous travel, buying sprees, foolish business investments, multiple relationships, unsafe sex, excessive use of drugs and alcohol
C. The episode is associated with an unequivocal change in functioning that is uncharacteristic of the individual when not symptomatic
D. The disturbance in mood and change in functioning are observable by others
E. Although the episode of hypomania, in contrast to mania, is not severe enough to cause *marked* impairment in social or occupational functioning or to necessitate hospitalization, there is clear dysfunctionality. The presence of psychotic symptoms defines mania and Bipolar I
F. Symptoms not due to a substance or general medical condition

Modified for Brevity

Note: A Dx of BP II requires criteria for a past or present hypomanic episode as given below AND criteria for a current or past MDE (Table 3.9)

Table 3.5 DSM-5-TR diagnostic criteria for Cyclothymic Disorder

A. Numerous periods of very mild hypomanic symptoms alternating with numerous periods of very mild depressive symptoms for at least two years (one year in children)
B. The mild hypomanic and mild depressive periods have been present for at least half of the two-year time period so that there has been no period without symptoms for more than two months at a time
C. Criteria for major depression, full mania, or hypomania are *never met* or the diagnosis is not Cyclothymia
D. The symptoms are not better explained by another psychiatric disorder
E. The symptoms are not explained by the physiological effects of a substance or another medical condition

Modified for Brevity

Note: The Cyclothymic symptoms cause significant distress or impairment in social, occupational, or other important areas of functioning

During depression, interest in sex is usually lost. This is confusing and frustrating to one's partner and warrants a sensitive discussion in therapy with the partner.

Since episodes of depression, rather than manias, usually predominate the lives of Bipolar individuals, identifying depression is an important initial step toward suspecting bipolarity. Table 5.1 offers brief screening questions for depression and for mania. If the initial results are positive, more detailed questions along with specific screening instruments will confirm the diagnosis (Sect. 5.3) (Table 5.2).

Bipolar II is distinguished by hypomania that is less severe than full mania and causes less life disruption and less risky behavior. It is easier to miss than mania and Bipolar I. The hypomania for Bipolar II must be clearly different from the client's baseline symptoms and must be present for a *minimum of four days*. Bipolar II must have at least *one lifetime MDE*. Again, both Bipolar Types I and II clients usually suffer multiple MDEs. According to Swartz and Suppes (2019), during Bipolar II depression, the risks for suicide, morbidity, and mortality are the same as for Bipolar I depression and MDD, with clients suffering equal severity of depressive episodes. They report that Bipolar II women are more likely to experience worsening menstrual cycle mood changes than those with Bipolar I or MDD. With pregnancy and delivery, women with Bipolar II are subject to a severe PPD or mixed episode recurrence.

Because of the predominance of depression and the need for only one lifetime occurrence of hypomania, a Bipolar II diagnosis is more often missed than Bipolar I. Despite successes, the lives of those with either Bipolar I or II are more chaotic than the lives of non-Bipolar individuals and they are more apt to seek psychotherapy (Tables 1.1 and 3.4).

Hypomanic symptoms of Bipolar II associate with both success and disaster (Sect. 2.1). Periods of increased focus and productivity characterize hypomania. A slight increase in severity, possibly related to a further increase in porosity of the brain's selective-attention filter system but still within the hypomanic range, allows outer-edge ideas to gain attention and possibly lead to brilliant successes. Greater filter porosity may portend poor judgments, decisions, and behaviors risking job loss, failure in school, relationship break-ups, and conflicts with law enforcement (Sect. 2.8). There can be successes even in the manias of Bipolar I especially as clients transition through hypomania into mania. There have been thousands of famous and successful people who have had Bipolar II or Bipolar I such as van Gogh (Sect. 4.3, Case 4.16; Table 1.1).

The average time that a manic episode lasts is about three months; hypomania averages a few weeks. An average MDE lasts six months. Unlike the severity of the manic/hypomanic episode, the severity of MDEs accompanying a Bipolar Disorder does not affect the diagnostic distinctions.

Cyclothymia is a difficult disease to recognize because the swings in mood are minimal to modest and can last for months. The ups are mild hypomanias, often associated with focus, accomplishments, and irritability, while the mild depressions can be borne without complaints. However, the changes in mood must exceed those in non-Cyclothymic individuals and must "…cause clinically significant distress or impairment in social, occupational, or other important areas of functioning."

Cyclothymia is a life-disruptive, chronic, persistent, lifelong but treatable Mood Disorder. It differs from Bipolar II because its highs are even milder than Bipolar II hypomania and *its depressions can only be mild, never with a Major Depressive Episode (MDE)*, or the diagnosis becomes Bipolar II. Cyclothymia associates with periods of increased enthusiasm, focus, and successes but it is not a benign condition. The DSM-5-TR diagnostic criteria for Cyclothymic Disorder are found in Table 3.5 and include the following:

There is ongoing cycling of mild hypomania and mild depression for at least two years and usually lifelong. During this two-year period, the mild hypomanic and depressive periods must have been present for at least half the time, and the cycling is never absent for more than two consecutive months (Fig. 3.1, Curve H). There may be brief periods of euthymia lasting for days or weeks interspersed with the mild hypomanias and mild depressions. Cyclothymia is treatable and clients with Cyclothymia seek psychotherapy more frequently than non-Bipolar individuals but typically do not recognize or acknowledge they have Bipolar. A trial of lithium may differentiate normal from Cyclothymic. This disorder does respond to weekly psychotherapy and mood-stabilizing medications (Chap. 6).

Seasonal Affective Disorder (SAD) is diagnosed when episodes of mania regularly occur in late winter and early spring and depressions in late summer and early fall. The change in the hours of daylight is the determining factor (Sect. 2.5).

Bipolar Type III (BP III), a more recent designation, is identified by a switch to mania or hypomania in a depressed client, given an antidepressant or stimulant medication. Typically these unrecognized Bipolar clients are misdiagnosed with MDD or ADHD and are either predisposed to Bipolar, or more likely, past episodes of mania or hypomania are not recognized and these drugs are stimulating a recurrence. The idea of *kindling* first proposed by Plater (1600) and redefined by Post (2009) postulates that Bipolar-predisposed brains may initially need an environmental stressor such as an antidepressant or stimulant to initiate a first manic episode but, thereafter, manic episodes can spontaneously occur without an outside stressor. Such switches from depression to mania may be welcomed by clients but are dangerous harbingers of rapid cycling and a worsening compared to the initial episode.

The presence of Bipolar II, Bipolar III, or Cyclothymia increases the risk for a full manic episode and a diagnosis change to a lifetime of Bipolar I. All Bipolar subtypes except for Bipolar I are provisional diagnoses because they are subject to change if a more severe episode of mania or, additionally in the case of Cyclothymia, a more severe episode of depression occurs.

Before making a Bipolar diagnosis, medications, street drugs, medical and surgical causes of manic symptoms must be ruled out (Sect. 3.7) (Tables 3.12 and 3.13). When medications, drugs, or medical conditions are thought to be causing the manic symptoms, the diagnosis is either (1) Substance/Medication-Induced Bipolar Disorder or (2) Bipolar Disorder due to another medical condition. These additional diagnoses apply to both Bipolar and Unipolar conditions.

To broaden descriptions and extend understanding of specific cases, the DSM offers specifiers and features which can be added to the Mood Disorder diagnoses, both Bipolar and MDD.

"With anxious distress" can be used in the presence of at least two of the following symptoms for the majority of days of the episode of mania, hypomania, or depression:

1. Keyed-up feeling or tenseness
2. Unusual restlessness
3. Difficulty concentrating because of worry
4. Fear that something awful may happen
5. Fear of losing control of oneself

Anxious distress associates with higher risk for suicide, longer episodes, and treatment resistance.

"Mixed states" is assigned when cases present symptoms of mania and depression at the same time. Such mixed states usually have predominant symptoms—either mania or depression—called mixed-manic or mixed-depressed Bipolar. A manic or hypomanic "mixed features" episode designation requires at least three of the symptoms of an MDE for the majority of its duration (Table 3.8). The diagnosis would be Bipolar I or Bipolar II, Manic with Mixed Features.

A depressive episode with "mixed features" requires at least three of the manic or hypomanic symptoms during the majority of its duration (Tables 3.3 and 3.4). The diagnosis here could be Bipolar I, depressed, Bipolar II, depressed, all with "mixed features." As with the "anxious distress" specifier, "mixed states" correlates with a less favorable prognosis.

"Rapid cycling" refers to the occurrence of four or more episodes of either mania or depression or both in a 12-month period in any combination or order. Rapid cycling can be Unipolar or Bipolar. "With rapid cycling" can be applied to Bipolar I, Bipolar II, or MDD. For rapid cycling MDD, only MDEs occur, never mania or hypomania. Ultra-rapid or ultradian cycling is described, especially in children, as mood changes occur daily if not hourly (Sect. 2.7).

"With melancholic features" is appropriate during an MDE of BP or UP/MDD when one of the following two symptoms is present:

1. A year with a complete absence of a capacity for pleasure
2. A lack of reactivity to usually pleasurable stimuli

In addition, at least three of the following six symptoms are required:

1. Profound despondency and despair and moroseness
2. Depression worse in the morning
3. Morning awakening earlier than normal by at least two hours
4. Marked psychomotor agitation or retardation
5. Significant anorexia and weight loss
6. Excessive and inappropriate guilt
   (Note: In MDD, this specifier of melancholic features is likely to associate with psychotic features that predict a change of diagnosis to Bipolar.)

"With atypical features" is added when the following symptoms or features predominate:

1. Mood reactivity is present when the mood brightens in response to positive events.
2. Two or more of the following are present:
   (a) Significant weight gain
   (b) Hypersomnia (sleeping 10 or more hours per day)
   (c) Leaden paralysis (there is heaviness in the arms or legs)
   (d) A pattern of interpersonal rejection sensitivity that results in significant social and occupational impairment

"With psychotic features" denotes the presence of hallucinations or delusions at any time during the episode. In MDD, psychotic features predict a diagnosis change to Bipolar.

"With peripartum onset" is used when mood symptoms occur during pregnancy or in the four weeks following delivery (Sect. 2.6).

3.3 The Wide Spectrum of Bipolar Characteristics

Diagnostic confusion in Bipolar clients derives in part from the challenge of recognizing the very wide spectrum of severity of symptoms from mild Cyclothymia to the overwhelming predominance of mood-incongruent, bizarre psychosis. Also confusing are the variabilities in course, cycle length, and outcome. Diagnostic mistakes are more often made at both ends of the symptom severity spectrum, so understanding Bipolar at its extremes enables better recognition and management (Chap. 4).

Rate of speech is an observable symptom in Bipolar that varies from a mild increase to non-stop and unintelligible; it is a clinical index of the severity of mania. The rate of speech in emerging hypomania may be slightly pressed and may be barely noticeable by others except for close contacts who talk with the client several times a week (Sect. 4.2; Case 4.6). There is a direct relationship between an increasing flood of thoughts and rate of speech from barely noticeable to incomprehensible word salad or speaking in tongues and the severity of the mania (Sect. 2.8; Cases 2.3, 2.4, and 2.5). This change seems to be regulated by an increasing porosity of a selective attention filter in the brain (Fig. 2.4). Severely depressed clients can be mute.

Activities range from minimally increased with increased productivity all the way to a frenzied state of purposeless hyperactivity (Sect. 2.8; Case 2.5). At the mild end, with increased confidence, ideas, energy, and drive, breakthrough successes are possible with fame and fortune gained (Sect. 4.3). With just a bit more filter porosity, too many stimuli reach consciousness and the manic brain is unable to prioritize them. This is observable as distractibility that takes a client inappropriately from one endeavor to the next before the last task was finished, so nothing is completed despite the potential for some successful projects (Sect. 2.8; Case 2.3). Finally the mind is so overwhelmed with incoming data that the client is dysfunctional (Sect. 2.8; Case 2.5). *Judgment* also decreases as mania progresses. In early hypomania, a slight decrease in judgment can allow for the acceptance of ideas that would have been rejected in euthymia but hold substantial potential for success. With worsening mania, healthy judgment is lost, and fully manic clients make terrible decisions sometimes with life-threatening consequences (Sects. 4.3 and 4.4).

The *age of onset* of Bipolar varies widely from in utero or infancy to the sixth or seventh decade of life. In addition to the wide disparity in severity of symptoms, judgment, and age of onset, other spectrums of divergency that confuse a Bipolar diagnosis are *cycle length*, *chronicity of course*, and *levels of achievement*, from CEO to living on the street. The discrepancy between dysfunctionality and success can be extreme and can occur in a single client.

In most cases, there are subtle signs of mania that increase in number and build in intensity during the days and weeks before a full manic attack. Therapists can help their Bipolar clients by emphasizing their clients' charting and self-recognition of premorbid symptoms that herald for them a manic or depressive episode (Chap. 5 and Sect. 6.4). In contrast, mania can have a rapid onset with a switch from months of normal mood to mania over night.

A first manic episode occurring after 60 years of age is more likely missed or misdiagnosed than a first episode before 60. Since Mr. T.C. denied any history of past episodes of mania or depression, Ms. T.C.'s input helped confirm the correct diagnosis, although his symptoms were classic.

The *course of Bipolar* rarely can consist of manic episodes without depressions; more common are five or more depressions to one mania. The frequency of episode occurrence, as measured by the cycle length which is the time from the start of one episode to the start of the next, also diverges extensively. There are cases of only one or two manic or hypomanic episodes during one's lifetime versus episodes monthly. An episode of major depression (MDE) can last days to several years to a decade or more with an average of six months. Manic episodes can last from hours in children to days, weeks, or months, or more in adults; average is three months. Usually a cycle is measured in months but can be as long as years or as short as minutes to hours in ultra-rapid cycling children (Sect. 2.7). In some adult cases, there can be decades of euthymia between episodes causing clients to be more likely to deny the Bipolar diagnosis and stop their therapy (Sect. 3.3, Case 3.2).

Case 3.2: Mr. T. C., Businessman

One end of the spectrum of episode occurrence is demonstrated by the case of Mr. T. C., who was a 64-year-old successful business and family man. He played competitive tennis at a 4.5 level three times a week. Normally a quiet, soft-spoken gentleman, he did not drink excessively or use street drugs. At 1:30 p m on a bright summer Sunday afternoon, he was at his club and on court number 1, playing singles with his regular Sunday game and close friend of 40 years. Within two games, it was clear that something was wrong with Mr. T.C. He was transformed by his long-dormant Bipolar into a loud, cursing, racket-throwing, intrusive, obnoxious, angry if not psychotic menace. After he hit the three new balls over the fence, cursing loudly and angrily accusing his opponent of cheating, his friend walked off court in disbelief. Mr. T. C. stormed to his car and squealed out of the parking lot. His wife drove him to the Emergency Department (ED) where the on-call psychiatrist diagnosed Bipolar Type I, Manic, Severe with Psychotic Features. He was admitted to the locked ward. Upon admission, he was unaware of his behavioral changes. He justified his fury saying that his opponent and friend had "cheated me blind." He denied any history of Bipolar episodes. His history, obtained from his wife, revealed several brief, mild, depressive episodes over 45 years and one manic episode in college that involved the police and caused him to drop out for one semester. Lithium had been prescribed, but he had discontinued it after a few months.

The case demonstrates one end of the pattern-of-recurrence spectrum, with only two manic episodes over 45 years. Including his episodes of mild depression, he may have suffered as little dysfunctional time as two months over his 64 years, but his manic symptoms on both admissions were severe with psychotic features. Bipolar can start abruptly, without warning, or can have a gradual onset of symptoms. Mr. T.C.'s second episode was unexpected and sudden in onset, demonstrating a rapid onset of psychotic manic symptoms worsening over the Sunday morning leading up to his tennis game. With treatment, Mr. T.C.'s episode lasted about three weeks. When asked, neither he nor his wife could identify any introductory symptoms such as decreased need for sleep or an increase in rate of thoughts or speech. On the day he was hospitalized, Mr. T.C. woke up manic about 4:30 a m, earlier than usual by about two hours, and his manic symptoms escalated rapidly through the morning. Mr. T.C. had little insight into his aberrant behavior. He denied any problems throughout his episode, despite his inpatient stay on a locked ward.

The divergence in *outcome* in Bipolar may be the most remarkable of its aspects of variability. A substantial percentage of the homeless and those incarcerated have Bipolar. In contrast, through the centuries, thousands of individuals with Bipolar have achieved success and fame (Table 1.1). A king with Bipolar episodes who "slaughtered the slaves" in a manic rage was recorded from some 2,000 years ago (Sect. 2.1; Table 2.1). See Sect. 2.8 and Chap. 4 for a sampling of Bipolar cases. Sometimes success and poverty occur in the same Bipolar client where an accomplished life deteriorates to on-the-street poverty when the disease causes a deterioration to a chronic irritable psychotic state (Sect. 3.3, Case 1.1).

Initially confusing, Bipolar is unique in the discrepancy of its symptoms between its two poles, mania and depression. No two conditions could be more different, close to opposites, and yet they are parts of a single disease (Table 3.6). A few symptoms superficially appear similar in depression and mania: irritability, weight loss, sleep disturbances, and delusions. Close scrutiny discloses that most of these symptoms are very different between the two. Manic clients lose weight and sleep less, if any, because they are too busy, highly energized, hypersocial, and motivated if not driven to complete the task at hand. Their delusions are usually grandiose with paranoia over fear that others want to kill them for their delusionally overvalued knowledge and possessions (Sect. 3.9).

Table 3.6 Contrasting symptoms between mania and depression, yet one disease

Mania	Depression
Euphoria; grandiosity	Sad; blue; down in the dumps; guilt
Little or no need or time for sleep	In bed 24/7
Hyperactivity; increased energy	Minimal activity; marked decrease in energy
Increased self-esteem; over-confidence; intrusiveness	No confidence; worthlessness; hopelessness; social isolation
Flight of ideas, some brilliant; racing thoughts; pressed speech	Thoughts slowed; no ideas; blunted cognition
Irritability; easy anger; violence	Irritability; anger; less acting out than in mania
Poor decisions with high chances of negative outcomes: spending, speeding, multiple relationships, unsafe sex, gambling, impulse travel	Minimal to no decisions; marked indecisiveness
When hypomanic, clear thoughts, focused activities, and brilliant successes can occur	Thoughts slowed; minimal to no follow-up activity
Loving life; on top of the world	Life not worth living; in the pits of depression; loss of interest and pleasure in life; suicidal ideations; thoughts of death

Depressed clients lose weight because they lose their appetites, enjoyment in life, energy, and motivation. They do not sleep but stay in bed too much because they worry about their "terrible" lives. Their delusions are self-persecutory, generating guilt and then paranoia over fear of "deserved" punishment. In states called mixed mania or mixed depression, there are *simultaneous symptoms of depression and mania.* Irritability and disturbances in sleep are common to both. Atypical symptoms are common in the Bipolar inpatient population (Table 3.7).

Table 3.7 Classic and atypical symptoms in 20 manic NIMH hospitalized patients[a]

Symptoms	Patients manifesting symptoms, %
Hyperactivity	100
Extreme verbosity	100
Pressure of speech	100
Grandiosity	100
Manipulativeness	100
Irritability	100
Euphoria	90
Mood lability	90
Hypersexuality	80
Flight of ideas	75
Delusions	75
Sexual	(25)
Persecutory[a]	(65)[b]
Passivity	(20)
Religious	(15)
Assaultiveness or threatening behavior	75
Distractibility	70
Loosened associations	70
Fear of dying	70
Intrusiveness	60
Somatic complaints	55
Some depression	55
Religiosity	50
Telephone abuse	45
Regressive behavior (urinating or defecating inappropriately; exposing self)	45
Symbolization or gesturing	40
Hallucinations (auditory and visual)	40
Confusion	35
Ideas of reference	20

From Carlson and Goodwin (1973)

Note: [a]These signs and symptoms are recorded from documented Bipolar inpatients. [b]About 50% of these Bipolar clients had paranoid delusions. Kraepelin, Bleuler, and Schneider and their followers counted many of these manic symptoms as indicative of "Schizophrenia"

3.4 Depressive Disorders

Unipolar depression or Major Depressive Disorder (MDD) is a subtype of the Mood Disorders (Table 3.2). Sometimes referred to as major or clinical depression, MDD is defined by two or more *Major Depressive Episodes (MDEs)*. Distinguished from Bipolar, the Unipolar or MDDs have only one pole, depression, *but their symptoms, severity, length of episodes, risk for suicide, and treatment are largely identical* to those in the depressions of Bipolar. Major Depressive *Episodes* occur in Bipolar and MDD. The occurrence of mania or hypomania rules out UP/MDD and all other Depressive Disorder diagnoses.

Depressive Disorders like Bipolar Disorders have subdivisions according to the DSM (Tables 3.2 and 3.8). Some of the most prominent are Major Depressive Disorder (MDD); Persistent Depressive Disorder (PDD), previously called Dysthymia; Disruptive Mood Dysregulation Disorder (DMDD) for children and adolescents (Sect. 2.7); and specifically for women, Premenstrual Dysphoric Disorder (PDD) and Postpartum Depressive Disorder (PPD) (Sect. 2.6).

MDEs typically occur in cycles with sometimes lengthy episodes of euthymia (normal mood) or of depression lasting months to years, even decades. MDEs that occur in Bipolar and Unipolar are indistinguishable one from the other.

Similar to Bipolar Disorders, over a lifetime of MDD, the time spent in depression versus euthymia can vary widely (Fig. 3.1, Curve C). Without treatment, an average MDE lasts about six months. Like Bipolar, a severe MDD can sometimes turn psychotic and chronic with persistent delusional depression and dysfunction without remissions to euthymia (Chap. 1, Sects. 1.3 and 3.3; Case 1.1). Major Depression (MDD), like mania, is also defined by the occurrence of a persistent complex of symptoms that are clearly different from one's baseline mood. Baseline can be difficult to establish after years of chronic depression. This set of symptoms that define a major or clinical depression (MDE/MDD) entails characteristic and persistent abnormal thoughts, feelings, actions, and behaviors.

Table 3.8 Subtypes of Depressive Disorders[a]

Major Depressive Disorder/Unipolar Depression (MDD)
Single episode
Recurrent
Disruptive Mood Dysregulation Disorder (DMDD)
Persistent Depressive Disorder (Dysthymia) (PDD)[b]
Premenstrual Dysphoric Disorder (PMDD)
Substance/medication-induced Depressive Disorder[a]
Depressive Disorder due to another medical/surgical condition[a]
Other Specified Depressive Disorder[a]
Unspecified Depressive Disorder[a]

[a]Depressive episodes can be associated with psychosis, i.e., hallucinations, delusions, disorganization, catatonia, paranoia

[b]Persistent mild depression, i.e., the glass half-empty person with symptoms lasting two years or more; often also associated with the occurrence of Major Depressive Episodes called double depression

The DSM diagnostic criteria for an MDE that both defines MDD and occurs in Bipolar depression are given in Table 3.9. For the diagnosis of an MDE, DSM symptoms must be present 24/7 for *at least two weeks* and be a clear change from one's normal feelings and behaviors. There must be either a *markedly depressed mood* and/or the *loss of interest or pleasure* in one's life. Severe MDEs can associate with significant weight change of at least 5% in one month, disturbance in sleep, *loss of energy*, agitation or retardation; feelings of *worthlessness*, *hopelessness*, excessive or *inappropriate guilt*; indecisiveness; loss of the ability to concentrate; and thoughts of death. Such symptoms must cause clinically *significant distress and impairment* in function and can occur with equal frequency in Bipolar and Unipolar (MDD) depressions. More than one MDE without a manic or hypomanic episode defines an MDD.

In the past, MDD was conceived as distinct from Bipolar but observations have identified non-manic Bipolar factors that, when at least three are present, suggest there will be a subsequent change of diagnosis to Bipolar. Thus, a provisional diagnosis of Bipolar is given (Sect. 3.5; Table 3.11). A Bipolar individual can be misdiagnosed with MDD because of suffering many MDEs over their lifetime but only a single hypomanic episode that is easily overlooked or denied (Fig. 3.1). Such an occurrence of only one hypomanic episode nonetheless determines the diagnosis of Bipolar.

Table 3.9 DSM-5-TR diagnostic criteria for a Major Depressive Disorder (MDD) (Modified for brevity)

A. Five or more of the following symptoms have been present during the same two-week period and are an obvious change from normal functioning; one of the symptoms is either (1) depressed mood or (2) loss of interest or pleasure in one's life:
1. Depressed mood 24/7 as indicated by either subjective report (feels sad, empty, or hopeless) or observations made by others (appears tearful). in children and adolescents, mood can be predominantly irritable
2. Markedly diminished interest or pleasure in activities and life
3. Significant weight change when not dieting exceeding 5% of body weight in a month; loss of appetite
4. Insomnia and /or hypersomnia
5. Psychomotor agitation and/or retardation
6. Fatigue and/or loss of energy
7. Feelings of worthlessness and/or guilt
8. Diminished ability to think and/or concentrate with decisiveness
9. Thoughts of death, recurrent suicidal ideation with or without a specific plan, or a suicide attempt
B. These symptoms cause clinically significant distress and impairment in social, occupational, or other important areas of functioning
C. The episode is not due to the physiological effects of a substance or another medical condition

As discussed in Sect. 6.2, the pharmacological treatment for MDD has changed and psychotherapists must be informed. For decades, the antidepressant drugs such as serotonin-specific reuptake inhibitors (SSRIs) have been prescribed, but these are no longer considered by some psychopharmacologists as treatment of choice for MDEs in either Unipolar or Bipolar depressions. Rather, the mood-stabilizing medications are recommended (Sect. 6.2; Table 6.1).

Persistent Depressive Disorder (PDD) is a new diagnosis similar to Dysthymia and replacing it. These are both defined by a *persistent mild to moderate depression* for at least *two years* without more than two consecutive months of euthymia. Symptoms are largely present 24/7, usually for life. PDD/Dysthymia is distinguished from MDD by its less severe symptoms, its persistence, with fewer and longer cycles and less euthymic time. Symptoms include a chronic low mood, poor appetite, sleep disturbance, low energy, low self-esteem, poor concentration, indecisiveness, and hopelessness. PDD/Dysthymia can coexist with MDD when MDEs occur and baseline is a chronic low-grade depression (PDD). For PDD there must be clinically *significant distress and impairment in one's life*. PDD/Dysthymia responds to psychotherapy which these individuals are also likely to seek (Table 3.10).

Two depressive disorders specific to women are *Premenstrual Dysphoric Disorder (PMDD)* and Postpartum Depressive Disorder (PDD) which are detailed in Sect. 2.6.

Disruptive Mood Dysregulation Disorder (DMDD) is limited to youth under 18 years and is detailed in Sect. 2.7 (Table 2.4).

Table 3.10 DSM-5-TR diagnostic criteria for Persistent Depressive Disorder (PDD, Dysthymia)

A. Mild to moderately depressed mood 24/7 for more days than not for at least two years (in children, at least one year)
B. Presence when depressed of two or more of the following:
(a) Poor appetite or overeating
(b) Insomnia and/or hypersomnia
(c) Low energy or fatigue
(d) Low self-esteem
(e) Poor concentration and indecisiveness
(f) Hopelessness
C. Never without the symptoms above for more than two months at a time
D. Criteria for an MDD may be present (double depression)
E. Criteria never met for mania, hypomania, or cyclothymia
F. Symptoms not caused by a substance or another medical condition
G. The symptoms cause clinically significant distress or impairment in social, occupational, or other important areas of functioning
H. The presence of criteria for MDD and PDD warrant the diagnosis of double depression

Modified for Brevity

Diagnoses of PDD/Dysthymia, MDD, PMDD, DMDD, and Bipolar II, as well as Cyclothymia, are provisional because, with the occurrence of a manic episode, each becomes Bipolar I.

Four additional DSM Depressive Disorders, below, have similar names and the same basic criteria as their four corresponding Bipolar diagnoses:

(1) Substance/medication-induced Depressive Disorder (Sect. 3.7)
(2) Depressive Disorder due to another medical or surgical condition (Sect. 3.7)

[Note: These substance/drug and medical/surgical potential causes given in (1) and (2) above must be ruled out before making any functional Depressive Disorder diagnosis.]

(3) Other Specified Depressive Disorder (OSDD)
(4) Unspecified Depressive Disorder (USDD)

[Note: The diagnoses above are new to the DSM-5 and the DSM-5-TR and allow for a diagnosis of a Depressive Disorder without fulfilling all criteria.]

The Depressive Disorder specifiers and features are similar if not identical to those discussed for Bipolar (Sect. 3.2).

3.5 The Bipolar-Unipolar Spectrum; Non-Manic Bipolar Factors in Depression

It had been thought that the Bipolar-Unipolar division was an either-or condition and that the absence of mania or hypomania ruled out a Bipolar diagnosis. However, data reveal that about 50% of subjects initially diagnosed as Unipolar or MDD convert to Bipolar over their lifetime. There have been major efforts to identify which depressed clients have or will have Bipolar and not MDD because clients misdiagnosed with MDD may be mis-served by physician-prescribed selective serotonin reuptake inhibitors (SSRIs) such as fluoxetine (Prozac) or serotonin-norepinephrine reuptake inhibitors (SNRIs) such as venlafaxine (Effexor). These may increase cycling of both Bipolar and Unipolar Disorders. Mood stabilizers and not antidepressants are recommended for both (Sect. 6.2).

More recently the concept of a spectrum linking them and the identification of the *non-manic Bipolar factors* has caused cases previously diagnosed as Unipolar to be considered as Bipolar (Table 3.11). An episode of abnormally elevated mood is no longer mandatory for a Bipolar diagnosis since the diagnostic therapist can now consider the non-manic Bipolar factors. These factors are not diagnostic of Bipolar but are rather indicators that there likely has been an unrecognized manic episode or that there will be one in the future based on long-term follow-up of clients with three or more of these factors (Table 3.11). One must consider a Bipolar diagnosis in a depressed client when at least three of these factors are positive.

Table 3.11 Non-manic Bipolar features suggesting Bipolar, not Unipolar depression

Likely Bipolar, not Unipolar (MDD), if there is/are:
A past personal or family history of manic or subthreshold manic symptoms
A past personal or family history of a psychiatric hospitalization
A past personal or family history of a diagnosis of "Schizophrenia" or "Schizoaffective Disorder"
A past personal or family history of a prescription for lithium or valproic acid/divalproex (Depakene/Depakote) (Sect. 6.2)
Several severe Major Depressive Episodes (MDEs)
Major Depressive Disorder (MDD) diagnosed at an early age
Postpartum and premenstrual MDEs
A personal history of serious suicide attempts or cutting
A family history of suicide or suicide attempts
MDEs unresponsive to several antidepressants
An antidepressant- or stimulant-induced switch to mania or hypomania

The use of the new diagnoses of OSBD or USBD allows for a tentative Bipolar diagnosis without the presence of a manic episode but with three of the non-manic Bipolar factors. Identifying such clients as having subthreshold Bipolar is supported by the *conversion of a substantial percentage of MDD clients with three factors but no manic episodes to Bipolar I and Bipolar II* (Tables 3.3 and 3.4).

3.6 Psychological Disorders Confused with Bipolar

A decision between Bipolar, normal mood cycling, and other psychological conditions can be subjective; there are as yet no objective laboratory or imaging tests to confirm (Sect. 2.4). While the diagnosis is clear in moderate to severe cases of Bipolar, in mild cases, it becomes a judgment call. For example, an active but non-Bipolar child can demonstrate non-stop motion, lack of impulse control, difficulty tolerating frustration, and a vivid imagination.

The severity of the symptoms and the degree of disruption in an individual's day-to-day life help distinguish a Mood Disorder diagnosis from non-clinical mood variations. *Time, observation, and a trial of a mood stabilizer* can determine the diagnosis. Scrutiny of the non-manic Bipolar factors is worthwhile because these individuals with ambiguous Bipolar symptoms are likely at risk of converting to a full Bipolar Disorder (Table 3.11). Since the mood-stabilizing medications and psychotherapy have a positive benefit-to-risk ratio and can reduce the risk for a conversion to clinical Bipolar, treatment is suggested.

Differentiating *non-mood psychological conditions* that cause mood symptoms from bona-fide Mood Disorders is also important. The training curricula of programs for therapists, social workers, and psychologists do not emphasize Bipolar; rather, Attention Deficit Hyperactivity Disorder (ADHD), Oppositional Defiant

Disorder (ODD), Intermittent Explosive Disorder (IED), Anxiety, Obsessive Compulsive (OCD), and Personality Disorders are diagnoses that are prioritized especially in children and adolescents (Sect. 2.7).

These psychological disorders have symptoms overlapping with Bipolar. One of the most important differential diagnoses in child and adolescent psychology is between childhood Bipolar and ADHD. This latter disorder has been the predominant diagnosis in hyperactive children. The symptoms of ADHD in children and adults must be differentiated both from normal limits and from Bipolar (Sect. 2.7). A correct diagnosis of Bipolar in children and adolescents is often more challenging than in adults but is of critical importance in both populations because the stimulant class of drugs prescribed to treat ADHD can make Bipolar worse.

The diagnostic criteria for ADHD and Bipolar overlap extensively (Sect. 2.7). For example, some of the DSM-5-TR (2022) diagnostic criteria for ADHD are "a persistent pattern of inattention and/or hyperactivity-impulsivity that interferes with functioning." Examples of this include the following: (1) often fails to give close attention to details, makes careless mistakes; (2) *difficulty sustaining attention and maintaining focus*; (3) does not seem to listen, *mind seems elsewhere*; (4) does *not follow through* and *fails to finish*; (5) difficulty organizing; (6) avoids tasks that require sustained mental effort; (7) loses things necessary for tasks; (8) easily distracted; (9) forgetful; (10) fidgets or taps hands or feet; (11) leaves seat inappropriately and runs about; (12) "on the go…driven by a motor"; (13) *talks excessively*; (14) blurts out answers inappropriately; (15) has difficulty waiting his or her turn, *interrupts*, or *intrudes*.

These symptoms overlap 100% with hypomania and mania of Bipolar. Such overlap of symptoms between ADHD and mania combined with other research data support the idea that some if not many of these childhood ADHD diagnoses may actually be early onset Bipolar. Current data show the typical onset of Bipolar is in early childhood (Sect. 2.7). Although Bipolar and ADHD have been considered separate if not mutually exclusive, there are clients still diagnosed with both. When an individual has a record of both diagnoses, it is most likely that they have Bipolar and do not have ADHD. Some consider a diagnosis of ADHD to be a misdiagnosis for Bipolar (Papolos and Papolos 2006). Geller et al. (2008) also believe that ADHD is overdiagnosed and misdiagnosed for mania and Bipolar. The most persuasive finding is the *frequency of a diagnostic change from ADHD to Bipolar* as the child reaches the teenage years to young adulthood (Sect. 2.7).

It is recommended that new and current clients with ADHD diagnoses, children and adults, be reassessed for Bipolar. Use of a daily mood-rating chart and mood-stabilizing medications may confirm the Bipolar diagnosis. There can be client resistance to giving up the ADHD diagnosis because the stimulant drugs used to treat ADHD are desired by clients for their stimulating effects. ADHD clients may refuse to give up their ADHD diagnosis so they can continue their stimulant medications (Sect. 2.7).

As documented in Sect. 2.7, the symptoms of *Oppositional Defiant Disorder (ODD)* and *Intermittent Explosive Disorder (IED)* also overlap with symptoms of mania and *Disruptive Mood Dysregulation Disorder (DMDD)*.

The importance of identifying Bipolar or DMDD in these clients is that the medications that stabilize mood are not given while those drugs most often prescribed are stimulants for ADHD and the SGAs for ODD and IED. These either make Bipolar worse or, in the case of SGAs, have the potential for significant side effects, especially in children.

Bipolar is also misdiagnosed as Major Depressive Disorder (MDD), Persistent Depressive Disorder (PDD), Dysthymia, or Disruptive Mood Dysregulation Disorder (DMDD) when there are multiple episodes of mild to severe, even psychotic episodes of depression but with only rare hypomanic or manic episodes that clients may not remember (Fig. 3.1, Curves D, E).

Delusional Disorders are of interest because their symptoms also overlap with mania and Bipolar. They are a rare but fascinating group of disorders, classified in the DSM with "Schizophrenia," not Bipolar where they belong. These clients display various non-bizarre delusions of *paranoia (persecutory type)*, *imagining an illness (somatic type)*, having some *great talent (grandiose type)*, *being loved by another at a distance (erotomanic type)*, and others. Delusional Disorder diagnoses may account for a small percentage of misdiagnosed Bipolar clients. For example, *Erotomania* suggests mania and a Bipolar Disorder. The erotomanic subtype involves the delusion that another person, typically of a higher social and economic status, is in love with the individual but cannot acknowledge their love. The client makes multiple inappropriate efforts to contact the desired person including stalking and house invasions. *John Hinckley*, who attempted to assassinate President Ronald Reagan in 1981, is an extreme example of a case of a psychotic Bipolar Disorder with Delusional Disorder, Erotomanic symptoms (Sect. 4.5, Case 4.38).

The Personality Disorders are commonly misdiagnosed in clients with Bipolar. There is again substantial overlap in symptoms that calls into question the presence of both diagnoses at the same time in the same client. In many clients diagnosed with a Personality Disorder, Bipolar alone may explain the symptoms. For example, the DSM diagnostic criteria for *Borderline Personality Disorder* include "…an instability of interpersonal relationships…marked impulsivity such as spending, sex, substance abuse, and reckless driving…recurrent suicidal behavior…affective instability…episodic dysphoria, irritability…chronic feelings of emptiness…intense anger…frequent displays of temper…" Bipolar relationships are fragile and unstable due to mood swings with *irritability*, *anger*, *impulsivity*, and destructive poor decisions that include inappropriate *spending*, *sex*, *substance use*, and *reckless driving*, all in mania. In Bipolar depression, there are *dysphoria*, chronic feelings of *emptiness*, *suicidality*, and more *irritability*. Phelps (2016) states that there is a 90% overlap in symptoms between Bipolar and Borderline Personality Disorder.

Similarly the DSM criteria for *Antisocial Personality Disorder* (APD) overlap with those for Bipolar. For example, APD is characterized as the "failure to conform to social norms…impulsivity…irritability and aggressiveness…physical fights or assaults…irresponsibility…failure to sustain consistent work behavior…" Manic clients can display all of these. The level of violence in some cases of mania that is severe with psychotic features is extreme to include murder, familicide, and mass murder (Sects. 4.5 and 4.6). Further evidence of symptom overlap is that the DSM does not allow the antisocial diagnosis if the symptoms occur during the course of a Bipolar Disorder because the symptoms of Bipolar account for the APD criteria.

To a similar degree, the symptoms of *Paranoid*, "Schizoid," and "Schizotypal Personality Disorders" overlap with those of Bipolar. If a Bipolar Disorder is misdiagnosed as a Personality Disorder, mood drugs are not given and the Bipolar may get worse. Therapists can help redirect such clients' diagnoses and treatment.

The *Anxiety Disorders* in children and adults also have a high comorbidity with bipolarity that has been described as "strong and indisputable." Anxious high school students are seven times more likely to have a Bipolar Disorder and over 50% of children and adolescents with a Bipolar Disorder also have an Anxiety Disorder. *When a comorbid Bipolar Disorder is treated, anxiety diminishes.* When the Bipolar diagnosis is missed in favor of the Anxiety Disorder, the danger is that Anxiety Disorders are medicated with antidepressants that may exacerbate Bipolar and the mood-stabilizing drugs are not given.

Obsessive Compulsive Disorder (OCD) co-occurs with Mood Disorders, especially MDD, because of a persistent loss of capacity and a discouraging chronic course of severe OCD. This leads to social withdrawal, sadness, loss of pleasure in life, marked dysfunction, and MDD. Of children with OCD, some 70% also have a Mood Disorder (Sect. 2.7).

The obsessions and global dysfunctionality of severe OCD have also been misinterpreted as psychosis and then "Schizophrenia." However, this observation may depend, in some cases, on the misinterpretation of obsessions as auditory hallucinations in OCD clients and by their evaluating physicians. The OCD client's dysfunctionality can be confused as MDD or "Schizophrenia" as demonstrated by the case summary given below.

Case 3.3: Mr. S. V.

Mr. S. V., a 36-year-old, never-married male, was so depressed and dysfunctional that he could not hold a job and was socially isolated and withdrawn, staying in his room in his parents' house. He was an inpatient at the state mental hospital on several occasions for months at a time because of his "psychotic" symptoms. His hospital summaries note that he "…talked to the television and to a tree in his yard" and he was severely depressed. He was diagnosed with MDD and "Schizophrenia" and was medicated with large dosages of *antipsychotic* drugs for years. He developed mild Tardive Dyskinesia (TD), a metabolic syndrome with marked obesity, but was considered so severely psychotic that the antipsychotic drugs were continued. He was not given a trial off his medications "for fear he would get worse." This decision was supported by his parents. He said his "voices were a little better" when he took these drugs but he was oversedated and was more dysfunctional.

During a "second opinion" interview at the hospital, his statement that he was *worse in the late spring and summer* stimulated the elucidating question, "Why"? He answered that he was worse in the spring because the *leaves came out on the large oak tree in his front yard* and when he tried to go out of his house, he saw the tree and *had to count each leaf before he could move*. He "spoke to the TV" when he heard or saw a number on the screen and then had to say that number, round to an even number, count by that number to 1000, "in a perfect voice," which took hours. When he counted, he formed the numbers with his mouth and was thus thought to be talking to the TV and the tree. He endorsed more than enough DSM symptoms to fulfill criteria for severe OCD and MDD. His diagnosis was changed, his SGA medications were tapered and discontinued, his *TD worsened*, and a high dose of an SSRI and lithium, coupled with psychotherapy, improved his daily function. It is most fortunate that he did not also develop Tardive Psychosis or his SGAs would have been continued for life (Sects. 6.2 and 6.3; Tables 6.7 and 6.8).

3.7 Drug and Medical Causes of Bipolar Symptoms

Certain drugs and medical diseases can present with Bipolar symptoms and must be ruled out before arriving at a Bipolar diagnosis. It is important to inquire about the use of alcohol and all drugs including prescribed medications, herbal remedies, over-the-counter, online, and street drugs. Consider the drugs in Table 3.12. Specific examples include the stimulant drugs such as methylphenidate (Ritalin) prescribed for ADHD, amphetamines, cocaine, and caffeine. Also relevant are occupational exposure and hobbies such as gardening which could entail handling chemicals.

It should be emphasized that mood and psychotic symptoms are associated with prescribed and *recreational anabolic steroids* often used in body building. Corticosteroid therapy alters mood in *75% of cases* with psychotic manifestations in about 5%. *Mania* is the most common mood state induced by steroids (35%), followed by depression (28%), mixed episodes (12%), delirium (13%), and psychosis (11%). After an initial episode, almost 50% of such clients have recurrent manic and depressive episodes without additional corticosteroid use. This means that the corticosteroids can activate a latent Bipolar Disorder that then cycles on its own. *Corticosteroids can kindle Bipolar.*

Clients with Bipolar are often inappropriately prescribed second-generation antipsychotics (SGAs) without mood stabilizers.

Table 3.12 Substances that can cause Bipolar symptoms

Alcohol[a]
Anesthetics
Anabolic steroids[b]
Antibiotics (ciproflaxin)
Anticholinergics[a]
Anticonvulsants (high doses)
Antihistamines: diphenhydramine (Benadryl), dimenhydrinate (Dramamine)
Antimalarial drugs (Mefloquine)
Antineoplastics (especially Ifosfamide)
Antipsychotic drugs[a]
Antituberculous drugs (D-cycloserine, Ethambutol, Isoniazid)
Antivirals: HIV medications: Efavirenz (at high plasma levels), Acyclovir
Cardiovascular drugs (antiarrhythmics, digitalis)
Corticosteroids[a, b]
Dopaminergic drugs (L-dopa, Amantadine, Ropinirole)[a, b]
Hallucinogens: bath salts (mephedrone and methylenedioxyprovalerone; sold under the names of Aura, Ivory Wave, Loco-motion, and Vanilla Sky); phencyclidine (PCP); Lysergic acid (LSD); ketamine
Interferon[a, b]
Miscellaneous (baclofen, caffeine, disulfram, cyclosporine)
Pain medications (opioids especially meperidine, pentazocine, indomethacin)
Stimulants (including illicit street drugs, over the counter, prescription, ephedra-containing diet supplements and food drugs such as caffeine)[a, b]

Modified from Freudenrich (2010)
[a]Substances particularly likely to cause psychosis
[b]Substances particularly likely to cause mood symptoms

Although several medical/surgical disorders can cause mood symptoms, they rarely do, with some exceptions, such as space-occupying brain lesions, pancreatic cancer, thyroid disorders, and Parkinson's (Case 3.4). Even though rare, the detriment to clients misdiagnosed with Mood Disorders or other psychological conditions when their symptoms are caused by a medical disease or a drug is high enough that it is worthwhile keeping these disorders in mind (Tables 3.12 and 3.13; Case 3.4).

Table 3.13 Medical disorders with potential Bipolar presentations

Autoimmune disorders
Systemic lupus erythematosus
Hashimoto's encephalopathy
Paraneoplastic syndrome
Rheumatic fever
Myasthenia gravis
Chromosomal abnormalities
Sex chromosomes (Klinefelter's syndrome, xxx syndrome)
Fragile x syndrome
Velocardiofacial syndrome
Chronic traumatic encephalopathy (history of head trauma)
Dementias and delirium
Alzheimer's disease
Pick's disease
Lewy body syndrome
Demyelinating diseases
Multiple sclerosis
Leukodystrophies
Schilder's disease
Electrolyte and fluid imbalance
Hypernatremia
Hypokalemia
Hypercalcemia
Hypomagnesemia
Endocrinopathies
Hypoglycemia
Insulinoma
Addison's disease
Cushing's syndrome
Hyper- and -hypothyroidism
Hyper- and hypoparathyroidism
Hypopituitarism
Pheochromocytoma
Epilepsy
Hydrocephalus (Case 3.4)
Infections
Viral encephalitis (e.g., herpes simplex, measles [including subacute sclerosing panencephalitis], cytomegalovirus, rubella, Epstein-Barr, varicella)
Neurosyphilis
Neuroborreliosis (Lyme disease)
HIV infection or AIDS
CNS-invasive parasitic infections (e.g., cerebral malaria, toxoplasmosis, neurocysticerosis)

(continued)

Table 3.13 (continued)

Tuberculosis
Sarcoidosis
Cryptococcus infection
Prion diseases (e.g., Creutzfeldt-Jakob disease)
Metabolic diseases (partial list)
Amino acid metabolism (Hartnup disease, homocystinuria, phenylketonuria)
Porphyrias (acute intermittent porphyria, porphyria variegate, hereditary coproporphyria)
GM-2 gangliosidosis
Fabry's disease
Niemann-Pick type C disease
Gaucher's disease, adult type
Tay-Sach's disease
Narcolepsy
Neuropsychiatric diseases
Huntington's disease
Wilson's disease
Parkinson's disease
Fahr disease (familial basal ganglia calcification)
Friedreich's ataxia
Spinocerebellar Ataxia 2
Nutritional deficiencies
Magnesium deficiency
Vitamin A deficiency
Vitamin D deficiency
Zinc deficiency
Niacin deficiency (pellagra)
Vitamin B_{12} deficiency (pernicious anemia)
Space-occupying lesions and structural brain abnormalities
Primary brain tumors
Secondary brain metastases
Brain abscesses and cysts
Tuberous sclerosis
Midline abnormalities (e.g., corpus callosum agenesis, cavum septi pellucidi)
Cerebrovascular malformations (e.g., involving the temporal lobe)
Pancreatic carcinoma
Chronic subdural hematoma
Stroke

Modified from Freudenrich et al. (2007)

When presented with abnormal mood symptoms or psychotic behaviors, the therapist's initial consideration must be to rule out usually treatable substance use and medical disorders, as given in Tables 3.12 and 3.13. This is accomplished with a thorough history and a referral to the client's primary care physician (PCP), requesting a physical exam, urine drug screen, a lab blood draw for toxicology, CBC, chemistries, and usually brain imaging. This is recommended for all new clients. An example is the individual in the case summarized below who received several psychiatric medications and *extensive psychotherapy for years*. She had hydrocephalus finally diagnosed by brain imaging before there was permanent brain damage, as discussed at the end of this chapter (Sect. 3.7, Case 3.4).

Some of the disorders more likely to cause psychological symptoms are briefly noted here. Autoimmune disorders include *Systemic Lupus Erythematosus (SLE)* which is a multisystem autoimmune disorder where in 11% of cases there are psychotic or mood symptoms. Appropriate treatment of SLE with corticosteroids causes symptoms of Bipolar in an additional 5%.

Chronic traumatic encephalopathy (CTE, chronic head trauma) is a risk factor for a chronic psychotic syndrome with paranoid features.

Demyelinating diseases include *Multiple Sclerosis (MS)* that is associated with symptoms of mania, depression, and psychosis.

Electrolyte and fluid imbalance is associated with depression, especially hypernatremia, hypokalemia, hypercalcemia, and hypomagnesemia.

Endocrinopathies, although systemic, typically affect the brain and can present with manic, depressive, and psychotic symptoms. *Thyroid disease*, *Cushing's Disease or Syndrome*, and *small cell lung cancer* can present with manic or psychotic features. *Addison's Disease* develops gradually and can present with severe depression of psychotic proportions.

Epilepsy, especially *temporal lobe*, has been misdiagnosed as Bipolar or "Schizophrenia."

Infections such as *HIV*, *neurosyphilis,* and any infection in the CNS can present with mania, depression, or psychosis.

Metabolic diseases such as *Acute Intermittent Porphyria* can present with psychotic features. GI symptoms and a peripheral motor neuropathy are typical. Fasting and alcohol can precipitate an episode.

Narcolepsy has been misdiagnosed as "Schizophrenia."

Neuropsychiatric diseases such as *Huntington's*, *Wilson's*, and *Fahr's Diseases* can initially present with manic, depressive, or psychotic features.

Nutritional deficiencies such as *vitamin B12*, *thiamin*, or *niacin* are associated with manic, depressive, or psychotic symptoms.

Space-occupying lesions and structural brain abnormalities such as *temporal lobe tumors* can present with psychosis. *Occipital lobe* lesions associate with visual hallucinations, while *frontal lobe* tumors can cause personality changes, a flat affect, and superficial euphoria. Parietal lobe tumors can cause sensory or agnostic symptoms as well as a lack of awareness that can be mistaken as depression. *Pancreatic carcinomas frequently manifest as severe depression*. Consider pancreatic cancer in a middle-aged male suffering from severe depression without any premorbid psychiatric history. Severe depression is common in *stroke victims*. *Normal pressure hydrocephalus* has been misdiagnosed as Bipolar or MDD and treated with psychotherapy and drugs for years.

Case 3.4: Ms. C. K.

Twenty-three-year-old Chloe R. Kral began college at the Fashion Institute of Technology, New York, in 2015, with a history of fainting, falling, anxiety, and possibly ADHD. She had had balance problems as an adolescent and had had to give up skiing because of frequent falls. She struggled in college, seemed depressed, and was prescribed antidepressants. Chloe did not improve on these meds and after several weeks in bed, she quit school, went home, and started therapy for severe depression. Her memory was undependable, causing her to forget to turn in assignments at the community college where she enrolled, as well as to lose jobs because she could not remember instructions. Four years later, in 2019, she demonstrated symptoms of *Bipolar Disorder*, including not sleeping, talking rapidly, and behaving aggressively. She also appeared to show signs of derealization, and began *dragging one foot* as she walked. She became *incontinent*, ceased to attend to her personal hygiene, and seemed increasingly depressed.

After a six-month stay at a private psychiatric treatment center, she suddenly became combative and threatened to kill herself or harm staff. In anticipation of a move to a long-term locked ward at a mental hospital, she was taken to an ED, incoherent and in restraints. There an alert ED physician ordered a CT scan of her head which disclosed "the most severe case of hydrocephalus" she had ever seen; she said, "How did no one figure this out?"

This case is a "…stunning oversight that resulted in years of needless anguish, hundreds of hours of psychotherapy, and multiple unnecessary psychiatric drugs with additional side effects." Chloe was immediately scheduled for lifesaving brain surgery (Boodman 2022).

Therapists are encouraged to remember this case at all times with their new clients as well as follow-ups. As an additional motivation to consider medical causes of psychological symptoms, consider that some of Ms. Kral's therapists and psychiatrists may have lost their licenses to practice.

3.8 Bipolar Can Be Overdiagnosed

The course in childhood Bipolar is considerably more variable than in adults and there are several other childhood disorders with overlapping symptoms. The Bipolar diagnosis has become acceptable with hyperactive, explosive episodes lasting only minutes to hours or days which may result in overdiagnosis in some childhood cases. There are questions between Bipolar and normal children who have a high level of hyperactivity. A hyperactive but non-Bipolar child can demonstrate nonstop motion, lack of impulse control, difficulty tolerating frustration, and vivid imagination. While the diagnosis is clear in severe cases of Bipolar, in very mild cases, it becomes a judgment call.

Despite some cases of overdiagnosis of Bipolar, psychotherapists will serve their child and adolescent clients well by considering a Bipolar diagnosis and addressing changes in diagnosis and medication recommendations with the prescriber when appropriate. Time and a trial of a mood stabilizer can help with the diagnosis. In general, *overdiagnosis of Bipolar is preferable* to underdiagnosis.

Bipolar can also be overdiagnosed in adults, undermining the acceptance of the Bipolar diagnosis. A common mistake is to elicit adequate DSM diagnostic criteria for Bipolar without assuring that the symptoms (1) occurred during the *same period of time*, (2) were outside of baseline range for that individual, and (3) were not better explained by another disorder such as episodic binge abuse of *speed or alcohol* (Sect. 3.7). Episodes of excessive spending, anger, insomnia, hypersexuality, and feeling especially "up" may occur, but if these symptoms do not occur together or if they are baseline behavior, they do not confirm Bipolar. Insomnia must be linked with increased energy and activities as well as additional DSM diagnostic criteria, all during the same hours and days (Table 3.3). The symptoms must also cause *significant life problems*. The symptoms of mania or depression must be persistent, 24/7 for at least several days but more often for weeks to months in adults (Tables 3.3 and 3.9).

The new *spectrum concept* of accepting *non-manic Bipolar factors* as diagnostic of Bipolar can lead to false positives (Sect. 3.5) (Table 3.11).

Certain medical/surgical conditions and drug and alcohol uses that can cause manic-like symptoms or depression must also be ruled out in order to prevent overdiagnosis of Bipolar (Sect. 3.7) (Tables 3.12 and 3.13). Most relevant is Ms. Kral, Case 3.4, misdiagnosed with MDD or Bipolar when she had hydrocephalus. Also important is abuse of street and prescribed stimulants or steroids that can cause manic-like symptoms that can result in a misdiagnosis of Bipolar allowing the substance abuse to go untreated. Overuse of weed can precipitate a psychosis (Chap. 4, Case 4.31) or cause symptoms of a chronic dysthymic or Persistent Depressive Disorder.

3.9 Psychosis in Bipolar: There Is No "Schizophrenia" or "Schizoaffective Disorder"

"Schizophrenia" and Bipolar, earlier known as Manic Depressive Insanity, are the most widely known and feared of all severe mental illnesses. However, persuasive data suggest that "Schizophrenia" is not an actual disease separate from a psychotic Bipolar Disorder, as all of the diagnostic symptoms of "Schizophrenia" are accounted for by psychotic mania or depression. "Schizophenia" is a misdiagnosis (Lake 2012). Since the 1970s, studies have accumulated showing complete overlap in clinical signs, symptoms, and course between clients diagnosed with severe, chronic Bipolar and "Schizophrenia." Some neuropsychiatrists have recommended discarding the diagnosis of "Schizophrenia."

The authors of the current Diagnostic and Statistical Manual (DSM-5-TR 2022) took a significant step toward the elimination of the diagnosis of "Schizophrenia" by dropping all of the subtypes upon which the diagnosis of "Schizophrenia" had depended for its existence for over 100 years. Curiously the DSM has retained these discarded subtypes as the symptoms and diagnostic criteria for "Schizophrenia."

The diagnosis of "Schizophrenia" was solidified in 1911 as a new diagnosis when Eugen Bleuler published his book titled *Dementia Praecox or the Group of Schizophrenias.* As he taught, "Schizophrenia" was different from Bipolar Disorder based on the misconception that psychotic features and chronicity of course were not consistent with Bipolar, so a new diagnosis was required. Bleuler dedicated his life to promoting his new diagnosis and his book had an enormous impact upon Academic Psychiatry and therefore on all mental health, medical, and legal professionals, the media, and the public. "Schizophrenia" was embraced as a valid diagnosis despite consistent descriptions for over 2,000 years of psychotic behavior in individuals with distinct mood cycling episodes (Goodwin and Jamison 1990). "Schizophrenia" became the predominant diagnosis for functionally psychotic clients to the marked detriment of these misdiagnosed Bipolar clients.

From the early twentieth century, for some 70 years, the rate of diagnosing Bipolar and Major Depression (MDD) declined as increasing numbers of psychotic clients with mood cycling were misdiagnosed with "Schizophrenia." These misdiagnosed mood-disordered clients were badly mis-served because they did not receive therapeutic mood-stabilizing medicines and did get years of SGAs in usually increasing dosages (Sect. 6.3). They were less likely to receive psychotherapy (Table 3.16).

Manic-Depressive Insanity (MDI) was the early name for Bipolar Disorder and the two are synonymous. That "insanity" was used for Bipolar clients confirms that such clients are capable of exhibiting insanity or psychosis. The term psychosis has replaced "madness" and "insanity" except in legal terminology where insanity frequently determines guilt or innocence (Sect. 4.7).

Dementia, madness, insanity, and psychosis were sometimes used interchangeably even into the 1900s; each reflects brain dysfunction. All have been associated with MDI or Bipolar Disorder.

Even into the twentieth century, MDI (Bipolar) was mistakenly thought to lead to Dementia because some MDI clients developed a chronic deteriorating psychotic state without further cycling (Case 1.1). Bipolar and Dementia are not directly associated, but both can deteriorate to a severe level of dysfunctionality (Case 1.1).

Dementia is a separate and specific brain disease. In dementia there are diagnostic characteristics of brain cell loss on imaging with cognitive decline and a gradual loss of memory, orientation, executive function, and the ability to carry out the activities of daily living (ADLs). Dementia is *progressive, irreversible, and incurable. Bipolar does not cause Dementia* and is treatable. Clients with Bipolar can develop Dementia in addition to Bipolar; the two are not mutually exclusive. The point here is that some Bipolar clients can deteriorate to a place of such dysfunctionality that dementia has been suspected. Yet these clients remain fully oriented.

Psychosis is a symptom complex caused by one of several diseases such as Bipolar, Dementia, a brain tumor, or psychotomimetic drugs; it is not in itself a disease and is usually not permanent. The challenge is to determine which disease has caused the psychosis. *Both acute and chronic psychoses do occur in severe Bipolar Disorders* (Sects. 4.3, 4.4, and 4.5). Another complication is that about 10% of healthy individuals apparently experience mild psychotic symptoms without consequences. If there are no medical, surgical, or drug causes, *psychosis is due to a severe Bipolar Disorder* (Sect. 2.8).

Acute psychoses usually occur during severe Bipolar episodes of mania but can also occur in severe depressions of Bipolar or MDD (Sects. 4.3, 4.5, and 4.6). Acute psychosis in Bipolar, in both mania and depression, is identified by a rapid onset over hours to a few days of psychotic symptoms that are strikingly different from the client's normal behavior. These symptoms are severe with regard to loss of touch with reality, are often bizarre, evidencing paranoia and fear for one's life, and are potentially dangerous (Sect. 4.5). Acute psychotic episodes are usually time limited lasting days to weeks, and such clients can fully recover and return to a productive existence in their work and family lives (Sect. 4.4).

Clients who have suffered a psychotic episode must be helped to realize that they are at substantial risk for another episode, and the more so without continuing psychotherapy and medications. Therapists can be most helpful by seeing such clients multiple times a week during such psychotic episodes in an effort to stabilize behavior and prevent hospitalization. This is not always possible, and admission is determined by the degree of risk for dangerous behavior. If there is an inpatient admission, therapists can identify an inpatient unit with a Bipolar-knowledgeable psychiatrist. Ongoing therapy sessions can be arranged.

An acute onset psychosis can become chronic or a persistent chronic psychotic state can begin in either Bipolar or MDD as early as the third or fourth decade of life, sometimes earlier. *Classic Bipolars can stop cycling and deteriorate to a chronic, persistent, non-cycling, dysthymic, irritable psychotic state without typical overt symptoms of mania or major depression* (Sect. 3.3) (Case 1.1). This state is characterized by a flat, emotionless affect except for irritability and anger. There is a major absence of motivation and marked dysfunctionality. Such clients are oriented to time and place but not their situation. They still may be able to carry on superficial conversations on a bus or in a bar, sometimes with an air of grandiosity and irritability but activities of daily living (ADLs) are marginal. These chronic, persistently psychotic Bipolars are difficult to diagnose without knowledge of a past or family history of cycles of mania and depression. An MRI of the brain is recommended. Once organic causes of the dysfunctional psychotic state are ruled out, the explanation is a chronic psychotic Mood Disorder that warrants a trial of more intensive psychotherapy and mood-stabilizing drugs with an SGA.

It is said that a psychotic Bipolar client is out of touch with reality because they adopt their "own reality" that is based on their delusions. These may begin with a seed of truth but as the psychotic state worsens, the initial reality is obscured, lost in the manic expansion into delusional paranoid grandiosity. Clients in such psychotic states do not recognize that their thoughts and beliefs are inaccurate or "crazy." They make decisions and act based on their delusions. If their psychotic delusions were accurate, their behaviors would make sense. Their decisions and actions are the best choices in the clients' minds despite appearances to the contrary to family, society, and law enforcement (Chap. 4).

When Bipolar II and Cyclothymia are included, only about 10–20% of all Bipolar clients have a severe manic episode with psychotic features but among selected severe Bipolar inpatients at the NIMH, as many as 70% suffered psychotic episodes. Some Bipolar I clients have only a few psychotic episodes in their lifetime that require hospitalization, although some have multiple such experiences. Many of these clients have productive, stable, and successful interepisode periods; some do not. Psychotherapy works to stabilize these clients with histories of severe episodes.

In psychotic Bipolar depression and MDD, the risk of suicide is between 15% and 25% and the morbidity is substantial with total dysfunctionality and tragic disasters in the worst cases (Sect. 4.6). A common psychotic theme in either MDD or Bipolar depression is the belief that life is not worth living and is hell on earth to be escaped only by suicide. Sometimes there are delusional beliefs of past sins and misperceived, exaggerated wrongdoings that deserve punishment in the mind of a delusional depressed client. This state of mind of delusional pessimism predisposes to suicide sometimes preceded by filicide by psychotically depressed mothers as well (Sect. 4.6) (Fig. 3.2).

It seems unimaginable that a parent could murder their children, but there are hundreds if not thousands of cases reported by the media and many go unreported. Such psychotic parents believe they are saving their children and themselves from the intolerable torture of life by murdering their children and attempting suicide themselves. These parents know what they are doing; they plan ahead in detail; *still they are psychotic* and should be deemed innocent by reason of insanity (Sect. 4.7).

After killing their children, a psychotically depressed parent usually attempts suicide to "join their children in a better place," but sometimes their attempt fails and in court they are wrongly deemed sane and charged with murder because "they planned ahead and knew what they were doing" (Sect. 4.7).

Like psychotic depression, acute psychotic mania also presents significant morbidity and mortality. Psychotic manic individuals can wreak havoc in their own lives and those of anyone unlucky enough to come in contact with them, sometimes by falling onto the manic person's paranoid delusional list of threats. Psychotic mass murderers are in paranoid manic states (Lake 2012, 2014a, b, c, d, 2022) (Sect. 4.5).

Bipolar and "Schizophrenia" are listed as separate diseases in the DSM based on the misconception that Bipolar is a disorder of mood while "Schizophrenia" is a disorder of thought. It should be clear that Bipolar is a disorder both of mood, and when severe, also a disorder of thought (Tables 3.14 and 3.15).

Such an understanding calls for the elimination of the diagnoses of "Schizophrenia" and "Schizoaffective Disorder." Further, there are substantial negative outcomes for clients misdiagnosed with "Schizophrenia" or "Schizoaffective Disorder" which also demand such a change (Table 3.16).

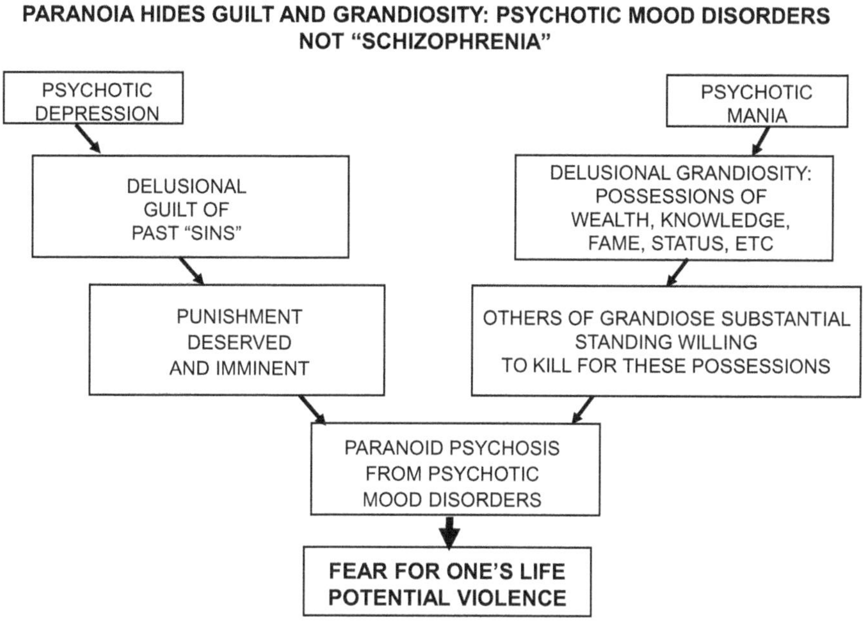

Fig. 3.2 Paranoia hides guilt and grandiosity: psychotic Mood Disorders, not "Schizophrenia"
Psychotic depression can cause delusions of exaggerated severity of past "sins" leading to delusional guilt. Such guilt stimulates thoughts that punishment is deserved and imminent. The fear of punishment, torture, and execution drives the depressive paranoid psychosis that consumes these clients' lives and instructs their behaviors (Sects. 2.8 and 3.9, Chap. 4).
Similarly, psychotic mania can cause delusional grandiosity of ownership of extremely valuable possessions. A logical result is the delusional belief that others want these possessions and are going to kill to get them, leading to a manic paranoid psychosis.
Since these patients, manic and depressed, present with complaints of fear for their lives, the core symptoms of their mood disorder may be overlooked and a misdiagnosis of "Schizophrenia" made. The paranoid psychoses and fear for their lives can result in violence (Chap. 4).

Table 3.14 Bipolar is a disorder of thought and speech; manic signs and symptoms explain the diagnostic criteria for "Schizophrenia" and "Schizoaffective Disorder"

A disorder of thought
Delusions
Hallucinations
Paranoia
Tangentiality
Circumstantiality
Loose associations
Derailment
Blocking
Disorganized thought and speech
Incoherence
Echolalia
Echopraxia
Clanging
Rhyming
Punning
Word salad
Ideas of reference
Ideas of influence
Ideas of control

Table 3.15 Psychotic Mood Disorders are

Disorders of thought
and
Disorders of mood

Table 3.16 Negative outcomes for Bipolar clients misdiagnosed with "Schizophrenia" or "Schizoaffective Disorder"

1. More likely to receive SGAs in larger dosages and for longer periods of time
2. As a result of long-term SGAs, more likely to suffer substantial and severe AEs including early death, tardive psychosis and any of several movement disorders (Sect. 6.3) (Table 6.8)
3. Unlikely to get needed mood-stabilizing drugs (Table 6.1)
4. In psychotic depression misdiagnosed as SZ, potentially life-saving ECT or mood-stabilizing drugs are not prescribed
5. Without mood-stabilizing drugs, BP disorders cycle faster and get worse
6. Without mood-stabilizing drugs, BP clients can be dangerous to themselves and others (Sects. 4.5 and 4.6)
7. The stigma of SZ is even greater than that for BP
8. There is hope for some successes in BP; in SZ the concept has been no hope
9. With SZ more likely to give up on life compared to clients with BP

Abbreviations: *SGAs* Second-generation antipsychotics, *AEs* Adverse effects, *SZ* Schizophrenia, *BP* Bipolar Disorder

References

American Psychological Association. Diagnostic and statistical manual of mental illness. (DSM-5-TR). Washington, DC. 2022.

Barth FD. The importance of your diagnosis: why your diagnosis matters and how to get the right one. Psych Today May 9, 2014.

Boodman SG. She was headed to a locked psych ward. Then an ER doctor made a startling discovery. Washington Post Feb 12, 2022.

Carlson GA, Goodwin FK. The stages of mania: a longitudinal analysis of the manic episode. Arch Gen Psychiatry. 1973;28:221–8.

Craddock N, Mynors-Wallis L. Psychiatric diagnosis: impersonal, imperfect, and important. Br J Psychiatry. 2014;204(2):93–5.

Freudenrich O. Differential diagnosis of psychotic symptoms: medical "mimics". Psychiatr Times 2010. XXVII, 56–61.

Freudenrich O, Holt DJ, Cather C, Goff dC. The evaluation and management of patients with first-episode schizophrenia: a selective clinical review of dagnosis, treatment, and prognosis. Harv Rev Psychiatry. 2007;15:189–211.

Geller B, Tillman R, Bolhofner K, Zimmerman B. Child bipolar I disorder. Arch Gen Psychiatry. 2008;6(5):1125–33.

Goodwin FK, Jamison KR. Manic-depressive illness: bipolar disorders and recurrent depression. 1st ed. Oxford: Oxford University Press; 1990.

Goodwin FK, Jamison KR. Manic-depressive illness: bipolar disorders and recurrent depression. 2nd ed. Oxford: Oxford University Press; 2007.

Lake CR. Schizophrenia is a misdiagnosis: implications for the DSM-5 and the ICD-11. New York: Springer; 2012.

Lake CR. Psychotic rampage killers: Mania, not schizophrenia—psychiatry's role in prevention. Psychiatr Ann. 2014a;44:213–4.

Lake CR. Rampage murderers, part I: psychotic versus non-psychotic and a role for psychiatry in prevention. Psychiatr Ann. 2014b;44(5):217–25.

Lake CR. Guest Editorial. Justification for breaking the Goldwater Rule: mass murderers' diagnoses. Psychiatr Ann. 2014c;44:211–2.

Lake CR. Rampage murderers, part II: psychotic mania, not schizophrenia. Psychiatr Ann. 2014d;44(5):227–35.

Lake CR. Bipolar. London: Elsevier Academic Press; 2022.

Love A. The diagnostic dilemma. InPsych 2018;40(1) On line.

Papolos D, Papolos J. The bipolar child. 3rd ed. New York: Broadway Books; 2006.

Phelps J. A spectrum approach to mood disorders: not fully bipolar but not unipolar – practical management. New York: W.W. Norton & Company; 2016.

Post RM. Etiology. In: Kowatch RA, Fristad MA, Findling RL, Post RM, editors. Clinical manual for management of bipolar disorder in children and adolescents. Arlington: American Psychiatric Association Publishing; 2009. p. 71–131.

Sartorius N. Why do we need a diagnosis? Maybe a syndrome is enough? Dial Clin Neurosci. 2015 Mar;17(1):6–7.

Swartz H, Suppes T, editors. Bipolar II disorder: recognition, understanding, and treatment. Washington, DC: American Psychiatric Association Publishing; 2019.

Chapter 4
Difficult-to-Diagnose Case Studies of Bipolar Demonstrating Wide Variations in Presentations

"*Public figures such as Cavett literally save lives* by advocating for mental health causes." (Fawcett et al. 2007)

"I've always hated sleep." (Mr. H.S.)

"I used as many as 30 Percodan per day to dial down the mania." (Carrie Fisher)

"Spade seemed concerned how hospitalization might harm the image of the happy-go-lucky Kate Spade brand…I'd come very close to getting her to go in for treatment but then she would chicken out by morning." (Reta Saffo, sister of Kate Spade)

"I was up two or three nights in a row…very alert and thinking quickly…I began to interpret people's postures and the flight patterns of birds as warnings to me." (Dr. K.A.)

"I did not sleep for six days…I was in jail to save the Pope and then I was the Pope…on an aircraft carrier…going to Ireland." (Mr. L.D.)

4.1 Case Studies Help with Recognition

Chapter 4 presents 60 clinical vignettes from the author's experience, from the literature, and from the media. Cases have been chosen across the extremes of symptom severity, some mild with hypomania and others with psychotic features. The cases presented aid in the recognition of atypical as well as mild cases. Other client profiles are provided in other chapters. See the *List of Cases* in the front matter at the beginning of this book.

Multiple professions are represented in Chap. 4 including medical doctors, psychologists, neuroscientists, nurses, business owners, CEOs, architects, scholars, artists, politicians, actors, designers of women's apparel, mothers, homemakers, lawyers, and professional athletes (Table 1.1). Bipolar touches all walks of life indiscriminately.

Many Bipolars succeed in their professional lives, some extraordinarily, at least for a time. A Wikipedia search for famous Bipolar individuals is long and impressive (Tables 1.1 and 2.1). Yet divorce, job and partner turnover, substance use, suicide, and other life crises are more common for them than for non-Bipolars. Striking successes are consistent with tragedy in the same Bipolar individuals (Sects. 4.3, 4.4, and 4.6).

C. R. Lake, *Bipolar for Psychotherapists and Their Clients*,
https://doi.org/10.1007/978-3-031-38750-0_4

In many cases, success and even fame have been achieved despite the occurrence of severe psychotic episodes characterized by paranoid manic delusions or severe suicidal depressions. Several successful Bipolar individuals summarized here were hospitalized on locked units and at least one was arrested and jailed before hospitalization in a psychotic manic state. Several individuals lost their jobs, most often during manic episodes. One spoke of losing 10 jobs by the time she was 32 and before she was accurately diagnosed and treated (Case 4.25).

An important feature in these cases is the paranoia involving grandiosity, as judged by the character of the delusions and the status of the feared threat (Sects. 3.9 and 4.5). There are delusional threats of endangerment from God, the Pope, the devil, and federal government agencies such as the CIA, the FBI, and Homeland Security. The grandiose status of the sources of such threats is diagnostic of mania and Bipolar I. Other symptoms of grandiosity included clients receiving secret messages of life-threatening importance meant for them only. These special messages were hidden in the numbers and letters on license plates, in the arrangement of the lettuce in a Panera Bread salad, in photographs on the fridge, in spinning gas pump numbers, in bird flight patterns, in cracks in the walls of the jail cell, and in random persons' postures. The grandiosity is appreciated by interviewers asking themselves questions such as "Is this client so important that they are getting special signals or being pursued by the CIA or the devil?" It is critical to recognize the *grandiosity of the paranoid delusions* as this aspect establishes the diagnosis of mania and Bipolar. In other cases, uncharacteristic *rage episodes,* conflict with law enforcement, Alcohol and Drug Use Disorders, and bizarre, usually paranoid delusions, support a Bipolar diagnosis.

Another feature of many of the individuals discussed in Chap. 4 is the *resistance to accept the diagnosis* of Bipolar and the *non-compliance* with medications. Such a reluctance to accept the diagnosis and treatment usually results in a deterioration. In some cases there are individuals who were initially resistant to accept their diagnoses, such as Kidder (Case 4.14) and Fisher (Case 4.15), who then accepted their Bipolar and publicly advocated for Bipolar recognition and acceptance. Both of these individuals struggled with long-term compliance and both may have taken their own lives during Bipolar depression. *Of the 12 very famous individuals described in Sect. 4.3, six suicided* and several others attempted. A majority had *positive family histories of Bipolar* including van Gogh whose sister was hospitalized for life with a diagnosis of "Schizophrenia." There are even more suicides among clients in Sects. 4.5 and 4.6.

Average age of onset in this group is the mid-teens. Alcohol and Drug Use Disorders were prevalent, occurring in 67% of these cases. ADHD (10%), "Schizophrenia" (10%), and MDD (80%) were misdiagnosed and these clients were inappropriately treated and medicated. *A positive family history was found in 65%* and all who had data available on premorbid function had had productive periods in their lives.

Bipolars tend to get *overconfident and stop their treatment*, putting themselves at increased risk for relapse. This occurred frequently in the cases reviewed in Chap. 4. At least two individuals probably demonstrate the concept of kindling. V. N. used potent weed before two of his psychotic episodes and J. S. took speed to study that seemed to coincide with her psychotic episodes; both clients' psychotic episodes required hospitalization. J. S. has incurred a second, milder episode without the use of speed. Kindling emphasizes the importance of avoiding illegal substances and alcohol, as no one knows whether they are predisposed to Bipolar.

Bipolar clients with psychotic or depressive symptoms are at high risk for misdiagnoses of "Schizophrenia" and Major Depressive Disorder (MDD) and then getting mismedicated with drugs that do not address a Bipolar Disorder, have an unfavorable risk-to-benefit ratio, or make it worse (Sects. 6.2 and 6.3). The antidepressants are no longer recommended by some psychiatrists for depression, either Unipolar or Bipolar (Goodwin 1989; Carlson and Goodwin 1973). The following cases are described in detail to help readers better identify and manage their Bipolar clients.

4.2 Cases of Subtle Bipolar II with Successful but Conflicted Lives

The following biographical sketches summarize the lives of mostly successful Bipolar II clients. Some of these clients in Sect. 4.2 had had symptoms and diagnoses of MDD and Postpartum Depression (PDD) for decades before Bipolar was recognized. The depressions in each had been severe and life disruptive, bringing one to a suicide attempt. The depressions had overwhelmed and obscured the brief episodes of hypomania and neither these clients nor their therapists had recognized *bipolarity*. All had been mismedicated with antidepressants. Knowledgeable therapists can influence medication changes.

Case 4.1: Mr. R. S. (b. 1963), Successful CEO and Business Person

Mr. R. S. is a 56-year-old male, married with a family. "I started my adult life at 14 years old with no financial support." Now he is very successful, owning at least four businesses, multiple other properties, and part of a bank. His net worth is well *over $10 million*. His family life is mostly satisfying. Mr. R. S.'s chief complaint was "I drink too much." What really brought him to medical attention, however, was a Major Depressive Episode (MDE). Although he denied suicidal ideations, he endorsed over two weeks of daily crying spells, sadness, loss of interest and enjoyment in usually pleasurable activities, helplessness, social withdrawal (*he would not answer his phone*), staying in bed or on the sofa 24/7 for over a week, not going in to work for two weeks, a marked decrease in energy, and debilitating indecisiveness. This was the worst episode he ever experienced. Since his twenties, at least once or twice a year he has suffered similar but milder episodes of depression. He saw a psychiatrist "on and off" in the past and was prescribed an SSRI/antidepressant.

After initial denials, he was prompted to consider Bipolar by detailed questions about symptoms of hypomania. He did admit that he also experienced brief episodes of feeling better than usual, even "on top of the world." His last episode was about three weeks before his most recent depression. He described himself as "*…going 90 miles an hour, up at 5 a m* after *only two or three hours of sleep* and ready to go, *talking non-stop*, multitasking with additional new activities taken on." His normal sleep is seven hours. He said, "It feels so good during those days… I'm unstoppable, I get a lot more work done but I am more irritable and into more conflict…*I make a lot of calls at midnight that piss people off*. Employees tell me they avoid me when they see I am up." His family and employees do not like his ups or downs. "When I miss my medicine, everybody knows it." The up episodes last three to five days and have occurred every two or three months for the past five years. Ironically, these hypomanic episodes may account for some of his successful business decisions.

He had increased his drinking during his high episodes and he says the alcohol can blunt his excessive highs and cause his mood to switch into depression. "When I really get to drinking, I can drink *one to two gallons of Jim Beam per week*." There is heavy use of alcohol on his dad's side of the family. Mr. R. S. said that his *dad is diagnosed with Bipolar* and that his mom may also have had undiagnosed Bipolar.

The diagnosis is *Bipolar II* since Mr. R. S. denies getting into extensive trouble during his hypomanic episodes. Medicated with lithium 600 mg/day, valproic acid/divalproex (Depakene/Depakote) 250 mg at bedtime and working in individual psychotherapy weekly, he is episode free for over two years; nor has he had a drink. He is the exception regarding compliance with therapy and alcohol abstinence.

Case 4.2: Mr. O. T. (b. 1998), College Student

Mr. O. T. is a 21-year-old college student who stopped going to his classes and left Merrymount College in L. A. after a year and a half because of a prolonged Major Depressive Episode. He moved back home. On presentation his affect was sad, down, and tearful. He said his mood has been consistently down and blue for the past two years. He could not do his class work at college because of his depression and could not even get himself organized to take withdrawals, so he received Fs. He endorsed a loss of interest in pleasurable things, described a feeling of heaviness, social isolation, and a *recent reluctance to answer his phone*, feeling like crying once or twice a week, and that life has not been worth living. He denied suicidal ideations but he said he has had *thoughts about dying for at least six months* and about the pain and suffering surrounding death. He said he remembers similar *episodes of depression since he was 10 years old* that got worse in high school. The current episode has been the longest and worst of all.

Upon detailed questioning, O. T. recalled that a year ago, he experienced an episode for several days to a week of "*feeling really good*." He had *no time to sleep* because of his increased activities and "*running around all over the place and impulsive decisions*." One example of a poor decision was getting *matching tattoos* with a new girlfriend on their first date. The relationship lasted less than a week. He said his *thoughts were racing* and "*... I couldn't stop talking*." He admitted that his thoughts at the time had been *grandiose* about the coming fame of his band. He endorsed another brief episode a year before that one, when he experienced *increased energy*, a *decreased need for sleep*, "*trouble keeping up with my thoughts*," *making calls in the middle of the night*, going out with friends more, and *up all night three days in a row*. His mom concurred that during that time he was much more upbeat, went out more, was more talkative, *could do "three things at a time*," initiated more activities, and thought his band would make a fortune.

In the past he had been prescribed an *SSRI* for a diagnosis of MDD which he recalled gave him a "burst of energy" for several days. He admitted drinking to *intoxication daily* a year ago but has cut back to two beers a week in the last six months. O. T.'s *family history is positive for Bipolar on both sides of the family*. Two cousins are diagnosed with MDD and a brother with ADD, possibly a misdiagnosis, given the strong family history of Bipolar.

O. T. initially did not accept Bipolar since his previous doctors had diagnosed MDD and prescribed antidepressants. After reading about hypomania, he did reluctantly agree to the diagnosis of *Bipolar Type II* and to a trial of lithium plus two anti-seizure mood stabilizers. His SSRI was tapered and discontinued. He continues to be ambivalent about having Bipolar and taking medicine; he stopped taking it for three days before restarting. With psychotherapy twice a week and the medicine, his mood has improved; he has increased his healthy activities such as enrolling in a local university, getting a part-time job, and exercising. He is more accepting of his diagnosis and the need for medicine but this could be week to week.

Case 4.3: Mr. S. M. (b. 1964), Tax Lawyer

Mr. S. M. is a 55-year-old single never-married lawyer. He graduated from law school and took a *Master's Degree at Yale* in tax law. He has been followed in therapy over the past 20 years. His most recent episode involves a Major Depressive Episode (MDE), intoxication with alcohol, and a likely *suicide attempt*. "I'm not sure how my car stopped in the middle of the railroad tracks." There he passed out due to alcohol and was by chance pulled out of his burning car, semi-conscious, by a good Samaritan. He was given his fourth Driving Under the Influence (DUI) and ordered to serve a year of intense supervised probation with daily community service, avoiding jail.

He initially presented some 20 years ago because of Major Depression and Alcohol Use Disorder. He was misdiagnosed by this author with Major Depressive Disorder and mismedicated with an *antidepressant*. He attended weekly psychotherapy sessions and his symptoms of depression resolved over a month. He discontinued his therapy thinking he was cured. He returned a year later in another Major Depression, restarted his antidepressant, added disulfram (Antabuse), and continued in psychotherapy for four months when he was lost to follow-up again. Disulfram (Antabuse) prevents alcohol intake by causing severe nausea and rarely death. The drug must be stopped for at least three days before drinking alcohol. This pattern of S. M. continued for some five years. After his fifth discontinuation of his therapy and medications followed by a relapse into severe depression, he finally resolved to never quit again.

He joined the Irvin Yalom-oriented group that met weekly. In group over several years he was observed to have brief periods when he *did not sleep as much for three or four nights* in a row, "*felt really clear*, saw life and what I needed to do; my *thoughts were going really fast…racing*, I'm much more talkative, *talk faster*, and feel more sexy." These symptoms were clear to the group as he uncharacteristically *talked non-stop and was irritable* when he was interrupted. His diagnosis was changed to *Bipolar Type II* and his medication was also changed to lithium, lamotrigine (Lamictal), and valproic acid/divalproex (Depakene/Depakote). His antidepressant was tapered and discontinued.

Overconfident yet again, he stopped his mood-stabilizing medications and his disulfram (Antabuse), and he continues drink and to cycle every six months but from a chronic baseline of depression. His initiative and motivation are low and he is delinquent on 10 years of his taxes, has lost his license to practice law and his driver's license.

Prior to his last DUI, Mr. S. M. had continued to drink on and off, did well for some years on disulfram (Antabuse) but discontinued it periodically and drank. He now has a year of sobriety and will finish his court-ordered urine drug screens soon.

Back on mood stabilizers and disulfram (Antabuse) and weekly psychotherapy, he has begun to accomplish some productive projects toward getting his taxes settled and his law license back.

He said that for years he never believed he had any psychological problems and explained that that is why he kept quitting his therapy. He calculated his rate of cycling and he admits that the medication and psychotherapy have reduced the frequency and severity of episodes of both hypomania and depression. He regrets the time he feels he wasted in his depressed states because he quit treatment. His diagnosis is *Bipolar II* with his persistent Bipolar depression resembling a *Persistent Depressive Disorder with MDEs*.

Case 4.4: Ms. K. J. (b. 1975), Mother and Homemaker

Ms. K. J. is a 43-year-old married female with a family. She presented saying, " I want to evaluate my medications." She was taking a *stimulant*, a benzodiazepine, and an SSRI. She said she was *diagnosed with ADHD in high school* and that her PCPs had continued her diagnosis and stimulant scripts for almost 30 years.

After the births of each of her two children, she suffered severe episodes of *Postpartum Depression (PPD)* that lasted one to two months. Her daughters are now 10 and 14 and she has had episodes of depression since their births with crying spells once or twice a day, loss of pleasure in usually enjoyable activities, feeling sad and down, social isolation, and decreased energy but she denied ever feeling like life was not worth living.

Her episodes of *depression began in college and resulted in a prescription for an SSRI.* About a month prior to presentation she said she had a "different" episode while she and her family were on vacation. She described herself as "hysterical, either crying or yelling, with *thoughts jumping in my head…I couldn't stay on subject or concentrate*." Ms. K. J. described increased activity such as *excessive cleaning* and *decreased sleep*. During her initial diagnostic interview she demonstrated *pressed speech*, making it difficult to ask her questions. A maternal cousin has been hospitalized because of paranoia and a maternal third cousin is diagnosed with Bipolar. There is a positive family history of alcohol use.

Ms. K. J. initially denied any possibility of having Bipolar because she had seen several psychiatrists and none had thought she was Bipolar but rather had diagnosed her with ADHD. She did not want to give up her dextroamphetamine (Adderall) or the ADHD diagnosis. She finally agreed to consider a diagnosis of *Bipolar Type II with Rapid Cycling and Mixed Features*. Lithium and lamotrigine (Lamictal) stabilized her mood and convinced her that Bipolar was the correct diagnosis. Her mood has remained stable for six months.

Case 4.5: Dr. G. S. (b. 1948), Successful in Two Professional Careers

A 72-year-old, three-times divorced male lawyer and PhD psychologist, Dr. G. S. has had an accomplished life. From a poor upbringing, he married young, raised his son as a single parent, graduated *summa cum laude* and *Phi Beta Kappa* from a large, well-known state university with over a thousand students in the graduating class. He continued his education with a *PhD in psychology* and landed an academic job where he *published and taught*. After retiring for four years, he entered and graduated from a top ten law school and practiced law for some 10 years. He presented in a moderate to severe depression and said he had suffered with depressions yearly for much of his life. He denied ever experiencing a manic episode, although his ability to drive himself for weeks with little sleep to meet deadlines was suspicious for Bipolar II. He was prescribed two antidepressants by his PCP and declined to consider lithium or a Bipolar diagnosis. Both his *father and brother had been diagnosed with Bipolar I* and his sister suffered recurrent major depressive episodes. His mood stabilized somewhat with weekly psychotherapy and careful mood monitoring.

This case is an example of how the stigma around the diagnosis of Bipolar and against lithium can prevent best treatment.

Case 4.6: Ms. H. L. (b. 1952), Successful Mother and Housewife

Ms. H. L., a 70-year-old widowed female, presented for psychotherapy because her best girlfriend told her she needed help. She has a B.S. degree and worked as a project manager at AT&T. She lives alone with her 54-year-old son living nearby. She has one sister and no known family history of any mental illness. She drinks occasionally, drinking to intoxication about one time per year.

According to her best friend, "I was not myself…I was *talking too fast and interrupting her*." In addition to talking too fast, she said that *she did not have time for sleep*, and averaged *only two or three hours per night for weeks*. She described her *thoughts as racing* with pressure to speak, increased confidence, *grandiose ideations*, increased irritability, increased interest in sex, and *decreased judgment*. She said that she *spent over $70,000 and did not need any of what she bought*. She bought a timeshare for about $50,000 that she said she not only did not need but also did not want. She also spent $10,000 to $15,000 on cosmetics saying she was "conned." She lost about $15,000 gambling in Vegas. She got out of the timeshare and returned the cosmetics. She said that during the episode *she had no idea that she was acting irrationally*.

Her first depression occurred many years ago. She averages three to four episodes of depression per year that last about a month, despite medications prescribed by her PCP. She said that during her depressions she feels hopeless, helpless, and sad; she isolates, has no enjoyment in walking her dogs, *tends not to answer her phone*, cannot get out of the chair, stays in bed more, and has had thoughts of life not being worth living but did not consider hurting herself.

Her PCP had prescribed olanzapine (Zyprexa), 10 mg qam, alprazolam (Xanax), 1 mg twice a day and had continued her on valproic acid (Depakene/Depakote) 500 mg, two at bedtime. Based on her history, the olanzapine (Zyprexa) was discontinued as was the alprazolam (Xanax), though it was tapered over a longer time period. Her valproic acid (Depakene/Depakote) was continued since she had no side effects; she was not oversedated.

Lithium was added at 300 mg with food, and lamotrigine (Lamictal) was also attempted but a *rash prevented its continuation* (Fig. 6.2). With weekly psychotherapy coupled with this medication regime, the frequency and severity of her episodes sharply decreased. She has had one or two brief week-to-ten-day depressive episodes, typically followed by three or four days of elevated mood no more than twice a year.

In such cases, with psychotherapy and review of her mood chart, she is able to identify slight changes in her mood. At the onset of early manic symptoms, the first approach by the psychotherapist is an increase in psychotherapy sessions to two times a week. If this does not resolve the episode, recommendations are made to the psychiatrist to increase her lithium as tolerated. Ms. H. L. also relies on her friend to give her feedback and now pays careful attention to what she herself thinks, feels, and says. She is more confident that she can identify and deal with her mood cycles. Her manic $70,000 spending spree warrants a *Bipolar Type I diagnosis*.

Case 4.7: Mr. T. E. (b. 1972), Successful Owner of a Small Tree-Trimming Company

Mr. T.E. is a 50-year-old owner of a small tree-trimming company. He works with his brother, daughter, son-in-law, and several other family members. His wife is a social worker. They sought help for couples work because there had been conflict and a substantial withdrawal by Ms. E. over the past six months. Ms. E. said that she was fed up with her husband's irritability and outbursts of anger "at the least little thing." She said that Mr. E.'s brother, son-in-law, and daughter agreed that Mr. E. was irritable, talked too much, and was a know-it-all. There had been discussions by Mr. E.'s brother and son-in-law of splitting off to form their own company to get away from Mr. E. During his session, when Mr. E. was made aware of his wife's and family's level of discontent with him, he was motivated to make whatever changes were needed to keep his marriage, family, and company intact.

Initially there was not an appreciation that this *irritability and anger were occurring in episodes*; the family believed this was just how Mr. E. behaved.

Couples therapy was undertaken and this included questions about the possibility of an episodic nature to Mr. E.'s anger. Questions about depressive episodes were met with ready acknowledgments that Mr. E. had four- to eight-week episodes when he was down in the dumps, sad, and blue…still irritable but not with the same degree of confidence and insistence on being right. Some of these episodes became severe so that he did not get out of bed for days to a week, attributing it to having the flu. He admitted that during these times he felt hopeless, worthless, and at times even felt that his life was not worth living. He denied that he ever tried to hurt himself but said that he had thoughts of taking his life. A first-degree relative had suicided.

The couple was given a mood chart to be filled out daily and over a year they gained an appreciation of episodic mood changes (Fig. 6.3). Outside of the two-month depressions, the episodes of irritability were found to be consistent with persistent *racing thoughts* and *loud, insistent speech.* During these times others could not speak because Mr. E. overrode them. His *sleep decreased* from eight hours a night to around four hours and yet he had *increased energy and activities*. He had *productive ideas* that, when incorporated into the business schedule, were beneficial and profitable. Upon questioning, he did admit that he drove more aggressively, spent more money on some things that he agreed he did not need, and may have taken on more jobs than he should have.

With therapy Mr. E. learned to recognize his propensity to talk over people, become easily irritated, and to lash out, alienating all around him. The couple agreed upon a signal that Mr. E. could recognize and attend. They picked "*quiet time*."

The couple reported over subsequent sessions that Mr. E. had become less abrasive. Ms. E. said that she was encouraged and felt closer to Mr. E. Once it was recognized that Mr. E. had episodes of depression followed by hypomania, a diagnosis of *Bipolar II* was determined.

Mr. E. was prescribed weekly psychotherapy, lithium 300 mg 1–3 qam with food, VPA (Depakote, Valproic Acid) 250 mg one to three at bedtime, and lamictal (Lamotrigine) 25 mg qam for one week before increasing to two for another week. Mr. E. has not had a depression or a hypomanic episode for a year. In the past he had suffered two months of depression twice per year and was hypomanic much of the rest of the time. This had been his pattern for 30 years and it was assumed to be "just how he was." Recognizing Bipolar II probably saved his marriage, his company, and possibly his life.

Case 4.8: Mr. C. R. (b. 1956), Successful Commercial Real Estate Agent

Mr. C. R. is a 66-year-old, married commercial real estate agent who had been successful at work and with his family for 40 years. He came to treatment during a second life-altering episode of severe depression. He was unable to work effectively but did try to continue to go in to the office. In the office he could not get much accomplished, which may have impeded future promotion. Initially he thought he could make it through on his own but finally sought therapy. He admitted to feeling down, blue, sad, hopeless, worthless, and helpless. With no motivation to follow through, he lost some potential clients. He wanted to stay in bed all day.

He saw his PCP who prescribed an SSRI and scheduled a follow-up six weeks out. This strategy was not sufficient and Mr. C. R. was urged by his wife to see a therapist.

His first episode of depression, five years earlier, had resolved after four to six weeks but now he was in a second episode that was detrimental to his job and family. Therapy twice a week was supportive, enabling Mr. C. R. to avoid hospitalization. The SSRI was tapered and discontinued and lithium, VPA (Depakote, Valproic Acid), and lamotrigine (Lamictal) were added for his MDD or possible Bipolar II. This combination with biweekly psychotherapy began to resolve Mr. C. R.'s depressive symptoms.

A confounding issue was Mr. C. R.'s alcohol intake. Initially Mr. C. R. thought that drinking to intoxication two or three times a week plus a couple of glasses of wine or beer on the other nights was inconsequential. He admitted he had made some bad decisions when intoxicated, such as driving. He had received one DUI but said he could have received several. He was able to hear that he must stop drinking alcohol and he has not had a drink in 10 years. Nor has he had another episode of depression.

He denied clear symptoms of a manic or hypomanic episode and yet has been very successful in his career. His diagnosis is *Major Depressive Disorder (MDD)* since he did not fulfill three non-manic factors (Table 3.11).

Case 4.9: Dr. S. D. (b. 1939), Medical Doctor

Dr. S. D., M.D., at 80 years of age and now retired, has had a long and successful career and family life as a pulmonologist and Medical Director at a large multidiscipline hospital. He finished his Bachelor's Degree with honors at the University of Michigan. Every fall at college he suffered the onset of depression that lasted until spring but it did not prevent him from doing well in his classes; he made *all As* and was *Phi Beta Kappa*. He was accepted to medical school and says those four years were some of his best.

He suffered Major Depressive Episodes during his residency and fellowship that hindered his progress. Still he completed his specialty training and accepted a position at a university medical center. Within two years, episodes of irritability and anger cycling with depression reduced his ability to adequately function for a time at work. He took a position at another major hospital where he worked for some 30 years and rose to *Medical Director*. Upon reflection on his career, he acknowledges the occurrence of several week-long episodes of increased irritability and inappropriate anger that alienated some on his staff and inhibited his professional advancement. He admits in retrospect that some of his issues were trivial and yet "*my anger was over the top*."

S. D. acknowledges a positive family history of Bipolar with his brother, uncle, and a nephew, all diagnosed and treated with lithium. His brother, a lawyer, had a diagnosis of Bipolar I with psychotic episodes. S. D. relates an incident when his brother called at about 4 a m demanding that S. D. immediately come down to his brother's office. His brother was talking very fast, non-stop, and *believed that the FBI was after him*. He had not slept for several days. He thought that the *license plates on the cars in the parking lot had special meaning* for him that related to the FBI. S. D. admitted his brother to the state hospital. Another episode involved his brother going to an automobile convention in Hawaii and hiring three "girls" to go with him. During this episode, he bought a new SUV at the car show. He stopped in Las Vegas on the way back from Hawaii to gamble. When he arrived home, he got into his car at the airport, having lost some $20,000, and *killed himself* with a shot to the head at 52 years of age. He left a family, although he was divorced. S. D. described his brother as very bright.

S. D. has a diagnosis of *Bipolar II*, has never been hospitalized, and has maintained a stable mood without depression for the last 10 years while doing psychotherapy and taking small dosages of lithium and valproic acid/divalproex (Depakene/Depakote). Prior to this combination, he typically had a moderate episode of depression every year and several three- to four-day episodes of heightened mood and irritability.

Case 4.10: Ms. J. P., R. N. (b. 1992), Student and Mother

Ms. J. P. is a 27-year-old nurse, married with a family who is studying to be a pediatric nurse practitioner. She is intelligent and successful in her studies. She presented in a severe depression that had lasted over a month. She reported regular depressive episodes once or twice a year since childhood beginning when *she was about 10 years of age* and lasting three to four weeks. She was sexually assaulted at 14.

She said, "I hated myself because of my weight." She cut herself when she was depressed. She suffered a severe *Postpartum Depression* (PPD) after the birth of her son three years ago. She wanted to die and *walked out onto a highway*. She also survived an *overdose*. She acknowledged the classic symptoms of a Major Depressive Disorder.

About five years ago *after starting night shifts and while taking an SSRI*, she incurred a manic or hypomanic episode that lasted for at least a month but *was not recognized* at the time. Her sleep decreased to *one to three hours* but she still had energy even after working a 14-hour night shift. *She tripled her workouts* in the gym and wanted to become a *professional bodybuilder*. She *studied for the MCATs* and planned on going to a top-ranked medical school; her activities increased and she experienced *racing thoughts*, *flight of ideas*, *pressed speech,* and *irritability*. During these days, she was *hypersexual*; she had an affair and considered getting a divorce. Ms. J. P. says she also has brief high episodes of two or three days, "maybe three or four times a year when …*I can't keep up with my thoughts*, I get much more work done on *one or two hours of sleep* and am much more irritable." After three or four days of hypomania, "I crash into moderate to severe depression." *Her euthymic episodes are rare and short.*

She denies drinking alcohol, using street drugs, or overusing prescription drugs. She is hypothyroid and takes replacement therapy. Family history is positive for alcoholism. She is stabilized now with lithium 1,200 mg/day, valproic acid/divalproex (Depakene/Depakote) 1,000 mg at bedtime, and lamotrigine (Lamictal) 200 mg/day. She *experienced a rash* and discontinued her lamotrigine (Lamictal). Upon presentation she had been taking olanzapine (Zyprexa, an antipsychotic drug) 300 mg/day "for depression;" this was tapered and discontinued since she was not psychotic.

It is unclear whether her earlier month-long episode was a full manic episode. Her hypomanic episodes last only a few days and were not initially recognized as unusual or abnormal. The hypomanias require careful questions to elicit adequate symptoms. Further evidence of Bipolar is the presence of at least three of the non-manic Bipolar factors found in Table 3.11. For example, she suffered *multiple severe depressive episodes since 10 years of age*, was *suicidal* with attempts, and had a severe *Postpartum Depression*. Ms. J. P. never recognized her mania as her depressions dominated. She accomplished more when hypomanic, even during the month-long manic/hypomanic episode. The symptoms and timeline meet criteria for Bipolar I but her life did not incur "major disruptions"; rather she became more accomplished leading to consideration of *Bipolar II*.

Case 4.11: Ms. C. J. (b. 1982), Schoolteacher and Mother

Ms. C. J. is a 37-year-old schoolteacher, married with two children, ages five and three. She is bright and successful in her job and with raising her children when not depressed. She sought help because of a severe Major Depressive Episode. She has been in the current episode for about six months and her symptoms had worsened over the past two weeks prior to presentation. Shc says of herself, "I am failing at work and I am failing at home as a mom."

She says she has been shutting down, *staying in bed,* and experiencing increased *apathy*, sad mood, *hopelessness*, helplessness, indecisiveness, *crying spells*, and *decreased interest* in previously enjoyable activities. Most striking, she says she *has not taken a shower in weeks*, which is highly unusual, as she normally showers daily.

She says her depressions *began in college if not in high school.* She remembers staying in bed and skipping classes, too depressed to get up. She saw three or four psychiatrists while in college and she has taken *SSRIs* since she was 18. She says she experienced a *Postpartum Depression* (PPD) with her second child that was severe.

Ms. C. J. also describes a persistent mild depression lasting years if not a decade or more that is constant and punctuated by more severe episodes of Major Depression. This description is consistent with diagnoses of both *Persistent Depressive Disorder (PDD) and MDD, known as Double Depression.* She has been treated by several psychiatrists in the past and consistently *diagnosed with MDD*. She has been prescribed bupropion (Welbutrin), fluoxetine (Prozac), other SSRIs, and alprazolam (Xanax).

She initially denied any symptoms of mania or hypomania. Her family history reveals evidence for bipolarity because her *father*, now deceased, had been *diagnosed with Bipolar II* in his forties. Her *maternal great-uncle was diagnosed with Bipolar I* and her paternal aunt, with MDD.

Ms. C. J. was asked to read about symptoms of hypomania and to report any positive history. On her third psychotherapy visit, Ms. C. J. recalled episodes characterized by decreased sleep to *only two to three hours, increased energy, increased motivation, "jumping from one task to another," distractibility*, and *racing thoughts*. She recalls that her dad "mocked my hyperactivity," indicating that he thought she also had Bipolar. She says these hypomanic episodes *occur every two to three months and last several days* during which she gets more done around the house and in her work for school. She says she spends more money during these episodes but not outrageously.

Ms. C. J. did not believe that she had Bipolar because all of her previous psychiatrists had diagnosed MDD. However, she was convinced by the questions about hypomania and her readings on the internet. With the change of diagnosis from MDD to Bipolar Type II, her medications were changed. Her weekly psychotherapy continued. She was supportive of discontinuing her antidepressants because she saw in the literature that they tend to make Bipolar cycle faster and get worse. Her 10 mg/day of fluoxetine (Prozac) was discontinued while her 300 mg/day of bupropion (Wellbutrin) was tapered and then discontinued. Simultaneously lithium was started at 300 mg/day. Two other mood-stabilizing medicines were also given in hopes of alleviating her cycling depressions. She experienced a *rash on lamotrigine (Lamictal)* and it was immediately discontinued without sequelae (Fig. 6.2).

Case 4.12: Ms. L.C. (b. 1978), Married with Six Children

Ms. L. C. grew up in the Mormon Church, married at 19, and had six children. She had been treated for anxiety in the past but sought treatment for depression with low mood, frequent *crying spells*, feelings of *hopelessness*, *helplessness*, *worthlessness*, social withdrawal, emptiness, guilt, and *shame*. She denied ever thinking of hurting herself.

Upon detailed questioning, she did acknowledge periods of about a week when she would *excessively buy expensive pets*. She has bought various exotic birds and reptiles for many hundreds of dollars. She bought several horses that she did not need or really want. She spent $15,000 on one horse and said she had *grandiose plans to travel to horse shows* after learning to ride and jump. During a recent up period she bought a $3,000 dog. In addition, she said that during these weeks when she buys excessively, "*I can't sit still...my mind races and I talk fast*." Also during these weeks she gets into multiple activities but loses interest and goes to the next. She said she sleeps less; "I pop up at 2 a m and *have gone several days without any sleep at all*. At the same time, *I'm wired and tired*." Her thoughts and plans are grandiose. She said she had ideas to start a "metaphysical store," to devise an energy-saving heating device, and to start a dog boarding business all at the same time.

She also said she is *hypersexual* during these times and met a woman online and drove three hours for a rendezvous with her.

Ms. L. C. did not recognize that there was anything medical about her condition to explain these behaviors and her ups and downs. Her diagnosis is *Bipolar I or II*, depending on the degree of life disruption, with *Rapid Cycling*. She has responded to lithium, valproic acid/divalproex (Depakene/Depakote), and weekly psychotherapy.

4.3 Chaotic Lives of Famous Bipolars

All of the individuals in Sect. 4.3 resisted the diagnosis of Bipolar for years to decades. Six suicided at the height of their careers. Before suiciding, two finally acknowledged their Bipolar and became mental health advocates; one never owned her Bipolar, was never treated, and hanged herself. The professional athlete apparently has not been compliant with treatment, likely remains in denial, and has lived a chaotic life. He is at high risk for suicide.

Case 4.13: Dr. Kay Redfield Jamison, PhD (b. 1946), Famous Neuroscientist

Kay Redfield Jamison has been named one of the "*Best Doctors in the United States*" and "*Hero of Medicine*." She received the *Suicide Prevention Research Award* and other awards for her advocacy for those with mental illness.

Jamison has written multiple books on her personal experience with her disease as well as co-authoring *Manic-Depressive Illness* (1990, 2007), the seminal textbook on Bipolar with Fred Goodwin, M. D. Having been awarded *lectureships at Harvard and Oxford*, she is currently a *professor at Johns Hopkins*. Jamison certainly qualifies as one of the most successful, famous, and accomplished of current individuals living with Bipolar despite a lifelong fight with it.

Her history is typical in that she retrospectively realized that she first struggled with Bipolar Disorder in late adolescence and during college. She took her *B. A., M. S., and Ph. D. degrees* at UCLA. Repeated manic episodes may have inhibited her early desire to become a medical doctor, but she achieved an equally challenging career through graduate school in psychology, specifically in researching the Mood Disorders. Jamison clearly acknowledged her Bipolar during her first position teaching psychology at UCLA.

Jamison has been married three times, the latter two marriages lasting many years. Her second was to Richard Wyatt, M. D., a leader at the NIMH who died prematurely of Hodgkin's Disease, surely a sad and depressing event in Jamison's life and for his other colleagues.

She writes of her own "mercurial" nature and of "essentially uncontrollable forces…moments of restlessness…maddened enthusiasms which, though disturbing, give meaning and color to one's life." She states that 15% of undiagnosed Bipolars may never experience depression but remain permanently "high." She was prescribed lithium but battled it, sometimes stopping it because it "impaired my motor skills." A more severe depression brought her back to the lithium, but then in a severe depressive episode she *attempted suicide* by overdosing on that very medication.

At one point in her early life, Jamison had resisted her diagnosis but works now with it and has made major contributions to the understanding and acceptance of Bipolar Disorder. Her paternal family history includes several individuals including her *father diagnosed with Bipolar Disorder*. Her diagnosis is *Bipolar II or Bipolar I depending on the severity of her worst manic episode.*

Case 4.14: Margot Kidder (1948–2018), Actor and Activist

Famous actor and activist Margot Kidder, best known for her role as *Lois Lane in the Superman films*, suffered publicly from Bipolar Disorder from 1996 until her *death by suicide* in 2018. Kidder was born and raised in Western Canada but became a US citizen in 2005 to participate in political and environmental activism. She experienced difficulties with mental illness as a young woman, expressed in *drug addictions, multiple marriages and divorces,* and many episodes of manic behavior. Kidder was formally diagnosed with *Bipolar Disorder in 1988* but her refusal of treatment for eight years allowed her Bipolar to get worse and cycle faster than if she had had psychotherapy and taken the medications at first diagnosis.

She finally accepted the diagnosis and treatment after her 1996 "nervous breakdown" at 48. Her manic paranoid psychotic delusional system involved her belief that her former husband and *the CIA* caused the loss in her computer of her autobiography she was writing. She also believed that they *were trying to kill her*. After *days wandering in L. A.*, probably in a delusional effort to escape capture by the CIA, she landed in a *homeless camp, was discovered, hospitalized, and then accepted treatment*. Her *paranoid psychotic delusions* are classic in Bipolar. Kidder recovered with treatment and never suffered another manic episode but she could not escape her depressions.

She revived her successful acting career, ultimately winning *three Canadian Screen awards* and *an Emmy*. Kidder served as an outspoken critic of the stigma mental illness brings upon clients and their families. She utilized medications, psychotherapy, and various holistic remedies, but despite apparent compliance with treatment, she suffered a severe Bipolar depression and *ended her life by an overdose of alcohol and drugs* in 2018 at her MT home. Another point to be made here is that even with treatment, disaster can strike. Proper treatment only reduces the risk. Her diagnosis was *Bipolar I, at times Severe with Psychotic Features*.

Case 4.15: Carrie Fisher (1956–2016), Actor and Advocate Against Stigma Around Mental Illness

Actress Carrie Fisher, daughter of singer Eddie Fisher (an undiagnosed manic-depressive according to Carrie Fisher) and actor Debbie Reynolds, began acting at 16 years of age, but made her name as *Princess Leia in Star Wars*.

Although she was not diagnosed with *Bipolar Disorder until she was 24*, Fisher began *therapy at 15* and had experienced episodes of *over-the-top drug and alcohol* use as a young woman. Fisher used drugs, including marijuana, acid, cocaine, and as many as *30 Percodan per day* to "dial down the manic in me." "I was lying to doctors and looking through people's drawers for drugs," she confessed. Fisher *resisted the diagnosis of Bipolar* until after she *overdosed* and was hospitalized at 28. Fisher tried various treatments including a year in a 12-step program, addiction support groups, and eventually the right psychiatrist, proper medications including *lithium* and a *support group for Bipolar*. She *periodically stopped her meds*, and on at least two occasions suffered *paranoid manic episodes*, going AWOL likely to escape her delusional perception of danger. In 1997 Fisher suffered what she called a "*psychotic break*," when she was in a severe depression and was again hospitalized.

This time she had five months' outpatient follow-up but relapsed again after stopping her meds.

After she finally accepted her Bipolar diagnosis, Fisher became a relentless advocate to reduce the stigma associated with mental illness. She believed that Bipolar Disorder can be handled if one accepts it and takes proper steps to manage the disease. Her manic and hypomanic periods were very productive: She *wrote three novels and multiple screenplays, as well as* edits of Hollywood film scripts. She raised a daughter as a single mom and had many close and loyal friends.

Her drug screen suggests that her death may have been a *suicide* by ingestion of *alcohol and multiple drugs* (Writer 2001; Serna and Winton 2017). Other data suggest she suffered a heart attack on a flight but this could have been drug related. Regardless, she suffered with *Bipolar I, at times Severe with Psychotic Features*.

Case 4.16: Mr. Vincent Van Gogh (1853–1890), Artist

The life of Vincent van Gogh has been analyzed with regard to several medical and psychological conditions that may have contributed to his suffering and demise. In 2006 an international conference of 30 medical experts on van Gogh's disorders concluded that "…one single thing cannot explain the entire picture of what happened to van Gogh" (*Amsterdam Telegraph* 2016 Conference in Amsterdam). Explanations given for his aberrant behaviors include his use of foxglove, lead poisoning from the oil paints, his consumption of absinthe, an early brain injury, epilepsy, Bipolar, "Schizophrenia," and Borderline Personality Disorder. "Schizophrenia" and Borderline Personality Disorder can be ruled out because both are accounted for by symptoms of Bipolar Disorder (Sects. 3.9 and 7.5).

Van Gogh may well have suffered from lead poisoning and temporal lobe epilepsy because of or in addition to his excessive use of absinthe. Epilepsy and poisoning are unlikely full explanations of other aspects of van Gogh's behavior that are consistent with a Bipolar Disorder. Four aspects of his history especially point to Bipolar: His cycles of depression and "*frenzied productivity*" are characteristic of Bipolar. He was *incredibly productive* and successful as a painter, though his work did not sell during his lifetime. His *family history is positive* for major psychological disorders, most likely psychotic Bipolar and, very important, he *committed suicide*. Suicide occurs during severe depression which is a central part of Bipolar. Lesser but multiple other characteristics also suggest a Mood Disorder: "His intense emotionality…" "I am…*prone to undertake more or less foolish things*…".

He became *deeply depressed at about 18*, lasting for months, when he "remained gloomy, renounced any social life, and communicated little with his family." Following this, he became "*...passionately involved in religion*." He was *an evangelist for four years*, was dismissed apparently because of his generosity, and suffered another Major Depressive Episode, abandoning religion. At age 27 "...he resolved to become an artist *with a passion* to produce works of art...with a *singular intensity*."

Between 1886 and 1888, van Gogh joined his brother Theo in Paris, and physical symptoms compatible with epilepsy are recorded at this time, potentially related to his heavy use of absinthe which has convulsive properties. It is written that he "*...often kept his brother up much of the night...*" Mania associates with less sleep and increased talkativeness, activities, and argumentative behavior. His brother described him: "It seems as if he were two persons: One, marvelously gifted, tender and refined, the other...always with arguments...he is his own enemy..." In Arles in 1888, at 35 years of age, he suffered an illness of "*psychotic dimensions*" for the first time. He wrote of "*...despair...*and *fatigue...heightened emotionality...would throw himself completely into his work...*became more disturbed. *Feverish, creative activity alternated with episodes of listlessness...*unpredictable *mood shifts of dysphoria alternating with euphoria* or with indescribable anguish...became more frequent." He wrote to his brother, "I have *attacks of melancholy* and of atrocious *remorse*...there are moments when I am *twisted by enthusiasm or madness or prophecy like a Greek oracle...and then I have great readiness of speech*."

Such descriptions of episodic mood changes from despair and dysphoria to "passionate involvement...a singular intensity...heightened emotionality...throwing himself into work...feverish creative activity [and]...euphoria..." are consistent with Bipolar. Additional descriptions of likely manic behavior are found below.

Gauguin's two-month visit with van Gogh ended poorly, after which van Gogh cut half his ear off, was found unconscious at his home, was hospitalized and "...lapsed into an *acute psychotic state* with *agitation, hallucinations, and delusions...*" He was diagnosed with epilepsy. Van Gogh wrote to his brother, "While I am absolutely calm at the present moment, I may easily relapse into a *state of overexcitement on account of fresh mental emotion*." Shortly after discharge from the hospital, he apparently continued to drink absinthe and suffered *two more psychotic episodes*.

He voluntarily entered the *asylum at St. Rémy* in May of 1889, remaining for a full year and experiencing *three psychotic relapses*. The last psychotic episode is said to have lasted from February to April of 1890. Van Gogh "experienced terrifying hallucinations...and he complained of the *religious content of his episodes* and wished to get away from the nuns who cared for him. The "psychotic" episodes could have been caused by alcohol, seizures, poisoning, or mania. While at St. Rémy, he *produced some 300 works of art…" in a single year*, making mania the most likely of these possible diagnoses.

He may have made *several suicide attempts* possibly related to his depression over his brother's engagement. He was discharged in May of 1890, judged by his physician to have been cured. "He abstained from drinking by now and remained free from confusional episodes." During the last *70 days of his life, he completed 70 paintings and 30 drawings*, many now famous. He admitted to "…sadness and extreme loneliness."

He shot himself in the lower chest on a Sunday and died two days later. He wrote, "I couldn't stick it any longer, *so I shot myself…*" That he produced 300 works of art while at St. Rémy in a year and 70 paintings and 30 drawings in 70 days suggests mania.

According to Blumer (2002), van Gogh "…experienced two prolonged episodes of reactive depression. Both episodes were followed by an extended period of manic or hypomanic behavior: first as an evangelist…and then as the quarrelsome and overly talkative artist in exciting Paris." This description implies Bipolar. Van Gogh's non-manic Bipolar features such as an *early onset of severe depression* (Table 3.11) and his *family history* suggest Bipolar.

Van Gogh's family history is persuasive for Bipolar. His youngest sister, Wilhelmina, "…was interned in a psychiatric asylum for life at the age of about 35…and was said to suffer from 'Schizophrenia'…" Van Gogh's youngest brother, Cornelis, "may have committed suicide or been killed in battle." As the current book documents, a diagnosis of "Schizophrenia" is most likely a severe, psychotic Bipolar Disorder. Van Gogh probably suffered with *Bipolar I, Mixed, with Rapid Cycling and, at times, Severe with Psychotic Features.*

Case 4.17: Mr. Jesse Jackson, Jr. (b. 1965), Politician, Elected Member from IL of the US House of Representatives, 1995–2013

Jesse Jackson, Jr., was treated as an *inpatient at the Mayo Clinic for Bipolar* Disorders for several weeks in 2012 after suffering a breakdown while serving as an Illinois Congressman. Having been an outspoken liberal lawmaker for 17 years, he also served as co-chair for President Barack Obama's first campaign. In addition to his *political activism for social justice and civil rights*, Jackson also *co-authored books* on personal finance and civil rights.

The Congressman was born in South Carolina and raised on the South Side of Chicago with four siblings. He was diagnosed as "*hyperactive*" and sent to a military school where he had to repeat ninth grade, was "paddled…for disciplinary reasons," and *suspended twice*. In high school Jackson was an *all-state running back* and he was *featured in a 1984 issue of Sports Illustrated.* He *graduated magna cum laude* from North Carolina A & T University in 1987. After a *Master's Degree from Chicago Theological Seminary*, Jackson took a *J. D. Degree at the University of Illinois College of Law*. He neither became ordained nor ever took the bar exam.

He never missed a vote in Congress. "He debated and voted with a contentiousness that made it difficult to view him as a team player." His fellow Congressmen described him as "*very energetic*, running *full-steam ahead, working six or seven days a week*." Jackson's *frenzied schedule* and the stress of legal entanglements took its toll on him. He resigned from the House in 2012, suffering from a sleep disorder, Bipolar depression, and gastrointestinal issues. He admitted to spending campaign funds for personal use and wire and mail fraud, and was sentenced to 30 months in federal prison (Gann and Parkinson 2012; CNN Wire Staff 2012; Wikipedia). Mania may have contributed to poor decisions. Mr. Jackson may suffer with *Bipolar I or II*, depending on the severity of his manic symptoms.

Case 4.18: Ms. Kate Spade (1962–2018), Designer, Entrepreneur, Business Woman

From Kansas City, MO, Kate Spade earned her *journalism degree* from Arizona State University and *rose to stardom*. She was *internationally known* as one of, if not the *most renowned designers of women's accessories* in the world. According to a commentary in the *Kansas City Star* by Jenee Osterheldt (2018a, b) who interviewed Ms. Spade in 2016, "Kate Spade was a *wunderkind… a dynamo* who positively impacted the fashion industry… she created clothes and accessories for the modern customer… She had it all… everyone said… Fame. Wealth. Friends. Family. A commitment to charity and helping others, she seemed happily married and [was] making *millions by her early 30s*. She continued to generate innovative and amazingly successful products for women. In 1993, after leaving her job as Accessories Manager at *Mademoiselle Magazine*, she started *Kate Spade New York* with her husband. She lived colorfully…her handbags had fun secrets to hide… The Kansas City girl celebrated her Midwest roots even as a New York woman of fashion" (Osterheldt 2018a, b).

The *Neiman Marcus group* bought a controlling stake of the company in 1999 and it was sold in 2006 to the *Liz Claiborne Co.* for *$124 million*. *Coach* then bought it for *$2.4 billion*. She returned to the fashion world yet again in 2016 with a new name. Spade won multiple awards from the Council of Fashion Designers of America and was named a "*giant of design*" *by House*

Beautiful Magazine. Spade was inducted into the *Entrepreneur Hall of Fame at the Henry W. Bloch School of Management* at the University of Missouri-Kansas City.

"On June 5, 2018, a housekeeper found Spade's body in her NY City bedroom *hanging from a red scarf* tied to a doorknob, police said. She was 55." After her death, Spade's older sister told the *Kansas City Star* that "…her famous designer sister suffered a debilitating mental illness for the last three or four years and was *self-medicating with alcohol*…Sometimes you simply cannot save people from themselves! *Spade seemed concerned how hospitalization might harm the image of the 'happy-go-lucky' Kate Spade brand*, …this was not unexpected by me [her sister]…Several times in the past three or four years [I'd tried] to help her get the treatment she needed (inpatient hospitalization). She was always a very excitable little girl and I felt all the stress/pressure of her brand (KS) may have flipped the switch where she eventually became *full-on manic depressive*… I'd come so very close to getting her to go in for treatment to the same place Catherine Zeta-Jones went for her successful Bipolar treatment program. She was all set to go but then chickened out by morning…We'd get so close to packing her bags but—in the end the image of her brand was more important for her to keep up. She was definitely *worried about what people would say if they found out she had Bipolar*."

"Depression doesn't have a face… It doesn't matter how much status you have, how much money is in your bank account, how many people love you. When people are depressed, sometimes they can lose themselves. Sometimes it's so difficult for them to process reality, and they get stuck. And sometimes they hide it because of the stigma attached to mental health. …People will look at your achievements and shame you for being in a low moment" (Adler et al. 2018; Adler 2018a, b; Osterheldt, 2018a, b).

It is possible that Ms. Spade suffered with Bipolar for 30 years or more before her death, not just three or four. Kate Spade exemplifies a typical case of Bipolar-promoted innovative brilliance and outstanding success. She also demonstrates a *reluctance to recognize* and accept treatment for Bipolar, which might have prevented her tragic early death. The current author's assumption of Ms. Spade's bipolarity is based on both her sister's report, Ms. Spade's striking successes, and the tragic suicide that substantiates the presence of Major Depression. The most likely diagnosis is *Bipolar II*.

Case 4.19: Mr. Kanye West (b. 1977), Musician, Fashion Designer, Record Producer

West, one of the most *awarded and best-selling musicians* of all time, has won *21 Grammy Awards* while maintaining a multifaceted career as a rap artist, fashion and clothing designer, and record producer. West's notorious conduct on social media, at award shows, and in other public venues such as his Oval Office visit has made him a source of controversy throughout his career. He also claimed he was *misdiagnosed with Bipolar Disorder* when he had "simply been sleep deprived."

Typical is West's visit with the President, described below, which suggests he suffers from a Bipolar Disorder. "In a rambling and disjointed monologue in the Oval Office which seemed to mystify even the President, rapper *Kanye West bounced among topics* as varied as politics, endorsement deals, Chicago violence, prison reform, mental health care, a hydrogen plane that he thinks should replace Air Force One, North Korea, and Hilary Clinton." West commented that one had to play 4-D chess to be able to talk with him. At the White House, West offered policy proposals, F-bomb expletives, and even a hug for the President. Also present were Jared Kushner, former NFL star Jim Brown, and an attorney who had represented a gang leader now in prison. West dominated, *not allowing anyone else an opening to speak*, including the President" (Lucey 2018).

Absent intoxication or a stimulant drug, this display of racing thoughts, pressed speech, loose associations, disorganization, and intrusiveness are consistent with mania. Mr. West's performance epitomizes moderate to severe mania which defines a Bipolar Disorder. Typical of Bipolar is his resistance to accept the diagnosis and treatment that might stabilize his racing mind and his grandiose and largely inappropriate ideas. However, some of his on-the-edge ideas likely relate to his incredible successes, which is also consistent with mania. The more time he spends untreated, the worse his disorder is likely to get. The most likely diagnosis is *Bipolar I or II.*

Case 4.20: Mr. Johnny Manziel (b. 1992), Professional Football Player
Johnny Manziel, recruited from high school as a "dual-threat quarterback," showed an astonishingly promising future in professional football. He was arrested in 2012 for disorderly conduct and has had other encounters with law enforcement. The *Texas A & M Heisman Trophy winner* and former *National Football League first-round pick* by the Cleveland Browns, he was nicknamed "Johnny Football." His earning potential was in the *tens of millions a year*. However, he has recently *forfeited his third professional football contract* due to "*unpredictable behavior*" related to his untreated and likely unacknowledged Bipolar Disorder. Manziel's most recent Canadian Football League (CFL) contract *required weekly therapy*, mandatory medical doctor visits, and *monthly lithium tests,* and while they declined specifics, CFL officials stated that the agreement has been "contravened" to the point that Manziel is *banned*

from playing for any Canadian team. His drinking, late-night partying, missed practices, and meetings had brought his firing by the Cleveland Browns (2014–2015), the Hamilton Tiger-Cats (2018), and the Montreal Alouettes (2018). It has been said, "… though at times Manziel looks under control, one never knows." According to *USA Today*, Manziel can draw crowds wherever he goes, perhaps less because of his football stardom than because he offers both a "good redemption story" and a "dumpster fire story"—irresistible to the American public. It was said upon Manziel's signing a 2019 contract to play for the Memphis Express of the Alliance of the American Football League (AAF) that, "Flirting with giving Manziel a chance could bring much-needed viewership, but his Bipolar could just as likely bring disaster." The AAF suspended operations later in 2019 making Manziel a free agent (Armour and Allen 2019).

He tried his old sport again with the Zappers, a team in the Fan Controlled League (FCL) in Texas, saying he had joined "out of boredom" and then played until he was pulled for poor performance (Wikipedia). In 2021 the former football star revealed that he planned a career as a professional golfer. He seemed to have chosen to leave football for golf, at least for a while. His golfing start was rocky but he planned to give himself 12 years to see if he could build a career, telling *USA Today* that it was a good opportunity to have a more structured life and to build business connections with a great group of men (Rivera 2022). Manziel announced he would serve as player-coach for the FCL for the 2022 season. It is unclear whether golf or football—or both or neither—remains in Manziel's future (Wikipedia 2022).

This story of Johnny Football shows how destructive unattended Bipolar can be despite so much talent. Manziel's resistance to accepting the diagnosis and treatment has had substantial consequences and may lead to even worse. The diagnosis is *Bipolar I.*

Case 4.21: Mr. Robin Williams (1951–2014), Celebrity Comedian

Williams gained his fame as an actor and stand-up comedian. "It's a brutal field…Man. They burn out. It takes its toll…If you're on the road, it's even more brutal." In the '70s he used cocaine and abused alcohol, probably as self-medication for the manias and depressions of his Bipolar disease.

Dick Cavett described an interview with Robin Williams: "*He was at full, manic, comic frenzy for an hour* without let-up. We even improvised a short Shakespeare play together… I caught his manic energy. It was exhilarating. And *exhausting*. When it ended, I was wet and spent. It took him a while to come partially down, and I thought, 'Can this be good for anyone?'" Cavett quoted Williams to say, "Isn't it funny how I can bring great happiness to all these people...but not to myself?"

Like van Gogh, Williams' medical history was more complicated than just Bipolar. He also suffered with Alcohol Use Disorder, Lewy Body Dementia, and Parkinson's. On August 13, 2014, he was found dead from *suicide by hanging*. His suicide may have resulted from a combination of Bipolar depression and the knowledge that his cognitive function and mobility would soon decline. Mr. Williams probably suffered from *Bipolar I or II*.

Case 4.22: Mr. Dick Cavett (b. 1936), Comedian and Talk-Show Host

Cavett has suffered all his life with depression and is diagnosed with *Bipolar Disorder*. Born in Nebraska of school teachers, Cavett was *bright, good at sports, and witty from childhood*. He was accepted on scholarship at *Yale*, where he experienced his *first major depressive event during his freshman year*. He describes himself as having lost interest in everything and feeling very sad. He had two Major Depressive Episodes later in life, one during his time writing for the Jack Paar late-night show when he *slept 14 hours a day* and could barely function.

Cavett has tried several forms of therapy, medical as well as *talk therapy*, but credits *ECT as his game changer*. He has been on regular medication and psychotherapy since those treatments and has apparently avoided additional downward spirals. Though he does not know much about his mother, who died when he was 10, he said that she also suffered from depression. He stresses the fact that Bipolar and other Mood Disorders are genetic. Cavett is active in educating the public about depression, particularly focusing on the stigma accompanying mental diseases. *Public figures such as Cavett literally save lives* by advocating for mental health causes (Fawcett et al. 2007). His diagnosis is *Bipolar I or II*.

Case 4.23: Mr. Kurt Cobain (1967–1994), Singer/Songwriter, Front Man for Nirvana

There is little question that high levels of creativity often accompany a diagnosis of Bipolar Disorder. Such is the case with *singer/songwriter Kurt Cobain, front man for the group Nirvana*. He suffered from *childhood with mood swings* extending from euphoria to *rage*. He was initially *misdiagnosed as a child with ADD and only later with Bipolar* (Sect. 2.7). This ADD/ADHD misdiagnosis likely worsened his Bipolar condition because of the use of stimulants for that disorder.

Cobain experienced extremes of mania as demonstrated by his high-energy performances on the music stage, his *prolific writing and drawing*, and his binges on *alcohol and drugs*. His mania expressed itself in *demolished stage sets and hotel rooms* when something angered him on tour. Just as frequently he created amazing numbers of *poems and paintings*, again during manic phases. His depressions became so intense that in an episode of delusional guilt he *committed suicide by gunshot at age 27.*

Cobain's *family history on both sides includes multiple suicides, alcoholism, and drug use*. He was accurately diagnosed as Bipolar late, underwent multiple treatments for his mental illness but *fell away repeatedly from regimens of therapy and medication* which might have extended if not saved his life.

This case demonstrates several informative lessons about Bipolar. It is a *disease of childhood often misdiagnosed as ADD or ADHD* and medicated with *stimulants that worsen the Bipolar Disorder*. Bipolar associates with both successes and rage during mania and suicidality in Bipolar depression. As Cobain did, Bipolars tend to resist the diagnosis, stop their treatment, and increase their risk for suicide. Mr. Cobain's diagnosis is *Bipolar I.*

Case 4.24: Mr. Dale Chihuly (b. 1941): Artist in Blown Glass, Businessman, Activist/Advocate with His Wife Against Stigma About Mental Illness

Famed artist Dale Chihuly, now 82 years old, has had an incredibly successful career renewing glass blowing as a fine art and creating nature-inspired works and exhibits worldwide. At the same time, he has suffered from Bipolar Disorder since his twenties, with big manic swings beginning in his forties. Chihuly and his wife Leslie had not spoken of his illness publicly until a former employee attempted to blackmail them, threatening to expose the artist's mental illness unless Chihuly credited him and paid him for work he claimed to have created as a part of his handyman position at Chihuly Studios in Seattle. While the Chihulys rebuffed the claims as baseless, they decided as a result of this experience to open up about the artist's mental illness. Leslie Chihuly explains that they believe they can help others face their mental health struggles by discussing Dale's.

Leslie Chihuly, whose mother also struggled with mental illness, has become the spokesperson for the family, appearing in videos and financially supporting organizations which work to eliminate stigma against those with mental illness. She states that the way she and her husband have successfully managed his Bipolar Disorder is by open communication between themselves and with their employees. They have structured their lives and the business around accepting and working with Dale's mood swings, understanding always that *the phases will pass*. When he is up they work together to utilize his energy and creativity; his down swings give the rest of them time to bring to fruition his ideas while he *nurtures himself by time in nature and by watching movies*—both of which provide him solace in those difficult times. He has benefited from psychotherapy and medications as well.

Born in 1941, Chihuly apparently had an uneventful life until his older brother was killed in 1956 and his father died in 1958. Shortly thereafter it became clear that he had Bipolar Disorder, though it is not clear whether he was officially diagnosed at that time. In a serious 1976 car accident in England, Chihuly went through a windshield and lost his left eye. Three years later, damage to his shoulder in a surfing accident prohibited his holding the pipe to blow glass. Around this time he began experiencing manic attacks.

The Chihulys met in 1992 and immediately began working together on his projects, first *Chihuly over Venice*. Ms. Chihuly states that because of her earlier experience caring for her mother, she was able to recognize the artist's needs in organizing his studio and his life. They have continued successfully with Chihuly, Inc. While protecting their privacy to a great extent, they both feel that by contributing financially and by speaking out, they can help diminish the stigma associated with mental illness. Mr. Chihuly probably suffers from *Bipolar I or II*.

4.4 Successful Bipolars Despite Psychotic Episodes

Case 4.25: Ms. R. C. (b. 1987), Mother and School Teacher

Ms. R. C. is a 32-year-old married female with a family. She works as a substitute school teacher. A year ago she presented a day after discharge from a three-day psychiatric inpatient stay. She was admitted in a severe paranoid state with psychotic features but was misdiagnosed with "*Schizophrenia*" and medicated with a needed SGA. *She was not given a mood-stabilizing drug*. Over the month before her hospitalization, her mood was *elevated*, she had time for only *three to four hours of sleep* per night but had a *marked increase in her energy and activities*, was hypervigilant, demonstrated *pressed speech, and talked non-stop*. Her *paranoid delusional system* initially involved beliefs that the sheriff's office was *reading her text messages* and then that the *FBI had tapped her cell phone*. She admitted to a similar episode a year previously when she actually had a job at the sheriff's office. At that time she had a diagnosis of Major Depressive Disorder and was taking *venlafaxine (Effexor)* prescribed by a previous psychiatrist. Upon starting the SNRI, she experienced an elevation in her mood for several days with less sleep and yet increased activities, "*my mind wouldn't shut off*," *racing thoughts*, *pressed speech*, *increased spending,* and poor decisions. That episode, apparently triggered by the venalfaxine (Effexor), lasted about two weeks and she was *fired* from her job. Ms. R. C. has such episodes at least once a year.

She has been taken to the *E D during mania four times* in the last two years. Three years ago she also had a psychotic episode and was fired from another job. She finished her college degree after attending over *six colleges*; she has *lost 10 jobs.*

She first saw a psychiatrist for depression at 18 and was *prescribed an SSRI.* She also began to *overuse alcohol.* About three months prior to her mania-induced hospitalization, she experienced a Major Depressive Episode. She said, "*I didn't want to get out of bed*; I was really down in the dumps; I *didn't enjoy anything* in my life. I felt discouraged, I didn't want to see friends, and I felt like *crying all the time.* I lost my appetite but I was not suicidal." This episode lasted three or four weeks. She suffers these depressive episodes at least twice a year.

She stopped drinking alcohol and smoking weed in 2019. One of her four brothers is diagnosed with Bipolar; a sister may have Bipolar and is prescribed an SSRI. Ms. R. C. is treated with three mood stabilizers and weekly psychotherapy. She has remained stable for over six months but has dropped her treatment. Ms. R. C. is diagnosed with *Bipolar Type I, at times Severe with Psychotic Features and Rapid Cycling* but she is now in partial remission.

Case 4.26: Mr. M. B. (b. 2003), High School Student

Mr. M. B. is a 16-year-old high school sophomore. He attends a parochial school and his parents are religious. He has a 3.8 GPA, runs varsity cross country, is popular with several close friends, and has a girlfriend.

He denies any psychological symptoms prior to six months ago when he began to have "*…hundreds of thoughts racing into my mind. They won't stop…*they fight against one another." These thoughts, that might be misidentified as "voices," involve *hyper-religious ideas* about God, the devil, and sin. The "bad thoughts" stimulate guilt, fear, and crying. "I love God…I have sinned. I was praying to the devil." His mind is overwhelmed with these thoughts that take the form of accusations of sin and arguments between God and the devil.

Mr. B's focus on God and the devil suggests grandiosity. These thoughts progressively increased and became more intrusive and predominant over the two months before his initial evaluation. His mom said that his speech became hesitant and he stopped talking. He said he *could not talk because he "had to attend to the racing thoughts.*" M. B. said, "I can't get through all the thoughts…I'm not functioning as well as usual…my energy is down and *I'm not enjoying life*. I'm not confident and I don't like being around people." His mom confirmed that there has been a marked increase in focus on Jesus, God, sin, and religion associated with a fear of going to Hell and delusional obsessions around past mistakes. She said he is more irritable and is subject to *uncharacteristic rages* since this all started. M. B. cried several times during the intake assessment. He appeared sad and blue and said, "I have lost my way."

M. B. volunteered an episode of "I got caught lying in the fourth grade." Since then he has "obsessed on a mistake I made." However, he denies a history of excessive checking, washing, orderliness, or arranging. His Yale Brown Obsessive Compulsive Score (YBOCS) score is low, ruling against OCD.

Mr. M. B. was read quotations from Kraepelin's books (1919, 1921) that involved intrusive, hyper-religious delusional thoughts of Bipolar from over 100 years ago.

> "...[There is] confusion with flight of ideas ... [when] they cannot concentrate or gather their thoughts together. The thoughts come of themselves, obtrude themselves, impose upon the patients. 'I can't grasp all the thoughts which obtrude themselves,' said a patient. ... 'I am not master over my thoughts, ... One thought chases the other; they just vanish like that,' ..." (Kraepelin 1921)

> "These delusions are frequently accompanied by ideas of sin..., he is a wicked fellow, the greatest sinner, ... has denied God, scorned the Holy Ghost, ... the devil dwells in him..." Kraepelin emphasized that "In connection with these ideas of sin, ideas of persecution are invariably developed..." Kraepelin gave examples that such patients believed that they "... must die, will be shot, beheaded, poisoned by the State..." (Kraepelin 1919).

M. B. said, "That's exactly what my thoughts are like!" (Fig. 3.2).

M. B. is waking up at 6 a m instead of 7 a m with these thoughts racing in his head. He said, "I'm paranoid...I'm not going to get any better...I'm afraid of the consequences with God..." During these times there are thoughts of killing himself that include picking a spot to run his car off a bridge. He said, "If I died, everyone else would be ok." He denies any current intent. Guilt over delusions of sinning against God, not doing the right things, and not being able to stop his sacrilegious thoughts is overwhelming for him. His affect is sad with tearing during psychotherapy sessions.

Despite carrying a 3.8 GPA through a year and a half, he is unable to effectively concentrate with these intensive thoughts and his GPA has dropped substantially. He continues to attend all his classes but struggles with his homework because of his intrusive thoughts. Also negatively affected is his social life as he is unable to interact with friends. Three of his close friends at school have noticed his distractibility and social withdrawal and asked him about it.

There has not been an obvious increase in energy, activities, pressed speech, detectable poor judgment, or a substantial reduction in sleep associated with the racing thoughts. There are signs of increased irritability, anger outbursts, and likely grandiosity. Symptoms of a Major Depressive Episode are simultaneously present.

A maternal great-grandmother *suicided with a shotgun*. A paternal grandmother is diagnosed with *Bipolar* and is prescribed *lithium*. A maternal second cousin is also diagnosed with *Bipolar*. There is a positive family history of alcoholism.

A trial of lithium, lamotrigine (Lamictal), and valproic acid/divalproex (Depakene/ Depakote) within two weeks reduced but did not totally eliminate his intrusive thoughts, supporting the Bipolar diagnosis. An SGA is under consideration. This case demonstrates severe symptoms of delusional paranoia consistent with his preliminary diagnosis of *Bipolar Disorder, Manic with Mixed Features and Rapid Cycling*. OCD, severe, remains a rule out.

Case 4.27: Dr. K. A. (b. 1985), Post-Doc Student in Molecular Genetics
Dr. K. A. is a 34-year-old married male with no children, born and raised in Turkey. He is a talented and successful PhD post-doc student in a respected molecular genetics laboratory. On his own, he generates important research questions and designs the experiments necessary to answer them. This is an unusually high level of function for a first-year post-doc student. He is already well published including a first-author *Nature* paper and will command a prestigious academic staff position upon finishing his post-doc training if he can stabilize his Bipolar Disorder.

About two years ago, K. A. experienced an "anxious" episode when he said, "*I was up two or three nights in a row…very alert* and *thinking quickly…* I began to *interpret people's postures as warnings to me*." This led to a suspicious, paranoid delusional system that involved a *grandiose plot* against him. He was even suspicious of his wife who was most concerned. He became increasingly "self-aware and began to see patterns," spending all night looking at pictures posted on his fridge and interpreting their *secret meanings specifically intended* for him. He thought there were *coded messages of life-threatening impact* contained in cards and photos on the fridge. He got messages from everything such as paintings and *movements of birds*. He denied racing thoughts but kept saying, "I got the message…is this world real?"

The effectiveness of his work in the lab decreased sharply as he could not concentrate. He thought he had been drugged. The previous year a neurologist had diagnosed anxiety and depression and *prescribed an SSRI* that caused acute psychotic manic symptoms resulting in *two trips to the ED*. At this time, he believed he was being *followed by the FBI*, woke up earlier than usual at *4 a m, did not sleep for four days* when "my mind was so clear…dark matter…" Then he slept only two or three hours per night for another several days, saw colors much more vividly, and thought his life was in danger due to a *plot against him.*

He related yet another incident that happened four or five years ago when he described a "*breakdown.*" He was "*up all night for several nights*, believed the *students in his lab were fakes and were put there as a test for him.*" He then entered a Major Depressive Episode for two months. He said that at this time he cried in front of his boss and simultaneously did not trust him. He took off three weeks from his research and had to get a letter from a psychiatrist to return.

He has been diagnosed with Narcolepsy and takes a small dose of a stimulant that is limited to only two or three days a week. This puts him at an additional risk for mania but he is aware of the danger. He does not know of any family history of Bipolar. There is no personal or family history of alcohol use or suicidality.

Lithium and lamotrigine (Lamictal) plus weekly psychotherapy have kept him stable for two years. He plans on organizing a Bipolar group made up of scientists that will meet at national and international scientific meetings. His diagnosis is *Bipolar Type I, Manic, at times Severe with Psychotic Features*, now in sustained remission.

Case 4.28: Mr. H. S. (b. 1991), Successful CEO, Business Owner

At 28, Mr. H. S. already owns his own business. He worked his way to ownership and has grown the business to four times what it was previously. He is engaged in beginning another business venture that is planned in detail. This is despite major episodes of *manic rage and severe, incapacitating depressions.*

In retrospect H. S. identifies what was likely a manic episode in the seventh grade when he gave "a stand-up talk in the school auditorium and brought the house down." He says he was "high as a kite" during those days. A propensity to *go manic before his performances* on stage and on the football field in high school through college and during his brief career in the NFL has remained consistent. He remembers a marked *increase in energy*, "*bouncing off the walls and talking too much.*" At 14 he was *misdiagnosed with ADHD* and prescribed *Adderall* through high school. This likely provoked his rapid cycling and worsened his manic symptoms which cannot be explained by Stimulant Use Disorder because he continues to cycle years after he stopped the Adderall.

A star linesman on the high school varsity football team, he describes rapid cycling mania triggered by Saturday game day excitement. Week after week during the football season he would not sleep at all on Friday and Saturday nights. He describes elation all day Friday and Saturday with a marked increase of energy and aggression on Saturday. He began to come down on Sunday and describes *depression* increasing during the early part of the week when he often stayed in bed 24/7. In high school, he overused *alcohol* and received a DUI that cost him a scholarship from a top division-one university. He *attempted suicide* by overdosing on six bottles of Nyquil after writing a suicide note but woke up with "no problem."

He received a football scholarship to a state college and his weekly cycles continued. He describes his depressions as the worst when in college, on one occasion staying in bed *every day for two weeks* and atypically missing an away game. He says when manic, "I was nuts…I would slam my helmet into my head, I threw my helmet at a coach, I threw a table at a graduate assistant coach and threw him down."

After college he made it to NFL training camp with the Cowboys. He describes this time as manic, going without sleep, *hypersexual with multiple women*, increased energy, and poor decisions such as taking a flight to another city to party and back the next morning in time for practice. He got injured on the field and was cut from the team. His manic rages in high school, college, and the NFL may have been excused by football mentality, but he describes several episodes that have occurred since his football career.

After football, he lost jobs because of both manic and depressive episodes. He developed a *gambling addiction* that fit with mania and alcohol. He said, "*I've always hated sleep*." Currently he describes his "*manic rages*" when he *breaks china, lamps, and furniture.* He head-butts the wall and doors, throws furniture (such as throwing a couch across the room) and feels hypersexual. Not unexpectedly, conflict characterizes his marriage.

He describes dangerous incidents of violence. "A guy on a Harley cut me off and I followed him for miles, screaming at him all the way to his house. I got out of my car and would have killed him. The Harley guy was terrified. A voice in my head said, 'Don't hit him.'" Mr. H. S. got back in his car and drove off. Another manic rage episode occurred more recently after his father called and criticized his wife. He said, "I was driving 90 miles an hour to my dad's house to kill him. I was lucky as I picked up my phone and allowed my wife to talk me down. I would have killed him. *Dad is also Bipolar but won't take his medicine*." A third near-disaster occurred on a pheasant hunt when another hunter who was drunk began to pick on Mr. H. S., finally pushing him. At this point, Mr. H. S., who had been restraining himself, "beat the guy to a pulp," but did not severely injure him because others pulled Mr. H. S. off.

H. S. describes more symptoms of mania: "*I'm grandiose*, I'm the smartest guy in the room, I get into *more activities, I sell more product, I spend more money*, I get into *new business deals*, such as flipping Airstreams, *I drive faster*, I'm much *more irritable* and easy to anger, my *thoughts race* and *I talk fast*; if anyone interrupts, I get irritated and angry."

Mr. H. S. has a *positive family history* of Bipolar. His father has untreated Bipolar, Type I. He says his father had been extremely successful, a millionaire, but then went bankrupt. His paternal grandmother also had symptoms of mood swings including depression and at other times "staying up all night."

H. S. has acknowledged his Bipolar, *stopped drinking,* and takes lithium, valproic acid/divalproex (Depakene/Depakote) and lamotrigine (Lamictal) and attends weekly individual and group psychotherapies. He continues to cycle every one to two weeks, but his cycles are less severe. His wife divorced him. The *Alcohol Use and Gambling Addiction Disorders* are in partial remission. He left his therapy. His diagnosis is *Bipolar I, Manic, Mixed with Rapid Cycling and at times Severe with Psychotic Features.*

Case 4.29: Mr. L. D. (b. 1962), Successful CEO and President

Mr. L. D. is a 57-year-old divorced male with a family. He was the *president and CEO* of a successful real estate company. Then, over three months prior to presentation, L. D. was *arrested and hospitalized on a locked psychiatric ward twice.*

His paranoid delusional system began with an angry tenant whom L. D. had justifiably evicted. The tenant did write a letter threatening Mr. L. D. and his family. L. D. began to believe he saw the tenant on the property in a car that resembled his daughter's car. L. D. was positive that "He [the tenant] bought a car identical to my daughter's so he could get on the property without raising suspicion." L. D. said he was "reacting…*getting restraining orders…calling the police* and private security." He was *not sleeping*, was very hyperactive, and became more and more *agitated and paranoid*, fearing for the lives of his family and employees. His waking hours, often 22 to 24 hours, became consumed with delusions and strategizing how to counter the tenant's imagined threats. One day he brought *his own handgun* to the office for protection as he thought that the tenant was coming to the office that day. In a panic state, he ordered all of his employees into the boardroom, locked the doors, and called the police numerous times. "My daughter thought that I was overreacting." One of the security guards told the police when they arrived, "We have a crazy guy over here holding hostages in the boardroom." *The "crazy guy" was Mr. L. D.* He said, "The police came in with guns drawn and *arrested me, putting on cuffs* but…the police recognized that I was keyed up…something was wrong, and they called an ambulance for me…I asked the ambulance guy if the ambulance was bullet proof." He was taken to the hospital ED where his blood pressure was 190/100. "I was a basket case." The psychiatrist threatened him with commitment if he did not voluntarily admit himself. He agreed to go into the locked ward.

Three days after discharge he was still psychotic, calling the police from home at all hours of the night, believing that "…something is going on in that building behind my house. I believe I was followed home." He was *not sleeping at all for six days*. The board of governors of the business told him to stay at home, not to go in to work. Within a few days he began to believe that the police were against him. He experienced *racing thoughts* and *wrote notes all night, filling an entire notebook*. His notes were largely incoherent. He soon concluded his ex-wife was in on the plot against him.

One evening, still in a paranoid manic psychosis, he went to his favorite bar. He said that after parking, he studied the *license plates* of the other cars in the lot and thought he had been followed due to the messages he interpreted from the numbers on the plates. Based on the license plates, "I believed that all the people there were *Homeland Security agents* assigned to detain me."

Once in the bar where he was well known, he said, "I thought my life was in danger. The shit hit the fan...I went crazy…*I threw over tables and broke glasses*. The bartender recognized I was not right and called the police. He is a friend. When the *police came, I felt I was in danger...I hit one* and was charged with a felony. *They took me down to the floor*, *cuffed me,* and *took me to jail* where they booked me, took a mug shot…I was incoherent and put in a *padded cell*. I thought I was in jail because I was the only one who could *save the Pope and then I was the Pope*…I thought I was *on an aircraft carrier* and that the *Pope had been kidnapped* to Ireland in an armored carrier with the number 37 on the side…We are knocking out terrorism…We are curing ALS." [L. D.'s brother had died of ALS.]

L. D. said that there were *dozens of messages* for him in his jail cell. These messages were hidden and disguised in the cracks in the ceiling, marks on the walls, and the shape of the tiles on the floor. He studied them thinking each message was of the utmost importance to the Pope's and his own life. From jail, Mr. L. D. was sent to the inpatient psych unit of a local medical center where he was screened for multiple organic causes for his psychosis. All tests including a spinal tap were unremarkable and a psychiatrist at the medical center said that "I did not have Bipolar," and another doctor diagnosed a "Stress Reaction."

Mr. L. D. does have Bipolar Type I, Manic, at times Severe with Psychotic Features. He was stabilized with aripiprazole (Abilify, an SGA), lithium, valproic acid/divalproex (Depakene/Depakote), and lamotrigine (Lamictal). When his psychotic symptoms resolved, the treatment plan included weekly psychotherapy and the down titration and discontinuation of the SGA.

L. D. lost his position as president of the company and was lost to follow-up. Hopefully he continues with his medicine and remains stable and retired in his Caribbean Island house. His diagnosis is *Bipolar I, at times Severe with Psychotic Features*.

Case 4.30: Ms. J. S. (b. 1998), College Student

Ms. J. S. is a 21-year-old, single, female student, a junior at a major state university. She denied experiencing any psychological symptoms before her recent episode. Her family confirmed that she had never had any previous mental health issues. About a week before final exams, her behavior became erratic and atypical for her, although at that time she did not recognize any changes. At the initial diagnostic interview, she said she *did not sleep for several days* and before that had only needed a couple of hours of sleep per night in contrast to her normal seven or eight hours. The changes in her behavior included the following: She wrote an *embarrassing, inappropriate e-mail* threatening suicide to one of her professors. She was hyperactive and *would not stop talking in a loud voice*. She pulled the emergency cord in a public restroom twice. Her irritability increased; unprovoked, she *screamed at a roommate, smashed her own cell phone* and drove off, "…turning the volume on my radio to the max." Her roommate said that she seemed "wired; her *speech didn't make any sense…was scattered*." J. S. felt she was getting *messages from the television* in Best Buy and Starbuck's. She went to Panera Bread, ordered a salad, and believed there were threatening *signals for her in the arrangement of the lettuce in her salad* so she "stormed out." She felt *car license plates were signaling* her. She became increasingly paranoid thinking the cameras in a store were tracking her for secret purposes and that the spinning numbers on the gas station pump had special meaning. While at the gas station filling her car, she crawled in the back seat and fell asleep. During this time of hyperactivity she was also having thoughts that her *life was not worth living* and of hurting herself. She did not.

J. S.'s roommate was worried and called J. S.'s mother who lives about four hours away; her mother drove to meet her daughter and recognized that she needed to go to the hospital where she was *admitted for a week* and diagnosed with *Stimulant Use Disorder*. J. S. admitted to smoking weed and to occasionally taking speed to study. This may be an example of a stimulant drug kindling the start of a Bipolar Disorder with future cycling, without further use of the stimulant. She took the spring semester off. Family history includes an older brother with Major Depressive Disorder or "Schizophrenia," which translates to psychotic Bipolar.

Because the stimulant may have kindled her first manic psychotic episode, she agreed to refrain from any further stimulants, weed, or alcohol use. Her SGA was tapered and discontinued once her psychotic symptoms resolved. She now takes lithium, two other mood stabilizers, has weekly or biweekly psychotherapy, and has remained stable for 10 months. She has returned to school with a lighter-than-usual class load and is doing well with the exception of another similar brief, mild episode about a year after her first one. It lasted for two or three days with less sleep, racing thoughts, suspiciousness, and increased irritability. She admitted that she was frightened. She denied taking any stimulants or smoking weed. Her diagnoses are *Bipolar Type I, Mixed, Severe with Psychotic Features*, now in remission, in addition to *Stimulant Use Disorder*.

Case 4.31: Mr. V. N. (b. 1991), Architect

Mr. V. N. is a 28-year-old married architect without children. A first episode, unrecognized at the time, may have been precipitated in architecture school when V. N. stayed up two or three nights with very little sleep in order to finish his project at the end of the semester. He said he fell into a *severe depression* at that time.

His most recent psychotic episode occurred in the *spring* about 18 months before presentation. He is normally a laid-back, quiet, and soft-spoken individual. This changed markedly over hours after smoking *weed with a bong*, a direct example of kindling from use of a psychoactive drug. He had smoked weed regularly.

His sleep reduced to one or two hours and even for several days, *no sleep*. He was terrified because he thought he was dying or *going to be killed*. He described his *thoughts as racing*; he *talked non-stop* and he was *hyperactive*. This hyperactivity rotated with several hours of not talking or eating and withdrawal into himself. Afterward he said he stopped talking because "I was trying to think of what to say…*my thoughts were flooding in so fast I couldn't speak*" (See Case 2.3). During this episode, which lasted about a month, he *lost 25 pounds* because he didn't have time to eat or sleep. He drew up plans to build "ideal houses" that would *make a fortune* and he believed he would win the Lotto. As his psychotic symptoms worsened, he spoke of *building a "mind temple*" and he felt he became the "*Green Power Ranger*." In addition he began to believe he was "…*Atlas* holding the world on my shoulders…too heavy…I was tricked…*Pandora…Chaos released…God and Jesus* trying to save me…Chaos got out of the box and I tried to get back in the box…*Chaos is threatening me…*The devil was crossing the river…He was fishing…There were snakes and dogs that equaled Cerberus protecting the gates of hell. The *devil is coming…*".

His *hospitalization* was precipitated around midnight when he began wildly running around, screaming, and was out of control because of his worsening paranoid delusions. He feared he was going to be kidnapped and killed. He admitted that he believed *his mom and wife were involved* in the plot against him. His mom and wife were terrified and called the police. *Six police officers* came and had to *physically struggle* to subdue and *restrain him*.

He took a medical leave from work. After the episode, he recognized the delusional grandiosity and paranoia of his plans and thoughts.

His first major psychotic manic episode had occurred about six months before this one, described above, also after smoking weed. He had smoked weed on an average of four days a week for several years and these were the first psychotic episodes he had experienced. He seemed to recover after this first episode but probably had not. These episodes necessitated *three inpatient hospital admissions* when he was misdiagnosed with "Schizophrenia" and given an SGA but no mood stabilizers.

Mr. V. N. said his older brother has been hospitalized at least twice, once at Vanderbilt, with symptoms of very little sleep, no time to eat, "flipped out." *The brother was psychotic and he has a diagnosis of Bipolar.* V. N. said that his brother had a diagnosis of *ADHD throughout kindergarten and grade school* and had been prescribed a stimulant for several years. *His brother does not accept his Bipolar diagnosis* and has stopped his therapy and his medications. A paternal great-aunt was also diagnosed with *Bipolar or "Schizophrenia."*

V. N.'s SGA was tapered and discontinued after his psychotic symptoms resolved. He was advised to keep the remaining SGA to be restarted if delusional symptoms reoccurred. Prescribed lithium, valproic acid/divalproex (Depakene/Depakote), and lamotrigine (Lamictal), Mr. V. N. has been symptom-free for over 18 months. He has abstained from weed since beginning therapy. He *developed a rash* during his up titration of lamotrigine (Lamictal), and had to discontinue it but has remained stable on the other two mood stabilizers plus regular psychotherapy, still without smoking weed. He has recently taken a new job in a very reputable architecture firm. Mr. V.N. suffers from *Bipolar I, Manic, at times Severe with Psychotic Features.*

4.5 Bipolar Paranoia Can Be Deadly

Section 4.5 offers descriptions of 15 cases of violence and murder, all committed by psychotic Bipolar clients during manic or depressive episodes. It is estimated that some *14%* of the psychotically mentally ill perpetrate violence within a given year. Such psychotic Bipolars are at increased risk for the most violent acts including suicide, murder, familicide, and filicide. Only 5–10% of all killers are psychotic, but they account for a surprisingly large percentage of murder victims annually because they can kill in large numbers.

Some of the same individuals, prior to their rampages, were very creative and successful at least for a time. For psychotic Bipolar clients, this risk for violence is considerably higher than for the non-Bipolar population.

Such acts have been recorded since CE 150 when Aretaeus wrote, “When the depressive phase is over, such [Bipolar] patients go back to being gay, they laugh, they joke, they sing…sometimes they laugh and dance all day and all night…sometimes they kill and slaughter the servants.” Although rare, some therapists may be confronted by such a client and will benefit from reading about some of the cases given below.

Cases in this section include Bipolar clients who have perpetrated violence or murder against strangers in the general population, their *own mental healthcare workers, US Presidents,* or federal establishments. Violence perpetrated on others by Bipolar clients is usually motivated by psychotic grandiose paranoid delusions. These clients delusionally believe they must take action first to protect themselves or save the world. Cases given in Sect. 4.6 are examples of clients murdering members of their families including their children.

Identifying such clients at risk for committing violence is critical to prevention. There are characteristics that differentiate psychotic from non-psychotic killers. (1) Psychotic killers are not intoxicated, radicalized, or members of a gang, (2) they are typically older, Caucasian, educated but unemployed males, (3) media scrutiny of the past histories of psychotic killers exposes a distinct deterioration in overall function, often episodically, accompanied with other periods of productivity, sometimes exceptional (Lake 2014a, b), (4) psychotic perpetrators have a bizarre personal, delusional, paranoid, grandiose logic, and motive for their attacks, (5) psychotic killers give warnings of their carefully considered plans about 75% of the time, but the decision to act can seem “spur-of-the-moment” (Goodstein and Glaberson 2000), and (6) about *half of psychotic murderers saw a mental health professional prior to their slaughter*. After a deadly act these clients more clearly differentiate from non-psychotic killers…but too late: (1) psychotic killers act alone, (2) they often kill in numbers, (3) the victims are usually innocent, seemingly chosen at random but may include their own therapists, children, and family, (4) they usually kill during daylight, (5) they do not try to escape the murder scene, (6) about half commit suicide after the rampage or are shot dead by others (“suicide by cop”) at a rate of 10 times that recorded after all homicides (Duwe 2010).

4.5.1 Strangers at Risk for Bipolar Violence

Case 4.32: Mr. Travis Reinking, 29, Killed Four in a Waffle House in Nashville, TN, April 22, 2018, at 3:25 a m

Travis Reinking, educated but unemployed, *without any obvious provocation, on April 22, 2018, killed four and wounded four others, all strangers,* with an AR-15 in a *Waffle House in Nashville, TN, at 3:25 a m.* A customer wrestled the rifle from Reinking as he tried to reload. He *wore nothing but a green jacket* which he threw off during his flight from the restaurant. *Naked*, Reinking stole a car and *remained at large for a day and a half* before being apprehended in a wooded area near his apartment. This behavior during and after the event is *exceptional* in two ways for psychotic rampage killers in that he *killed at night* and *fled the scene*. Reinking had a loaded handgun and ammunition in his possession at the time of arrest but surrendered without incident (Blinder 2018; Vera 2018).

Reinking had had several previous episodes in which he demonstrated psychotic manic behavior. In *May of 2016* in IL where he was then living, Reinking drew law officers to a parking lot where he was disturbing the peace, yelling that "*Taylor Swift* was stalking him and hacking his phone and his family was also involved…".

In *June of 2017*, still psychotic or psychotic again, he "…marched into a community swimming pool in Tremont, IL, and jumped into the water wearing a *pink woman's coat over his underwear*." Officers were called and it is believed that he had in his trunk at that incident the AR-15 he would later use in Nashville.

In July 2017, he drove from Tremont to Washington, DC., where he was *arrested* for crossing a security barrier at the *White House*, *seeking a meeting with President Trump*. After this incident in Washington, DC., Reinking moved from IL to Nashville, TN, when the *family expressed concern* for his welfare because he was *exhibiting delusional behavior* (Blinder 2018).

Mr. Reinking was certainly psychotic with *grandiose delusional episodes* recorded in May, 2016, and in June and July of 2017. Grandiosity is documented by his delusions involving *Taylor Swift* and *President Trump*. These grandiose themes of relationships with a famous performer and the President of the United States are strikingly consistent with the case of Mr. Hinckley (Case 4.38). Mr. Reinking's inappropriate naked or near-naked episodes reinforce the diagnosis of a psychotic manic state. His family documented their son's delusions. That he attacked at 3:25 a m is consistent with manic hyperactivity and lack of need for sleep. Mr. Reinking is *Bipolar, Type I, Manic, at times Severe with Psychotic Features*.

Case 4.33: Stephen Paddock, 64, Killed 58 and Wounded Hundreds in Las Vegas, NV, October 1, 2017, Between 10:05 and 10:15 p m

Stephen Paddock grew up in Sun Valley, CA, and attended California State in Northridge before working as a postman, an IRS agent, an auditor, a real estate investor, and later a professional gambler. His father was a convicted bank robber. Paddock was seven years old when his father was convicted of "robbing banks with a machine gun."

At the *Mandalay Bay Hotel, Las Vegas*, NV, on *Sunday, October 1, 2017*, just after 10 p m, Paddock executed a well-planned mass shooting from windows 32 stories above the huge *Route 92 Harvest Country Music Festival where 22,000 people had gathered*. Seemingly unprovoked, he indiscriminately *murdered 58 and wounded over 400, all strangers*, with 1,100 rounds. He *killed himself as law enforcement closed in*.

He had spent months to years gathering firearms and ammunition, as well as arranging a system of cameras to monitor the area around his rooms at the hotel. Police found *47 weapons* in the hotel, many with bump stocks (Glenn et al. 2018).

Paddock had no prior identified mental condition and his only medication was diazepam (Valium) prescribed for anxiety. Paddock owned several homes in different states but mostly lived gratis in one casino or another, repeatedly *gambled all night*, betting as much as a *million dollars in one night*. He does not seem to have been in financial difficulty, although he lost big at times. His girlfriend Marilou Danley said that he was *extremely generous* with those he loved. On the day of the shootings, he had wired her $100,000 in the Philippines where he had sent her earlier to visit her family. Employees at the hotel said he was a good tipper. He kept to himself, and no one but his brother and Danley seem to have known him very well. Even they were totally shocked by his actions in Las Vegas.

Paddock had previously rented rooms or condos overlooking other big events in Chicago, Boston, and Las Vegas before moving into the Mandalay Bay six days before the country music festival he chose for his massacre. Police said that he "appeared to be living a secret life and had spent decades acquiring ammunition and weapons…He had 50 pounds of Tannerite as well as ammonium nitrate and 1,600 rounds of ammunition in his vehicle" parked at the hotel (Glover et al. 2017; Olmstead 2017a, b; Medina et al. 2017).

His motive is critical but unknown. It may be revealed when and if his delusional system is discovered from his records, if any. Enlightened speculation is warranted. Such perpetrators are either sane (non-psychotic) or psychotic and Mr. Paddock's actions fit the profile of psychotic (Sect. 3.9). He acted alone, suicided at the scene, was not intoxicated or radicalized, was a Caucasian male, educated but unemployed/retired, and had been successful. Mr. Paddock's girlfriend said, "He seemed to be mentally and physically deteriorating in recent months." This suggests the onset of an episode of severe mental illness. The question is which one.

The paranoid delusional systems that reveal the motives and manic diagnoses of other similar psychotic mass murderers reviewed here invite consideration of a manic diagnosis for Mr. Paddock. His paranoia in some way involved a threat from attendees to large concerts that in his mind called for such a slaughter. In another case reviewed below (Case 4.39), Mr. Alexis believed that the US Navy was attacking his mind with ELF waves and Ms.

Carey (Case 4.40) believed that President Obama was stalking her. Both suffered with Bipolar. These delusions were revealed by research of the media that has determined diagnoses of *Bipolar I, Manic*.

Mr. Paddock's behavior is psychotic and not due to an organic disease; the autopsy CT of his head and his labs were normal. Last, it is unlikely that the symptoms were caused by a substance, based on his autopsy results showing positive only for the prescribed benzodiazepine, diazepam (Valium) (German 2018). His suicide is another factor indicative of a psychotic Mood Disorder such as Bipolar (Glover et al. 2017; Olmstead 2017a, b; Medina et al. 2017). Thus the most likely explanation for his murderous rampage is *Bipolar Disorder, Type I, Manic, at times Severe with Psychotic Features*.

Case 4.34: Mr. James E. Holmes, 24, Killed 12, Shot 70 at a Movie Theater, Aurora, CO, July 20, 2012, at Midnight

While *dressed as the Batman comics character*, "*The Joker*," and wearing a protective vest, James Eagan Holmes, *unprovoked, murdered 12 and injured 58, all strangers*, in an Aurora, CO, theater during the Friday midnight premier showing of a new Batman movie. His apartment was bizarrely decorated with Batman paraphernalia, hardly appropriate to his academic program. Both before and after his rampage, he made *grandiose, disorganized, incomprehensible, and delusional statements* to a number of people, including the owner of a gun club that he tried to join. Mr. Rotkovich, the gun club owner, said that "Mr. Holmes' voice mail, in hindsight, sounded like the Joker … it was like somebody [Mr. Holmes] was trying to be as weird as possible." Consistent with a psychotic killer, after his assault, Mr. Holmes seemed to *wait by his car* for the police to arrest him (McLean 2012; Wikipedia).

Mr. Holmes is "… the son of a registered nurse and a mathematician working as a senior scientist. His father has degrees from Stanford, UCLA, and Berkeley." In high school, Mr. Holmes *played soccer and ran cross country*. "Beginning in 2006 he attended the *University of California, Riverside,* and, in 2010 received his undergraduate *degree in Neuroscience* with the *highest honors*." He was invited to join *Phi Beta Kappa* and Golden Key. He graduated with a *3.949 GPA* in the top 1% of his class. In 2011, he enrolled in a *PhD program in Neuroscience* at the University of Colorado Medical Campus in Aurora on full scholarship.

Rather *abruptly, his academic performance declined during the spring semester and he dropped out of his studies in early June, 2012,* probably in a severe mixed Mood Disorder. He *was seen by "… at least three mental health professionals* at the University of Colorado prior to the massacre" and was *misdiagnosed with "Schizophrenia."* Some of his peers suspected that "…Holmes suffered from mental illness and could be *dangerous*." Similar to Alexis, Loughner, and Cho, he was frightening.

His *hyperactivity* included the purchase at least *four firearms, over 6,000 rounds of ammunition*, a black urban assault vest, and a knife in the two months prior to his rampage. He had *dyed his hair red.* That *his attack occurred at midnight*, not during the day, is an exception but suggests the lack of need for sleep as was the case with Misters Reinking (Case 4.32) and Paddock (Case 4.33).

Holmes' academic successes and psychotic violence are similar to those of Mr. Laudor (Case 4.48). Based on the plans, activities, calls, purchases, timing (midnight), premorbid successes, specifically exceptional performance at a high academic level that abruptly changed to psychotic grandiose delusions, anger and violence, he fits the profile of *Bipolar I, Manic, at times Severe with Psychotic Features*.

Case 4.35: Mr. Anders B. Breivik, 32, Blew Up a Building in Downtown Oslo and Murdered 77 on Utoeya Island, Norway, July 22, 2011, During the Day

During the day on a Monday, Anders Behring Breivik, 32 years of age, while wearing a *fake police uniform*, executed his *carefully considered grandiose and politically motivated plans*. Unprovoked, he *blew up a government building* in downtown Oslo before driving to another site on Utoeya Island where the *Labour Party Youth Camp* was being held. There he *killed a total of 77 people*, mostly teenagers and young adults, *all strangers*. He was arrested at the site and is in prison. Breivik stated his motive saying that the "… attacks were necessary to stop the 'Islamization' of Norway." Breivik referred to himself as "… the *future Regent of Norway, Master of Life and Death* … and '*Europe's most Perfect Knight* since World War II.'" Previously he had distributed electronically "a [massive] *compendium of [bizarre] texts* entitled: '2083: A European Declaration of Independence'" demonstrating a grandiose, paranoid, psychotic, politically based delusional system. This is similar to that of Mr. Cho (Case 4.36). Such excessive writing is symptomatic of mania.

He was *educated* and held a demanding professional position. In 1997 at the age of 18, while employed as an investment banker, *he lost the equivalent of $369,556 in the stock market*. Mr. Breivik had suffered past *states of depression,* withdrawal, and isolation, according to media reports. Despite this, he was subsequently misdiagnosed with "*Schizophrenia*." Premorbid success followed by episodes of depression, politically based psychotic, paranoid, and grandiose delusions in a violent psychotic mass killer are compatible with psychotic mania. Others have opined that Breivik is a sane terrorist but his grandiose delusions of being the *Regent of Norway, Europe's Most Perfect Knight,* and others contradict the terrorist motive (BBC 2012; Lambert 2011). He has *Bipolar I Disorder, Manic, at times Severe with Psychotic Features.*

Case 4.36: Mr. Seung-Hui Cho, 23, Murdered 30 in Classrooms on Campus at Virginia Tech, Blacksburg, VA, April 16, 2007, at 7:15 a m
"Around 7:15 a m EDT on a Saturday, … Seung-Hui Cho, 23, *without obvious provocation, killed two students...* [in their] dormitory [rooms]… Cho returned to his room to re-arm himself and *mailed [an excessively extensive and grandiose] package to NBC News [similar to the grandiose e-mail written by Mr. Breivik].* At approximately 9:45 a m…Cho then crossed the campus to Norris Hall, a classroom building where, in a span of nine minutes, he *shot dozens of people,* [*at random,* mostly students] *killing 30 of them.* As police breached the area of the building…Cho committed *suicide*…with a gunshot to his temple…Cho…had left a note in his dormitory which contains a *rant referencing Christianity*…he stated that '*Thanks to you I died like Jesus Christ,* to inspire generations of weak and defenseless people.'"

Prior to the rampage, some of Mr. Cho's professors and fellow students at Virginia Tech found him "*menacing*" and became *concerned for their own safety,* similar to Mr. Loughner's and Mr. Holmes' classmates (above) (Cases 4.41 and 4.34, respectively). On a previous occasion Cho told another student during a telephone call that he [Cho] was in North Carolina "… *vacationing with Vladimir Putin,*" the President of Russia. He sent another message with the words, "I might as well kill myself now." Alerted by campus authorities, the *police escorted Cho to the Virginia Mental Health Agency* serving Blacksburg, VA. He was misdiagnosed with "*Schizophrenia" and Major Depressive Disorder.* Outpatient treatment was recommended but it seems neither Mr. Cho nor the Mental Health Agency followed up. Apparently there was not adequate concern regarding a potential for danger.

The package Cho *mailed to NBC News in New York* is diagnostic of mania when considered along with his actions noted above. It contained *25 minutes of video, 43 photographs, 23 pages of bizarre, disorganized written material, and 23 PDF files* that were last modified at 7:24 a m after the first two murders. In his writings sent to NBC, Cho "…[sent] *threatening messages to then US President George W. Bush, Vice-President Dick Chaney and Secretary of State, Condoleezza Rice*…in another video he compared himself to *Jesus Christ…*".

Specifically threatening the President and Vice President of the United States defines grandiosity, psychosis, mania, and Bipolar (Chap. 3).

An autopsy revealed the absence of any drugs or alcohol (Wikipedia). Note that the activities of Misters Alexis, Holmes, Breivik, Loughner, and Cho include making and executing detailed plans, inducing fear in their teachers and classmates (especially Holmes, Loughner, and Cho), psychotic, grandiose, and politically flavored delusions that together define mania and a diagnosis of *Bipolar I, Manic, at times Severe with Psychotic Features.*

4.5.2 Political Leaders at Risk for Bipolar Violence

Case 4.37: Mr. John Patrick Bedell, 36, Shot and Wounded Two Pentagon Police Officers Before They Shot and Seriously Wounded Him at the Pentagon, Washington, DC, March 4, 2010

Mr. John Patrick Bedell lived in CA before shooting two Pentagon police officers who then shot and seriously wounded him at the Pentagon. He had "*crisscrossed the country* in a frenetic and sometimes doped-up state that had *his parents so worried that they alerted the police* that he might be armed…He had been *slipping into increasingly disturbed thinking for years* but his behavior became uncharacteristically disturbed in recent months [before the shootings]." Bedell had made what appeared to be a spur-of-the-moment decision to move to Austin, TX, to live with a woman he had met at a bookstore at UC Davis. At one point, he became interested in *developing a different currency for the US.*

A few months before the shootings, he was *stopped for speeding.* He was *traveling erratically*, told his parents he was heading from TX to the East Coast, but instead, drove 1,500 miles in the opposite direction to his CA home. In February, 2010, he drove to Reno, NV, and posted on the internet a suggestion that "after the 1963 assassination of President John F. Kennedy, the United States had been infiltrated by a *cabal of gangsters he called the 'Coup Regime.'*" He believed songs on the *radio gave him special messages* and warnings that "they" were watching him and his father [a former CA Deputy Attorney General]. His father said that he likely had "*Paranoid Schizophrenia* (Klein et al. 2010)."

Mr. Bedell's erratic, spur-of-the-moment decisions, multiple trips, speeding, his frantic state, grandiosity, delusional paranoia, and violence are diagnostic of *Bipolar Disorder I, Manic, at times Severe with Psychotic Features.*

Case 4.38: Mr. John Hinckley, 25, Attempted to Assassinate President Ronald Reagan at the Washington Hilton Hotel, Washington, DC, Monday, March 30, 1981, at 2:27 p m

In the days before his rampage, *Mr. Hinckley's parents had asked his doctor to hospitalize their son* but he would not. Mr. Hinkley flew from his home in CO to CA and then took a bus to Washington, DC. CA was a bit out of the way and fits with manic poor judgment, a spur-of-the-moment decision, and his trips. He arrived at the Washington Hilton Hotel at about 2:27 p m ET, as *President Reagan* walked out to his waiting armored limousine. John Hinckley, Jr., 25, *single and unemployed*, opened fire, getting off six shots in 1.7 seconds, missing the President with all six shots. The sixth bullet ricocheted off the armored side of the limousine and hit Reagan under his left arm lodging in his lung and stopping about an inch from his heart.

Mr. Hinckley was misdiagnosed with "*Paranoid Schizophrenia*," but his grandiose delusion of winning the attention and love of the actor, *Jodie Foster*, by assassinating a President of the United States, is compatible with grandiose psychotic mania. Hinckley wrote that his shooting of Reagan was "...the greatest love offering in the history of the world..." It seems that any President would have sufficed, as Hinckley had *stalked former President Carter* around the country while carrying a firearm, looking for an opportunity to assassinate him.

As a teenager he had suffered *episodes of major depression* but he had been a *well-adjusted child* and adolescent playing *team sports* and being *elected class president* twice. In 1976, he *spontaneously left home for Hollywood "...hoping to become a famous song writer*." He reportedly saw the movie *Taxi Driver 215 times* and fell in love with the star, Ms. Foster. During his years in prison, he has demonstrated the *ability to organize and write numerous and extensive legal motions* (Wikipedia).

A healthy premorbid life, cycles in mood that include episodes of depression and episodes of focused, grandiose, paranoid, psychotic delusions with less need for sleep, as well as irritability, anger, and violence are compatible with a *Bipolar Disorder I, Manic, at times Severe with Psychotic Features. Erotomania* has also been applied.

Case 4.39: Mr. Aaron Alexis, 34, Shot and Killed 12 at the Navy Yard, Washington, DC, September 16, 2013, at 8 a m

Just after 8:00 a m on a Monday, Mr. Aaron Alexis, a former Naval Reservist and a Navy contract employee, drove his rental car to his work assignment and, with his *DOD security clearance* and newly purchased Remington pump-action shotgun, entered the Washington Navy Yard on the banks of the Anacostia River, a few miles from the White House, and unprovoked killed 12

Navy personnel, *all strangers*. Mr. Alexis was killed by police after a gun fight, likely a suicide by cop.

According to the media, "... federal and local authorities have interviewed hundreds of people and are poring through the contents of Alexis' Yahoo email account." Mr. Alexis' past history suggests *cyclic episodes of poor judgment, violence, and likely psychosis* as well as euthymic years when he was stable, productive, and *successful* as shown by his holding DOD security clearance and a demanding technical government job.

When he was on active duty in the Navy, he was AWOL for two days that he spent in jail for a fight in a Georgia bar. In 2004 he was *arrested* in Seattle, WA, "*... for shooting out the tires of another man's vehicle* in what Mr. Alexis later described to detectives as an *anger-fueled 'blackout*.'" It is likely both of these episodes were during times of irritable mania. In 2010 he was investigated in Ft. Worth, TX, "...for *discharging a firearm [through his ceiling*] after his upstairs neighbor said he [Mr. Alexis] had confronted her in the parking lot about making too much noise ..." A friend in Ft. Worth said that Mr. Alexis "...went *three days without sleep...*" around that time. All together these behaviors suggest mania.

A month prior to his rampage (August 7, 2013), while on another job for the Navy, Mr. Alexis "... *called the police* in RI to complain that he had *changed hotels three times* because he was being *pursued by people [Navy personnel] keeping him awake* ... and harassing him ... *by sending vibrations through the walls ... with a microwave machine"*.

He researched, located, *called, and told a DC area Electronic Surveillance and Mind Control Support Group* that the *Navy was "targeting his brain"* with a new experimental weapon that transmitted *Extremely Low Frequency (ELF) waves* that caused him to hear "... *voices speaking to him through the wall, flooring and ceiling*." He believed the Navy ELF research was being conducted at the DC Navy Yard where his next assignment was. The grandiosity to these delusions and auditory hallucinations is based on his belief that the Navy had specifically singled him out for harassment and is diagnostic of psychotic grandiose mania that defines Bipolar. There is more.

"On Aug. 23, Mr. Alexis went to the Veterans Affairs Hospital in Providence [RI], where he had been working as a Navy contractor, complaining of *insomnia* ... Mr. Alexis said he could not sleep ... Doctors there *prescribed him an antidepressant* commonly prescribed for insomnia, trazodone (Desyrel)... Five days later, Mr. Alexis went to [another] Veterans Affairs Hospital after driving to Washington, D. C., where he had traveled to work on another job at the Navy Yard." Mr. Alexis told "... medical personal in D. C. that he was *still having trouble sleeping* and the doctors prescribed *more trazodone (Desyrel)...*" (Shear and Schmidt 2013; Goldstein and Schmidt 2013; Woodruff 2013; Dupree 2013).

Such focused hyperactivity of changing hotels three times over three days, calling the police, going to two hospitals, finding and calling the Mind Control Support Group, his reported paranoid and grandiose delusions, insomnia, past episodes of poor judgment and violence, and his murderous rampage interspersed with times of competent functionality are consistent with Bipolar. The diagnosis is *Bipolar I, Manic, at times Severe with Psychotic Features.*

Case 4.40: Ms. Miriam Carey, 34, Drove from CT to the White House and Tried to Ram Her Way in to See President Obama in Washington, DC, October 3, 2013

Ms. Carey made an apparent spur-of-the-moment decision on a Thursday morning to *drive 265 miles* from her home in CT directly *to the White House in Washington, DC.*, with her *18-month-old daughter strapped in the back seat.* Ms. Carey's mother said that she thought her daughter was taking her toddler to a doctor's appointment in CN on Thursday and her sister said, upon hearing of the rampage, that Ms. Carey "...would not be in D. C.... She was just in CT...I just talked to her."

However, the idea to *confront President Obama* had been considered by Ms. Carey for weeks if not months. Although insomnia, racing thoughts, and excessive speeding during the trip to DC and before were not documented, reckless speeding and likely racing thoughts certainly occurred at and between the White House and the Capital.

Arriving by about 2 p m at the White House, *unprovoked* and without apparent explanation, she recklessly attempted to *break her way into the White House* grounds by trying to drive through a metal barricade. *She struck a uniformed Secret Service Officer*, refused to stop or exit her car, and then *sped off down Constitution Avenue toward the Capital Building at 80 mph*, ignoring red lights and efforts by trailing Secret Service officers to pull her over with their lights flashing, sirens blaring, and guns firing. An observer said of the procession that he thought it was the President's motorcade; he did not noticc thc gunfirc. Her actions and behavior can be described as frantic and she was likely terrified sustaining at least two episodes of gun fire into her car. Near the capital her car became stuck and *she was shot to death* in a hail of gunfire. This bizarre episode is entirely compatible with psychotic mania based on her history, detailed below. Miraculously no one else was injured including her 18-month-old in the back seat. This was not a case of suicide by cop.

Her recent and past histories demonstrate manic psychosis, grandiosity, and paranoia. *There was warning* prior to her rampage; her *boyfriend* was so concerned that he *called the local police in CT* reporting her *delusions that*

President Obama had bugged her apartment and was stalking her. He added that she thought she was a *prophet*. These paranoid and grandiose delusions explain her flight to the White House. About 18 months before, Ms. Carey was *hospitalized with Post-partum Psychosis* that can initiate a Bipolar episode. Her mental health status over the preceding 10 months is described as "*… ups and downs*, [a] *serious degradation in her mental condition*." A few years before, a neighbor observed Ms. Carey "inappropriately…outside her mother's Brooklyn apartment clutching a *Bible and wailing at the sky*." She was said to have been quoting scripture. In August 2012 she was fired from her dental hygienist position because "… she *had a temper* and was not getting along with her coworkers." A Homeland Security investigation of Ms. Carey's medical record revealed that she had been misdiagnosed and treated for "*Schizophrenia*." *Antipsychotics but no mood-stabilizing medications* were found in her apartment which was otherwise unremarkable.

She had performed on a high level in *college and as a dental hygienist* and according to others did not appear to be unstable. A neighbor found Ms. Carey "… likeable, *very well spoken and obviously educated*." Another neighbor noted that "… she kept her shiny black Infiniti very clean and in good shape" (Zapotosky et al. 2013; Tucker and Christoffersen 2013; Kleinfield and Rashbaum 2013).

Her episodic psychotic episodes, marked with grandiose and paranoid delusions, reckless, frantic activities, coupled with past episodes of severe depression, irritability at work, and stable time during which she functioned quite well are consistent with a cycling *Bipolar I Disorder, Manic, at times Severe with Psychotic Features*.

Case 4.41: Mr. Jared Loughner, 22, Killed Six, Shot 19, at Congress Member Gabrielle Giffords' Political Rally, Tucson, AZ, January 8, 2011

During the day on Saturday, Jared Loughner, without provocation, *shot 19 people, all strangers,* including then-Congress member Giffords at her political rally in Tucson, AZ. *Six died* including *a nine-year-old girl*.

According to media reports, on the night before his rampage, Loughner may have gotten *little or no sleep*. Media research indicated that he *posted incoherent writings* on MySpace through the *middle of the night*. At 7:04 a m, he drove to buy more ammunition and was stopped by law enforcement for *running a red light* but not detained. Back at home, a *heated argument with his father* prevented him from driving the family car to his rampage; he took a cab. These actions demonstrate poor judgment (running a red light) and irritability (argument), and yet he was able to maintain focus on his mission of the day. His father described his behavior during these days as "*out of control.*" His actions at the site of the massacre were described in the media: "Mr. Loughner kept up his fatal barrage, *dancing up and down excitedly*, turning from Ms. Giffords before *firing, apparently indiscriminately*, at her constituents, staff, and the random passers-by." He *did not try to flee* and was taken down by survivors as he tried to reload to kill more people. Insomnia, excessive incoherent writings, hyperactivity, politically motivated grandiosity, and violence by a rampage killer indicate psychotic mania, as did his past and family histories.

"Over the years before the rampage, his high school and college teachers described '... a pattern of *inappropriate disruptive behavior* [during classes] marked by *hysterical laughter, bizarre non sequiturs, and aggressive outbursts...*'" Episodically both in high school and at Pima Community College, *police were summoned multiple times* when Mr. Loughner disrupted the classroom. Loughner instilled fear in others as did Cho, Alexis, and Holmes. At least one classmate, who sat by the door when Mr. Loughner attended the class, and one of his instructors said they were *fearful of him.*

Mr. Loughner has a *family history of Bipolar Disorder*. Yet, after his arrest, two medical evaluations concurred in the misdiagnosis of "*Paranoid Schizophrenia.*" During treatment in prison, he admitted he had "harbored a grudge against Ms. Giffords for years" (Becker et al. 2011; Gardner et al. 2011; Sulzberger and Carey 2011) (Sect. 4.7). Mr. Loughner is now inappropriately serving *seven consecutive life sentences* despite suffering with a psychotic Bipolar Disorder at the time of the murders. His diagnosis is *Bipolar I, Manic, at times Severe with Psychotic Features.*

4.5.3 Mental Health Workers at Risk for Bipolar Violence

"According to the Department of Justice (DOJ) National Crime Victimization Survey for 1993 to 1999, the annual rate for nonfatal violent crime for all occupations was 12.6 per 1,000 workers. For physicians, the rate was 16.2, and for nurses it was 21.9. But for *psychiatrists, psychologists, psychotherapists, and other mental health workers, the rate was 68.2 [per 1,000 workers]*" (Rosack 2006). Undiagnosed, misdiagnosed, and mismanaged psychotic Bipolar clients, especially when manic, are a *threat to doctors, therapists, counselors, and caretakers* as shown in the five cases below (Table 4.1).

Table 4.1 DOJ National Crime Victimization survey for 1993 to 1999; annual rate for nonfatal violent crime[1]

Occupation	Rate of Violent Crime per 1,000 Workers[2]
All Workers	12.6
Physicians	16.2
Nurses	21.9
Psychologists and Other Mental Health Professionals	68.2
Mental Health Custodial Workers	69

[1]Rosack (2006)
[2]Violence upon workers in the mental health fields are assumed by the current author to be perpetrated by psychological clients primarily suffering from acute psychotic mania or psychotic from drug intoxication (stimulants such as cocaine, crack, and methamphetamine or hallucinogens such as PCP or "bath salts") or organic brain syndromes

Case 4.42: Mr. Deshawn James Chappel, 27, Murdered His Counselor in Revere, MA, in January 2011

Ms. Moulton was working her solo shift as the counselor of Mr. Chappel's group home. The other residents had left the house to attend programs while she was scheduled to accompany Mr. Chappel to a therapy session. Believing *Ms. Moulton was communicating about him to President Obama*, Mr. Chappel *beat her, stabbed her repeatedly,* and then dumped her partially nude body in a church parking lot. Mr. Chappel stole some clothes to replace his bloody ones and then called his grandmother.

Mr. Chappel was the oldest of five, a *running back in high school, outgoing,* and *churchgoing*; his mom thought he would be a *minister*. He *took a girl with a prosthetic leg and arm to the senior prom because nobody else would. Then he changed.* He began *neglecting his appearance*, stopped talking about God, and started *talking about the devil.* He would say the *devil was telling him what to do*; he talked about curses and hexes and *by 21*, "...the voices in his head *prevented him from sleeping...*" His inability to sleep was likely due to racing thoughts, also compatible with mania (Sontag 2011). He asked his mom to take him to the hospital and he was admitted to Mass General Hospital (MGH), misdiagnosed with "*Schizophrenia,*" and prescribed SGAs. He was *hospitalized at least four additional times* and *arrested several more times on assault charges* over the following couple of years. In 2007 "he seemed to be *doing better*." He talked about going back to school and getting a college degree. Instead he suffered depression and stayed in his room. He got second-generation antipsychotic *(SGA) injections* every other week but no mood-stabilizing medicines. By Thanksgiving, 2010, he was talking about *people watching* him, felt too uneasy to leave the house, *began inappropriately phoning relatives* and making *delusional statements*. He began to believe his counselor, Ms. Moulton, was sending his personal information to *President Obama*. Mr. Chappel told his psychologist that he "…hailed from TX and rooted for the Washington Redskins and that he *wanted 'a lawyer from UCLA with a 3.5 grade point average*.'" He murdered Ms. Moulton less than two months later.

Such a grandiose and paranoid delusional system after a healthy premorbid period is typical of psychotic *Bipolar I, Manic, at times Severe with Psychotic Features.*

Case 4.43: Mr. Vitali Davydov, 19, at the Office of Dr. Wayne Fenton, Bethesda, MD, Sunday Afternoon, September 3, 2006, the Day Before Labor Day

Of the murders involving mental health professionals, one of the most notable occurred in Bethesda, MD, just south of the NIH *on Sunday*, September 3, 2006, the day before Labor Day. Dr. Wayne Fenton, a psychiatrist and expert in "*Schizophrenia*" from the NIMH, agreed on an emergency basis to see his new 19-year-old client named Vitali Davydov. He saw Mr. Davydov *alone in his office while Mr. Davydov's father waited for him in the parking lot.* Mr. *Davydov beat Dr. Fenton to death with his fists* saying that "… he had killed Fenton in self-defense. He was *afraid that Fenton was about to sexually assault him*." Mr. Davydov believed he had received *messages from the television* about this. In another explanation for the murder, Mr. Davydov said that "Dr. Fenton had asked him [Davydov] to kill him because he had been the victim of a rape and wanted his soul to leave his body…" Several different psychiatrists had misdiagnosed Mr. Davydov with "*Schizophrenia*." He was also diagnosed with Bipolar but Mr. Davydov refused any medications because he thought medicine would allow the psychiatrists to control his mind.

Such delusional paranoia, intense aggression, and violence are in keeping with an acute manic episode. Dr. Fenton did not have the opportunity to treat him (Rosack 2006). This tragic case emphasizes the importance of *including a significant other* in sessions with new clients, especially delusional ones. Mr. Davydov has *Bipolar I, Manic, Severe with Psychotic Features.*

Case 4.44: Mr. J. Carciero, 37, Boston, MA, Stabbed His Psychiatrist on October 26, 2009

Mr. Carciero was *a client in the Bipolar Clinic* near the Mass General Hospital (MGH). During a therapy session, he *stabbed his psychiatrist*, Dr. Astrid Desrosiers, an MGH psychiatrist. *Mr. Carciero was shot dead* by an off-duty security guard and Dr. Desrosiers survived. Based on his actions that day and his treatment in the Bipolar Clinic, Mr. Carciero has *Bipolar I, Manic, Severe with Psychotic Features* and was in a delusional, paranoid psychotic state (Ward 2009).

Case 4.45: Mr. Thomas Belanger, 18, North Andover, MA, Fatally Stabbed His Social worker in February 2008

Mr. Belanger had a knife in his hand when his social worker showed up to make a house call. She was apparently unable to persuade him to give up the knife and he stabbed her to death in the back and then *slit his own throat but survived.*

Four years earlier Mr. Belanger, then 14, was charged with *multiple assaults* with a knife. He was *stable as a young child*, based on a neighbor's saying that they watched football games together and describing Mr. Belanger as a "*lonely, gentle kid*."

Mr. Belanger carried a diagnosis of previous trauma to the head *and Bipolar Disorder I, Manic, at times Severe with Psychotic Features.*

Case 4.46: Mr. David Tarloff, 39, Murdered His Psychiatrist's Partner, Dr. Kathryn Faughey, PhD, 56, Upper East Side, New York City, February 2008

Mr. Tarloff developed a *grandiose delusion* that he was *sanctioned by God* to take his incapacitated mother out of her nursing home and on a vacation to Hawaii. He carried a *meat cleaver* to his psychiatrist's suite of offices to rob Dr. Shinbach, his psychiatrist, but found Dr. Faughey alone in her office, so he murdered her instead. Dr. Shinbach heard her screaming, came to her office, and was himself attacked, robbed, and cut badly.

Mr. Tarloff had attended *Syracuse University*, but when he came home, *he was different, changed*. He became severely paranoid and mute. He could not hold a job for longer than a day and also dropped out of *St. John's University and the University of Miami* without completing an entire semester. Mr. Tarloff had been previously misdiagnosed with "*Paranoid Schizophrenia*" *at the age of* 22.

He was *committed more than a dozen times* and *treated with lithium, valproic acid/divalproex (Depakene/Depakote)*, haloperidol (Haldol), quetiapine (Seroquel), and olanzapine (Zyprexa). The two mood-stabilizer medications suggest a diagnosis of Bipolar was also considered. When he began to feel stabilized, he would *stop taking his medication*. It is recorded that he made spur-of-the-moment decisions that involved travel, compatible with mania. His diagnosis is most likely *Bipolar I, Manic, Severe with Psychotic Features*.

This section summarizes the cases of five psychotic Bipolar clients who, during a paranoid psychotic manic episode, murdered or attempted to murder their mental health caretakers. When the delusional systems were exposed in the media, the clients were shown to be psychotic, grandiose, and manic. For example, Mr. Chappel believed his therapist was sending his personal information to *President Obama*. Mr. Tarloff believed *God* had given him a mission to rob his psychiatrist for money to take his invalid mother to Hawaii on vacation. Mr. Davydov who murdered Dr. Fenton in his office believed that he was receiving *messages from the TV* and that Dr. Fenton was about to sexually assault him.

Most of the individuals reviewed here were misdiagnosed with "Schizophrenia." A few were also diagnosed with *MDD*. These diagnoses can be explained by one disorder, Bipolar, Manic, Severe with Psychotic Features. These perpetrators with Bipolar but misdiagnosed as "Schizophrenia" or MDD are unlikely to have been prescribed first-line mood-stabilizing drugs (Sect. 6.2). Such an error increases the risk of deterioration, violence, suicide, homicide, and incarceration.

4.6 Bipolar, Familicide, and Filicide

"Psychiatric patients are assaulting and murdering their loved ones at an alarming rate, with family members the victims in three out of four killings committed by the mentally ill…" (Mandal 2002)

The families of psychotic Bipolar individuals are at increased risk for violence and murder. Mandal (2002) notes, "…family members are the victims in three out of four killings committed by the mentally ill…" Among clients with Bipolar Disorder, one report found that more commit homicides of family members, especially in filicides, during the depressed rather than during the manic phase (Kroft 2013; Fazel et al. 2010). Examples of both follow.

Familicide is the murder of one family member by another. *Filicide* is the deliberate murder by a parent of his or her children; it derives from the Latin words *filius* (son), *filia* (daughter), and *cide* (to kill). *Filicide is the third leading cause of death in children aged five to 14 in the United States* (Friedman et al. 2005). Filicide by psychotic perpetrators occurs during psychotic mania or depression, usually Bipolar depression, MDD, or Post-partum Depression (PPD). The 14 cases of family murders presented in Sect. 4.6 are a small sample of hundreds if not thousands of such tragic cases (Mandal 2002).

Eighty-eight per cent of the killers among the family and filicide cases presented here had been under mental health care before or during their rampages. Appropriate diagnoses and more frequent follow-up with psychotherapy might have changed some of these tragic outcomes. All of the aggressors considered in this chapter were psychotic. Their murders were *not due to family arguments* or substance abuse but were typically planned well ahead and motivated by bizarre and grandiose delusions that had no basis in reality. These delusions are powerful motivators.

The perpetrators firmly believe they are doing the right thing such as saving the world from WW III or their children from torture on earth. Commonalities that point to a diagnosis of Bipolar Disorder include their grandiose and paranoid delusions, hyperactivity, mood swings, suicide, and attempted suicide. Perpetrators of filicide are more likely to attempt suicide because of the delusional belief that the family will be reunited in a better place and escape the hell on earth. Another common delusional motive for killing family is the psychotic belief that the devil or God has told them to kill for the betterment of the world, or that the devil has taken over the family member, who therefore must be killed.

Across these cases, the majority had had successful premorbid lives, some spectacularly successful (Mr. du Pont, Case 4.47, Mr. Laudor, Case 4.48; Ms. Yates, Case 4.51). In 25%, an abrupt change in "personality" was noted. These "changes" usually represent the onset of episodes of severe, psychotic Bipolar, sometimes mania and other times depression, along with an unshakeable paranoid delusional system.

Case 4.47: Mr. John du Pont, 57, Murdered His Friend at the du Pont Mansion in Suburban Philadelphia, January 26, 1996, in the Afternoon

An example of a manic, paranoid, psychosis-driven murderer is Mr. John du Pont, 57, who at various times, believed that he was the *Dalai Lama*, the *last Russian Czar*, the *CIA's top consultant*; that his wife was a Russian spy; and that international conspirators would break into his house and kill him. He placed razor wire in his attic, "*ghost-finding cameras*" in his house, and had his house's columns and walls x-rayed to prevent anyone tunneling into his house to attack him. In 1996 Mr. du Pont *murdered his house guest and long-time friend*, the *US Olympic wrestling coach*. Despite this description of grandiosity and paranoia, his diagnosis was "*Paranoid Schizophrenia*."

Mr. du Pont was described as "…a shy, gawky teenager who never had a girlfriend and avoided school dances…" After high school his life was characterized by cycles of "…throwing himself into a series of passions over which he at first would take total control but then would totally withdraw…" *His cycles occurred at four-year intervals.*

"He earned a *B.S. in biology at the University of Miami*, has *two bird species named after him* because he first identified them, earned an *M.S. at Villanova University*, won the *1965 Australian National Pentathlon Championship*, became an *accomplished wrestler*, and *housed the US Olympic wrestling team on his estate*." *Forbes Magazine* in 1987 estimated his worth at *$200 million* (Gladstone 1987). Yet he was described as an unhappy man.

Mr. du Pont believed his long-time friend and the Olympic wrestling team coach, *Mr. Schultz*, was part of an *international conspiracy to kill him*. On the day of the murder, Mr. Schultz was "…repairing his car radio in the driveway when Mr. du Pont drove up and shot him *without provocation*…Mr. Schultz's' last words were 'Hi, Coach,' to which Mr. du Pont replied, 'You got a problem with me?' and shot him...Du Pont used hollow point bullets and fired the last shot into Schultz's back while he was bleeding to death from a gunshot wound in his chest and crawling face-down in the snow, trying to get away…" (Longman 2010; Wikipedia 2011). Such grandiose delusions and psychotic episodes involving violence are diagnostic of mania and *Bipolar Disorder I, Manic, at times Severe with Psychotic Features*.

Case 4.48: Mr. Michael Laudor, 35, Yale Law School Faculty, 1998

Mr. Michael Laudor, a *Summa Cum Laude graduate of Yale University* Undergraduate and Yale Law Schools, was a member of the *Yale Law School faculty* and he held *a $2.1 million contract for his biography*. He was engaged to be married and living in New York City with his fiancée in the apartment they shared on the banks of the Hudson River.

In 1998, he incurred a psychotic episode and *murdered her, believing she was involved in a conspiracy to kill him*. He stabbed her 10 times in the back and neck in their kitchen. After the murder, for no apparent reason, Mr. Laudor then *drove to Binghamton, NY*, and from there took a *bus to Ithaca, NY*, where on the campus of Cornell University he flagged down a patrol car and told the officer that he had hurt his girlfriend…he was covered in blood but assured the police he was not hurt and the blood was not his. He was alternatively calm and agitated and *assaulted law enforcement some three times*.

His misdiagnosis is "*Schizophrenia*" although he was described as "…unbelievably charismatic, unbelievably bright, someone you'd never forget...He is handsome, kind, spiritual, a wonderful conversationalist, [has] a wonderful sense of humor and was destined for what everyone thought was greatness... The golden boy…" (Berger and Gross 1998; Foderaro 2000).

Such a description of brilliance and success is somewhat similar to that of Dr. John Nash, a senior research mathematician at Princeton University whose work in game theory and partial differential equations earned him a Nobel Prize in Economics and the most prestigious international prize in mathematics, the Abel Prize. Nash, like Laudor, was also misdiagnosed with "*Schizophrenia*" but displayed symptoms consistent with a Bipolar Disorder. Nash's life inspired the film "*A Beautiful Mind*." Such characteristics as charisma, leadership, brilliance, success, the ability to excel with only two or tree hours of sleep a night coupled with psychotic episodes and other episodes of major depression with reduced productivity suggest a *Bipolar I Disorder, Severe with Psychotic Features*.

Case 4.49: David Patten, 45, Toronto, Canada, 2000, Beat His Parents and a Nurse to Death to Avert WW III; Believed He Was the Commanding General of the British Army

Mr. Patten is a 45-year-old, single Caucasian male with a diagnosis of "Schizophrenia."

According to the media, "…he thought he was the leader [general] of the British Army, heading into the Third World War and that he could avert the conflict by killing the *devil possessing his parents…*" Mr. Patten "…bludgeoned to death his parents…and a retired nurse, with whom Patten lived. He *beat them to death in their driveway with a red-handled spad*e…He thought he was killing the devil inside his father and that while his father was still alive, the devil was then transferred to his mother, so he killed her" (Mandal 2002).

Mr. Patten's grandiose delusions of being a general in the British Army and his ability to stop World War III along with his violence suggest psychotic mania and a *Bipolar I Disorder, Manic, Severe with Psychotic Features.*

Case 4.50: John A. Okie, 22, Augusta, ME, July 10, 2007, Murdered his Girlfriend and Father Because He Thought They Were Reading His Mind

Mr. Okie was a 22-year-old single male with a steady girlfriend. Misdiagnosed with "Schizophrenia," Mr. Okie began to believe that his girlfriend "…was part of an evil group and that she could read his mind because 'it was exposed to her'." So he killed her. He believed that by killing her on July 10, 2007, "the world would thank him."

Six days later, Okie *killed his father* because his delusion expanded to the belief that his father had actually been the reason he *couldn't use his mind* and was part of the evil group.

"[His sister] described him as distant, distracted, and often unresponsive in conversations…We called him 'the Sloth'…He was always tired." [This might be explained by depression or SGA medications.]

"…Okie told his sister he was convinced he had to use cocaine to prevent cancer." He also insisted his *mother was raping him in the night*, and injecting heroin into his feet to kill him. "He reasoned to protect himself he would have to kill her to save himself."

Therefore he was hospitalized in 2004 and described as "…*quite depressed*, and distant, and very much different." It was reported that in a "…2005 incident, *Johnny 'took off' to New Hampshire and Massachusetts*, and was locked in a woman's restroom. He was arrested but *not charged due to his mental status*. "Another incident involved his driving to visit his sister in Boston following a tonsillectomy surgery…and he arrived covered in blood. [Taken to the ED], Okie was admitted for blood loss" (Fletcher 2008).

Such violence, paranoid delusions, poor judgment, spontaneous trips, and odd behavior are likely the result of his paranoid delusional system consistent with a psychotic *Bipolar I Disorder, Mixed, at times Severe with Psychotic Features*.

Case 4.51: Ms. Andrea Yates, 37, Austin, TX, June 20, 2001, Drowned Her Five Children One by One in Her Bathtub and Attempted Suicide to Escape This Earth. Successful in High School and College

One of the most infamous examples of multiple filicide is the case of Ms. Andrea Yates, who at 37 *killed her five young children by drowning them one by one in her bathtub* at their home in Austin, TX, on June 20, 2001, an hour after her husband left for work. The children ranged in age from six months to seven years old.

In high school, Ms. Yates was class *valedictorian, captain of her swim team,* and an officer in the *National Honor Society*. She graduated in 1986 from the *University of Texas School of Nursing* in Houston and worked as an RN from 1986 until 1994 at the University of Texas, *M. D. Anderson Cancer Center*. She was misdiagnosed with *"Schizophrenia" and accurately with Post-partum Depression with psychotic features* after the birth of her first son in 1994 when "*…she felt Satan's presence* shortly after Noah's birth and '*heard Satan's voice* tell her to pick up the knife and stab the child.'…The symptoms of 'Schizophrenia' [psychosis] didn't resurface until Yates' fourth son, Luke, was born in 1999…Yates *attempted suicide* twice that year" (CNN Justice 2002; Anderson 2002).

She reportedly first spoke of suicide and *experienced depression at the age of 17* (Wikipedia 2011). She suffered *numerous psychotic episodes*, most associated with misdiagnoses of "Schizophrenia" and psychotic MDD. Her diagnosis of Post-partum Psychosis and MDD were likely part of her Bipolar Disorder, Depressed or Mixed, with Psychotic Features. After hospitalizations in 1999, she was medicated with "… a mixture of medications …" but *no mood-stabilizing drugs were mentioned* and the several antidepressants might have worsened her Bipolar Disorder (Wehr and Goodwin 1987; Goodwin 1989). "After being discharged [in late 1999 or early 2000], her condition worsened. 'Staying in bed all day… she experienced visions and voices. She would hear *commands: Get a knife!* Get a knife!'" (Walsh 2002).

She seemed to *recover and in between episodes, she apparently functioned fairly normally* as is typical of Bipolar. Although warned against another pregnancy by a psychiatrist based on the fear of another psychotic post-partum episode, "The Yates' conceived their fifth and final child approximately seven weeks after her discharge [from a psychiatric inpatient stay and she]… gave birth to Mary Yates on November 30 of that year [2000]. She seemed to be coping until the death of her father on March 12, 2001."

Although she avoided a psychotic episode after Mary's birth, her father's death and the *miscarriage of her sixth pregnancy* caused episodes of *psychotic depression* resulting in two additional hospitalizations in March and May of 2001. Ms. Yates "…then *stopped taking medication*, mutilated herself, and *read the Bible feverishly*… believed that *the children would be tormented and perish in the fires of hell unless they were killed*" (Walsh 2002). "She believed her children would suffer in hell because *the mark of the devil was hidden under her hair*. She was evil; possessed by Satan. She had to kill her children before it was too late for them to get to heaven" (Sable 2002). Reading the Bible "feverishly" like Ms. Carey (Case 4.40) is a sign of mania indicating a psychotic episode of Bipolar. She murdered her children in June, 2001.

Deemed sane because she planned ahead, Ms. Yates was inappropriately *convicted of capital murder* and sentenced to life in prison; she was *denied the insanity plea*. In *2006, this verdict was reversed* and she was found *not guilty by reason of insanity* and sent to the Kerrville State Hospital in Kerrville, TX. This hospital is a low-security mental health facility and is a cross between a hospital and a prison. Guards do not have firearms and there are no razor wire fences. Treatment is emphasized, not punishment "…for doing something they did not know was wrong…" Clients/inmates are not free to leave. There, "patients learn to take their medication; *90% of them are on antipsychotic medicine*…The ultimate goal here is to move them out of the hospital and into the community." Nevertheless, according to the media, Ms. Yates "is likely living out the rest of her life at Kerrville State Hospital…" (Chan 2016). Ms. Yates has waived her annual reviews and passing the review is the only way she can be released. This case raises the judicial versus psychological interpretation of insane or psychotic (Sect. 4.7).

In prison, Ms. Yates continued to have psychotic episodes, at one time during a severe depression refusing food and losing more than 20 pounds. She has been placed on suicide watch at least four times in prison. She said that "…she could not destroy Satan and that '*Gov. Bush would have to destroy Satan*.'" Ms. Yates was psychotic and grandiose and needed psychotherapy and the short-term prescription of an SGA plus mood-stabilizing drugs that she did not receive.

Her episodic course, onset of a Major Depressive Episode at 17, her accomplishments, her episodes of Post-partum Depression and psychosis, her grandiosity marked by the delusion that she was possessed by Satan, and belief that Governor Bush was involved in her life and could kill Satan in her as well as a reference to her "reading the Bible feverishly" assure she has a *Bipolar I Disorder, Mixed, at times Severe with Psychotic Features*.

Case 4.52: Ms. Marilyn Lemak, 41, Naperville, IL, April 4, 1999, Smothered Her Three Children and Attempted Suicide to Escape Hell on Earth

A 41-year-old *surgical nurse*, Ms. Marilyn Lemak, *drugged her three children with lorazepam* (Ativan), which doctors had prescribed for her, and *smothered them*. She first killed the two younger children, aged three and six, while the oldest child played downstairs. She made him a peanut-butter and jelly sandwich, sprinkled it with crushed Ativan, and then smothered him as well. The next morning Lemak called 911 to report that she had killed her children. When police arrived they found her lying near her daughter's body, having *slit her wrists and swallowed medications in an unsuccessful attempt at suicide*.

Lemak confessed to police that she had killed the children and attempted suicide to join her children and "*escape the pain brought on by depression*." She was *psychotically depressed*. Her family said that she had suffered with depression for the previous four years. She had divorced the children's father in what had initially appeared to be an amicable parting. When she learned he was dating, her depression had worsened.

The prosecutor stressed that "the goal in this case was to prove that despite the depression, Lemak was sane at the time of the killings..." Ultimately Lemak was "*found fit to stand trial and convicted*." She was committed to a *life sentence* rather than execution as the family did not want to "deal with all the challenges that would occur in a capital case" (Baker 2019).

This is another example of the disconnect between psychology and the judicial profession (Sect. 4.7). Ms. Lemak was psychotic and insane; she suffered with *Major Depression (MDD) or Bipolar I or II, Depressed, at times Severe with Psychotic Features*.

Case 4.53: Ms. Aubrianne Moore, 28, Solon Township, MI, February 18, 2019, Shot Her Three Daughters to Death with a Hunting Rifle and Suicided

A 28-year-old mother, Ms. Aubrianne Moore of Solon Township, MI, was *involuntarily hospitalized based on a social worker's petition in mid-September, 2018*, because of fear that she and her family were in danger of harm because of Ms. Moore's *paranoid delusions. One day Ms. Moore believed that the television had warned her* that there would be a school bus accident that day so she kept the children at home. On another occasion she had ceased to eat because she believed her *food had been poisoned*. She *feared sleeping* as she thought someone was going to break into their home. In the hospital, Ms. Moore was misdiagnosed with "unspecified '*Schizophrenia*' and psychosis." She was psychotic but her delusional paranoia and not sleeping are more likely due to a psychotic Mood Disorder. She was *held for 10 days* and "discharged on deferral status."

The hospital recorded no violent tendencies toward others and there were no court records of abuse by her. However, social workers had noted that *Ms. Moore was experiencing delusions, visual and auditory hallucinations, and mood swings*. They had specified that she *was a risk for self-harm or harm to others* because of her *disconnection from reality* and inability to grasp her need for treatment. She did eventually agree to another hospitalization for no more than 60 days and treatment by a private physician not to exceed 90 days. It is unclear whether she followed through with that hospitalization or treatment.

On February 18, five months after her 10-day commitment, *using a fake doctor's appointment note, Ms. Moore removed her three daughters, aged 2, 6, and 8, from their grade school and took them to a wooded area* on land owned by their great grandparents. She took them *one by one into the woods and shot them* with a bolt-action hunting rifle. She then drove the dead children to her boyfriend's house where she *shot herself* outside her car (Kranz 2019; Aaro 2019).

Typical motives in such cases are the delusion that the children must be saved from the continuing misery on earth and that after the perpetrator's suicide, they all will meet in heaven. The diagnosis is a *Bipolar Disorder, Type I or II, Depressed or Mixed, at times Severe with Psychotic Features.*

Case 4.54: Ms. Otty Sanchez, 33, San Antonio, TX, July 20, 2009, Murdered Her Infant Son and Ate Parts of His Body

Another example of filicide by a psychotic mother is the case of Ms. Otty Sanchez, 33, who *murdered, mutilated, and ate parts of her infant son* in July, 2009, at 4:30 a m. The autopsy on the infant showed that Ms. Sanchez must have spent a considerable amount of time mutilating him, certainly consistent with a psychotic state.

She seemed to have a *healthy life until about five years prior to the murder* when "… *her behavior became erratic*. She had trouble staying employed, bouncing from one low-paying job to another." Such a work history is typical of rapid cycling Bipolar Disorders. In 2008 she was *seen at a mental health clinic* and was described as psychotic, paranoid, and depressed. She had been admitted to psychiatric *inpatient units multiple times in the previous five years*. The year before the murder, while psychotic, Sanchez may have made a spur-of-the-moment decision to *travel to Austin, TX*, from San Antonio, TX (about 80 miles) with a friend. Ms. Sanchez became separated from her friend and was finally *found in a CVS store after wandering around for seven hours "... shopping for an imaginary trip to China*." The Austin police took her to the *State Mental Hospital* where she spent the next 16 days. She was misdiagnosed with *"Paranoid Schizophrenia"* and was prescribed needed antipsychotic medication but *not mood stabilizers*. She returned home to San Antonio and stopped this medication during her subsequent pregnancy, possibly related to manic hypersexuality. She began taking the medicine again after her delivery but stopped it again nine days before the murder. She had paranoid delusions that *other women were trying to breast feed or take her baby away*. She believed "... *the devil made me do it*" (Mann 2009, 2010). She was correctly judged innocent by reason of insanity.

Such delusional paranoia and grandiosity in considering a trip to China, violence, and hyperactivity in traveling to Austin are compatible with mania and a *Bipolar I Disorder, Manic or Mixed, Severe with Psychotic Features.*

Case 4.55: Ms. Dena Schlosser, 35, Plano, TX, November 23, 2004, in a Psychotic Religious Frenzy Cut Her Baby's Arms Off

Ms. Schlosser "... 'euphorically' told a 911 operator she had *cut off the [10-month-old] baby's arms*; police found Schlosser *covered in blood* and holding a knife *while listening to a hymn*." Earlier, 911 had called Ms. Schlosser because a day care worker had called them with concern for the baby's welfare.

Neighbors described Ms. Schlosser as "....*a loving, attentive mother*...The children had always been happy and cared for...[Then she changed.] In January the *child protective agency* was called to the home after Schlosser was reported running down the street with one of her daughters bicycling after her...The child told them her mother had *left her six-day-old sister alone in the apartment*. She was hospitalized and diagnosed with *Post-partum Depression*. In a conversation with her mother the day before the slaying, Ms. Schlosser seemed *oddly 'euphoric'*." Her mother said, "It bothered me a little...*She wasn't herself*." Her attack was described as a *religious frenzy*.

She had had at least two psychotic episodes involving hyperactivity. She interpreted a television news story about a boy being mauled by a lion as a *sign of the apocalypse* and heard *God commanding her to remove the baby's arms* and then her own (*USA Today*, Nov 23, 2004; *Wikipedia* 2011).

She was correctly *deemed insane* and has been in state-run mental hospitals. When she has been released, she has relapsed into religious delusions and been readmitted. A state of "religious frenzy, euphoria," a delusion about the apocalypse, hearing God's voice commanding her, and violence are consistent with *Bipolar I, Manic or Mixed, Severe with Psychotic Features*.

Case 4.56: Ms. Christina Marie Riggs, 26, Sherwood, AK, November, 1997, Smothered Her Two Children and Attempted Suicide

"Ms. Riggs *smothered her two children*, two and five years of age, with a pillow. She then *attempted suicide* by *swallowing 28 Elavil tablets* and *injecting enough potassium chloride to kill five people*." She lived. "…She requested and *…fought for her right to die by lethal injection…*[She said,] I'll be with my children and with God. I'll be where there's no more pain. Maybe I'll find some peace." She was *executed by lethal injection* on May 3, 2000, in Pine Bluff, AK (Anonymous Children Murdered by their Christian Parents, Memorial Page 2006).

She should have been deemed insane by the court and not executed but rather rehabilitated. She likely suffered from a psychotic Mood Disorder, either *Post-partum Depression, MDD, or Bipolar I or II, Depressed, Severe with Psychotic Features.*

Case 4.57: Ms. Magdalena Lopez, 29, Dyer, IN, July, 2005, Beat Her Two Sons to Death with a 10-Pound Dumbbell

"Police reported that Ms. Lopez *beat her two sons [nine and two] to death with a 10-pound dumbbell* because she thought they would be better off in heaven…They're in a much better place now" (Anonymous Children Murdered by their Christian Parents, Memorial Page 2006). Ms. Lopez had *Bipolar Disorder that was Severe, with Psychotic Features.*

Case 4.58: Deanna Laney, 39, New Chapel Hill, TX, May, 2003, Beat to Death Two of Her Children with Heavy Rocks

The crime scene video showed her *eight- and six-year-olds lying dead* in the yard near Garden signs that read, "Mom's Love Grows Here," and "Thank God for Mothers." The boys were found in their underwear with *heavy rocks on their chests.* The video also showed a large spot of blood in a baby bed where Ms. Laney severely injured the youngest son, 14 months old at the time.

Ms. Laney was a stay-at-home mother who home-schooled her children and was *deeply religious. She "…believed God ordered her to kill her children* last Mother's Day weekend. She struggled over whether to obey God or to selfishly keep her children…She [believed she] saw Aaron with a spear, then throwing a rock, then squeezing a frog, and believed God was suggesting she should either stab, stone, or strangle her children...She would *read everyday events or objects as messages from God.* When her baby had abnormal bowel movements…she thought it was a message from God that she was not properly 'digesting' God's word…A previous psychotic episode occurred several years earlier when she thought she smelled sulfur and believed that this was God's warning that the devil was near" (Anonymous Children Murdered by their Christian Parents, Memorial Page 2006).

Her diagnosis is a psychotic Mood Disorder, either *MDD, PPD, or Bipolar I or II, Depressed, at times Severe with Psychotic Features.*

Case 4.59: Mr. John Allen Rubio, 23, Brownsville, TX, May, 2003, Cut the Heads Off His Three Children

Mr. Rubio "…allegedly *strangled, stabbed, and cut the heads off of his and his common-law wife's three children* [three years, fourteen months, and two months] …" and has remained on death row at the Polunsky Unit in Livingston, TX, for about 20 years.

"Mr. Rubio believed that *an ultimate battle between good and evil* would take place… *Rubio believed he was killing demons* when he committed the murders…He *secluded himself with his family during the three days in the house* before the murders, [when] Rubio allegedly *cleaned the place with bleach* in an effort to keep evil away…when Rubio's hamsters got agitated, Rubio took it as a sign of demonic possession and *killed them with a hammer…*When he choked the children and they gasped for air, Rubio interpreted that as a further sign of possession…After the murders, Rubio told his wife that no one would understand their actions and he *persuaded her to have sex one last time…*His regular [illegal] drug use made the condition worse" (Brezosky 2010). Mr. Rubio has *Bipolar I, Manic or Mixed, at times Severe with Psychotic Features.*

Mr. Rubio's case has been reopened (2022) and he is appealing his death sentence on the basis of insanity (Puentez 2022).

Case 4.60: Mr. Geoff Fertuck, 35, Montreal, Canada, May, 2001, Stabbed His Parents to Death and Suicided

Mr. Fertuck *stabbed to death his mother and father* and then threw himself *in front of a freight train* in a successful suicide.

His psychological history included a misdiagnosis of *"Schizophrenia" and MDD.* In 2000 he was being treated for MDD, and in 2001 his psychiatrist told Fertuck's parents that "It would be *dangerous to keep him at home.*" No action was taken to move him out of the home.

A family friend described Mr. Fertuck as "*…cheerful, witty, unassuming…*He was so *tender and gentle* and full of self-doubt that he didn't realize what a *terrific person he was*."

The change from "tender and gentle" to a person committing a vicious murder with a knife is typical of Bipolar when a paranoid delusional system takes over. Absent more detail about Mr. Fertuck's delusions, his likely diagnosis is *Bipolar I, Manic or Mixed, at times Severe with Psychotic Features.*

4.7 Psychotic Killers Inappropriately Deemed Guilty

It is unfortunate that in the US judicial system, violence committed during a psychotic episode does not necessarily entitle that person to a successful insanity defense. From a mental illness standpoint, *psychosis is insanity*, and psychotic perpetrators of violence are not guilty by reason of insanity, even if they planned ahead, knew that their act was illegal, and had some areas of clear thinking. However, the legal and medical definitions of insanity should be but are not synonymous in court. These terms can mean the difference between life and death or at least long-term prison time versus mental health treatment and rehabilitation. Moreover, a therapist is merely an expert witness. The judge and/or jury will make the sanity/insanity judgment and therefore determine the consequences meted out on the perpetrator.

Psychotic murderers can usually be identified by characteristics discussed in Sects. 2.8 and 3.9. In general psychotic murderers are males in their 30s or older, *educated* but unemployed, *act alone*, *rarely try to get away, kill during the day,* and are not intoxicated or radicalized. About *half suicide*. Many *kill in numbers*, typically *strangers*, family, political leaders, or family and often *without obvious provocation or motive* such as Mr. Paddock (Case 4.33). A majority had stable if not successful premorbid periods and often suffer an identifiable point of personality deterioration earlier in their lives before their rampages (Sects. 4.5 and 4.6). Despite premorbid stability, a history of contact with law enforcement and mental health personnel is common. Motivations are usually obscure, but when documented, involve bizarre, grandiose, paranoid delusions that induced the perpetrators' fear for their lives, such as Mr. Alexis (Case 4.39). Most if not all planned their rampages for weeks to years. Spur-of-the-moment murders by psychotic killers are more rare than those planned ahead. This ability to logically plan is what the judicial system considers indicative of sanity and therefore guilt.

The court first decides whether the defendant is "competent" to stand trial; that is, do they understand the charges against them and are they capable of assisting their attorney? Unless the *psychotic delusional system and racing thoughts are severe* and persistent, a psychotic murderer often *can understand the charges and can assist the attorney,* so psychosis does not always establish incompetence. Further, if found not competent to stand trial, the defendant may be detained or forcibly treated until such time as they become competent. This can result in long incarceration times comparable to being found guilty.

At trial, psychosis alone is not sufficient to support a finding of "not guilty by reason of insanity." There are several *legal tests* for making this determination. The relevant legal standard is a matter of statute and case law; accordingly, it varies depending upon the jurisdiction. The focus is on whether the defendant knew "right" from "wrong." Commonly any amount of *planning will bar an insanity defense*. The basic law school example of criminal insanity is that the defendant was so crazy that he/she thought he/she was shooting a pumpkin.

This "example" sets the bar for insanity much too high. Legally if a parent kills their children because they believed the devil was in them and they were killing the devil, this should be interpreted as insanity. If a parent kills their children because God or the devil told them to do so, this also should be interpreted as insanity. Psychologically, these parents are equally psychotic. A client can be psychotic and at the same time plan ahead and know what they were planning is wrong. In the court they could be deemed sane and guilty despite delusionally believing they were doing the right thing overall.

A particularly terrible subtype of mass murder involves killing family (Sect. 4.6). Filicide, usually committed by psychotic mothers, is most tragic. The tragedy is compounded when these cases become entangled in the legal system where *a person may be deemed both psychotic and legally sane*.

As discussed above, the legal and medical understanding and definitions of insanity are sometimes incompatible. Because of this, legal outcomes are usually unfortunate for both the defendants and for society at large. Psychotic defendants are frequently imprisoned and some are executed, both at great expense, such as the case of Ms. Riggs who was executed in AR in 2000. The better outcome for both defendants and society would be appropriate inpatient psychiatric care (Case 4.56).

Some of these mothers sincerely believe that by killing their children they are doing the right thing and saving them from the devil or further torture on earth. They usually attempt to kill themselves in order to join their children in heaven. When they survive and it is shown in court that they planned ahead, their chances for being found not guilty by reason of insanity are reduced if not eliminated.

An example is Ms. Andrea Yates. At 37, suffering with Bipolar Disorder that involved severe psychotic episodes of mania and depression, she was misdiagnosed with "Schizophrenia" and MDD (Case 4.51). In *2002* Ms. Yates drowned her five children, ages six months to seven years, in her bathtub. Her delusional system involved messages from Satan and believing she had to kill them to save them from evil. She had grandiose delusions that involved TX governor George Bush. She was initially found *sane and guilty of murder* because she had carefully planned her attack for weeks to months. She was sentenced to *life in prison. In 2006* this verdict was reversed and she was deemed *not guilty by reason of insanity* and sent to a locked-down state hospital. It is unclear if she will ever leave because she has not put herself up for release. She had had a successful premorbid history in high school, college, and her career as a nurse.

Ms. Christina Marie Riggs, 26, smothered her two small children to death and then took an overdose of Elavil and injected a lethal dose of potassium chloride but survived (Case 4.56). She had intended to "…be with my children with God." She was deemed sane, convicted, and *executed by lethal injection in AR* as she wished. She was psychotic and should have been sent to a locked-down state mental hospital and treated for her MDD or Bipolar depression.

Another example is Ms. Marilyn Lemak, a 41-year-old *surgical nurse*, who murdered her three children by drugging them with a benzodiazepine and then smothering them (Case 4.52). After this she *slit her own wrists* and swallowed medications in an unsuccessful attempt to join her children and live happily ever after. She had planned the event and was found competent to stand trial, convicted, and *committed to a life sentence for murder. She was psychotic during the weeks and months leading up to and through her attack* and afterward.

It would seem that the discipline of psychology that studies mental health, including "insanity," (renamed psychosis over a century ago), would be the source for setting the standards for the mental status of such clients, rather than the judicial system. Detailed planning ahead or knowing right from wrong does not rule out psychosis or insanity. Hopefully this will change because there are many such psychotic murderers incorrectly deemed sane by the court who are now serving life sentences, some on death row or some that have even been executed. This sad and irrational state of affairs is much in need of change.

References

Aaro D. Michigan mom who killed her children used fake doctor's note to get them out of school, investigators say. FOX News. 2019 Feb 24.

Adler E. Spade's father: death could shed light on mental illness. K C Star. 2018a June 7.

Adler E. Kate Spade suffered years of mental illness, sister says. KC Star. 2018b June 8.

Adler E, Smith J, Osterheldt J, Williams MR, Saffo R. Kate Spade, dead at 55, always said Kansas City helped shape her life and career. Kansas City Star. 2018 June 5.

Amsterdam Telegraph. Van Gogh was not psychotic or bipolar when he cut off his ear, medical experts decide. Amsterdam Telegraph. 2016 16 Sept.

Anderson J. Witness testifies Yates was insane. Assoc Press. www.beliefnet.com/news/2002/03/Witness-Testifies-Yates-Was-Insane.aspx. 2002.

Anonymous Children Murdered by their Christian Parents, Memorial Page, 2006.

Armour N, Allen K. AAF Teams will need answers from Johnny Manziel. USA Today. 2019 Mar 1.

Baker S. 20 years ago Marilyn Lemak killed her three children in their Naperville home. The case still haunts law enforcement. Naperville Sun. 2019 Mar 2.

BBC. Timeline: how Norway's terrorist attacks unfolded. 2012 Apr 17. On line.

Becker J, Kovaleski SF, Lou M, Barry D. Jigsaw picture of an accused killer. NY Times. 2011 Jan 16.

Berger J, Gross J. From mental illness to Yale to murder charge. NY Times. 1998 June 19.

Blinder A. Waffle House suspect once had his guns taken away. NY Times. 2018 Apr 23.

Blumer JD. The illness of Vincent van Gogh. Am J Psychiatry. 2002;59(4):519–26.

Brezosky L. Jury sentences Brownsville man to death. San Antonio Express News. 2010 July 29.

Carlson GA, Goodwin FK. The stages of mania: a longitudinal analysis of the manic episode. Arch Gen Psychiatry. 1973;28:221–8.
Chan M. Revisiting Andrea Yates 15 years after she drowned her children. Time. 2016 June 20.
CNN.com/Justice. Yates sentenced to life in prison. CNN. 2002 Mar 15.
Dupree D. Navy Yard shooter had mind control group contact. Examiner.com. 2013 Oct 26.
Duwe G. Opinion: the rise and decline of mass shootings. AOL News. 2010 May 1.
Fawcett J, Golden B, Rosenfeld N. New hope for people with bipolar disorder. New York: Three Rivers Press; 2007.
Fazel S, Lichtenstein P, Grann M, Goodwin GM, Langstrom N. Bipolar disorder and violent crime: new evidence from population-based longitudinal studies and systematic review. Arch Gen Psychiatr. 2010;67:931–8.
Fletcher K. Schizophrenia drove Okie to murder, psychiatrist says. Lincoln County News, Augusta, MA, 12/17/2008.
Foderaro LW. Man who killed fiancée is sent to mental hospital. NY Times. 2000 May 12.
Friedman SH, Hrouda D, Holden C, Noffsinger S, Resnick P. Filicide-suicide: common factors in parents who kill their children and themselves. J Am Acad Psychiatry Law. 2005;33(4):496–504.
Gann C, Parkinson J. Stress of life in the public eye might have fueled Jackson's mood disorder, doctors say. ABC News Medical Unit. 2012 July 12.
Gardner A, Fahrenhold DA, Fisher M. Loughner's descent into a world of fantasy. Wash Post. 2011 Jan 13.
German J. Las Vegas' shooter's autopsy gives no clues. Las Vegas Review-Journal. 2018 Feb 9.
Gladstone R. The Richest, Says Forbes, Got 41% Richer. Forbes Magazine. 1987 Oct 13. On Line.
Glenn C, Peter J, Johnson K, Madhani A. Who is Steven Paddock? Police say he killed 59 in Las Vegas rampage. USA Today. 2018 Oct 2.
Glover S, O'Neill A, Lah K, Ortega B. Sources: Vegas killer paid cash for property and privacy. CNN. 2017 Oct 5.
Goldstein DB, Schmidt S. Genic intolerance to functional variation and the interpretation of personal genomes. PLOS genetics on line. 2013 Aug 22.
Goodstein L, Glaberson W. The well-marked roads of homicidal rage. NY Times. 2000 Apr 9.
Goodwin FK. The biology of recurrence: new directions for the pharmacologic bridge. J Clin Psychiatry. 1989;50:40–4.
Klein A, Williams C, Weil M. 2 officers shot at pentagon's main entrance. Wash Post. 2010 Mar 5.
Kleinfield NR, Rashbaum WK. Miriam Carey was in car when police fired, official says. NY Times. 2013 Oct 4.
Kraepelin E. Dementia Praecox *and Paraphrenia*, E & S Livingstone, Edinburgh Scotland 1919 Thoemmes Press, 2002.
Kraepelin E. Manic depressive insanity and paranoia. 1921/1976.
Kransz M. Mother who killed 3 kids was hospitalized with paranoid delusions months before shooting. mkransz@mlive.com 2018, updated Feb 20 2019.
Kroft S. Untreated mental illness an imminent danger? [transcript] 60 minutes. 2013 Sept 29.
Lake CR. Psychotic rampage killers: Mania, not schizophrenia—psychiatry's role in prevention. Psychiatr Ann. 2014a;44:213–4.
Lake CR. Rampage murderers, part I: psychotic versus non-psychotic and a role for psychiatry in prevention. Psychiatr Ann. 2014b;44(5):217–25.
Lake CR. Personal interview with Mr. Andy Loya. Jan 22 and 29, 2014c.
Lambert R. Was Anders Breivik a psychotic spree killer or a calculating terrorist? RUSI Analysis. 2011 Aug 18.
Longman J. John E du Pont, 72, dies; killed athlete. NY Times 2010 Dec 10.
Lucey C. Kanye West delivers jaw-dropping performance in oval office. Assoc Press. 2018 Oct 12.
Mandal V. Families of mentally ill pay terrible toll: psychiatric patients are killing and assaulting their families at an alarming rate. Vancouver Sun. 2002 Oct 7.
Mann D. The case of Otty Sanchez: StandDown Texas Project. 2009 Dec 1.
Mann D. Gone baby gone. Texas Observer. 2010 Jan 13.

McLean H. James Holmes – schizophrenia could be a game changer. HarryMcLean.com. 2012 July 28.
Medina J, Burns A, Goldman A. No manifesto, no phone calls: Las Vegas killer left only cryptic clues. NY Times. 2017 Oct 5.
NBC News. Mother confesses to severing baby's arms. 2004 Nov 23. On line.
Olmstead M. What we know about the Las Vegas shooter. Slate.com. 2017a Oct 2. Online.
Olmstead M. Las Vegas gunman's brother describes a high-roller life at the casinos. Slate.com. 2017b Oct 4. Online.
Osterheldt J. Superwomen like Kate Spade smile to hide the pain. Time to hang up the cape and live. Kansas City Star. 2018a June 5.
Osterheldt J. Time to hang up the cape, seek help and live. KC Star. 2018b June 7.
Puente N. Case reopened for Brownsville man convicted of killing three children. Valley Central. com. 2022 Mar 2.
Rivera K. What is Johnny Manziel up to now? 2022 Feb 23. NickiSwift.com on line.
Rosack J. Patient charged with murder of schizophrenia expert. Psychiatr News. 2006;41:1.
Sable. 2002 Sable K. Parents who murder. http://karisable.com/Parentmur.htm. Captured 3/20/20.
Serna J, Winton R. Carrie Fisher's autopsy reveals cocktail of drugs, including cocaine,opiates, and ecstasy. Chicago Trib. 2017 June 19.
Shear MD, Schmidt MS. Gunman and 12 victims killed in shooting at D.C. Navy Yard NY Times. 2013 Sept 16.
Sontag D. A mental patient, a slain worker, troubling questions. NY Times. 2011 June 17.
Sulzberger AG, Carey B. Getting someone to treatment can be difficult and inconclusive, experts say. NY Times. 2011 Jan 19.
Tucker E, Christoffersen J. Slain motorist reportedly suffered delusions. Associated Press, KC Star. 2013 Oct 5.
Vera A. Waffle house shooter was once arrested by secret service for trespassing near White House. CNN. 2018 Apr 22.
Walsh D. The murder conviction of Andrea Yates: a tragic case, a barbaric verdict. World Socialist Web Site. 2002 Mar 15.
Ward B. Dr. Astrid Desrosiers talking to investigators at MGH. Boston.com/news. 2009 Oct 27.
Wehr TA, Goodwin FK. Can antidepressants cause mania and worsen the course of affective illness? Am J Psychiatry. 1987;144(11):1403–11.
Woodruff J. How did Aaron Alexis get security clearance to be a defense contractor? PBS Newshour. 2013 Sept 17.
Writer. 2001.
Zapotosky M, Horwitz S, Morello C. Miriam Carey, driver shot near U.S. Capitol, likely struggled with mental illness, police say. Wash Post. 2013 Oct 4.

Chapter 5
Preparations for Treatment for Therapists and Clients

5.1 Client Preparations for Treatment: Find the Right Professionals

For individuals unsure whether Bipolar could explain some of their mood changes and life conflicts, get opinions of those who know you well and listen to them. Read in depth about Bipolar and its symptoms. Here are some questions to ask yourself that can help determine the presence of a Mood Disorder (Table 5.1). "How has your life been going over the past months to a year? Has there been a general deterioration from a previously successful life? Would you describe your mood as steady or up and down? Consider how up and down; question if these heights and depths in your mood are substantial and beyond your past average and for others in general. Have there been episodes lasting days or weeks that were persistent 24/7 when you were 'high as a kite,' mind racing, 'on top of the world,' into multiple activities, and you did not have time to sleep as much? You may have been overly suspicious, afraid for your life, or felt you had lost touch with reality. Because of increased irritability and anger during such episodes, have you lost jobs, friends, or family or failed courses in school after doing well earlier in your life?" Compare your symptoms to those in Tables 3.3, 3.4, 3.5, and 3.11.

"Have there also been different episodes when you were so down that you felt life was not worth living? Were you feeling sad, hopeless, helpless, worthless? Had you lost enjoyment in your life, felt socially withdrawn, all lasting weeks to months and present 24/7 (Table 3.9)? Do these different episodes in mood cycle back and forth?" These are questions that your therapist will be asking upon your first or second meeting (Sect. 5.3).

Such symptoms may define Bipolar that could be responsible for some of your conflict and dysfunctionality in life. It is treatable. Talk about your concerns and recognize that rationalization, resistance, and denial, which means blaming others or circumstances for one's problems, are typical of Bipolar.

C. R. Lake, *Bipolar for Psychotherapists and Their Clients*,
https://doi.org/10.1007/978-3-031-38750-0_5

Table 5.1 Initial brief screening questions for Mood Disorders

A. *The four-question "90-second depression screen"*
1. "Over the past few weeks (or months), have you been getting less enjoyment out of your life and/or feeling more down in the dumps, sad, or blue?"
2. "Out of the blue have you felt weepy or like crying more often than is usual for you?"
3. "How often have you woken up in the morning wishing you had not woken up?"
4. ("How often") or "Have you recently thought that your life is not worth living?"
B. *Mania screening question*
"Have you ever in your life experienced an episode lasting three or more days when you needed much less sleep than normal for you yet had more energy and activities than usual, felt wound up or on top of the world, and had racing thoughts?"
C. *Dysthymia screening question*
"For most of your life, have you and others considered you someone who more often than not is negative about things, i.e., looking at a 'glass as half empty rather than half full'?"

A definitive diagnosis will be determined by a mental health professional, but your preparation before the meeting can help facilitate accurate assessment and treatment (Chap. 3, Sect. 5.3). To gain confidence of your diagnosis, daily chart your symptoms, mood, hours of sleep, and level of irritability on a form, like the one in Fig. 6.3, or on an online mood charting app. Record dates of historic episodes with similar symptoms you have experienced or observed. Include the most outrageous, striking actions atypical of the individual's normal behavior.

With the availability of so much information through the internet, considerable research about Bipolar can be accomplished by anyone and his or her significant others. If you are a significant other, compare the symptoms exhibited by the person you are observing with those diagnostic of Bipolar from Chaps. 2 and 3. Use Tables 3.3 and 3.4 for help with the diagnosis of Bipolar when it is unclear whether manic behavior is occurring. Investigate the *family history*, including all blood relationships, for any mental health contacts, such as hospitalizations. Find out about those individuals' diagnoses, symptoms, treatments, and medications.

When the suspected Bipolar client does not recognize a problem or take responsibility, as a significant other, chart the symptoms yourself, enlisting help from others who have observed the individual's aberrant behavior and speech. The chart becomes a daily journal of recorded abnormal mood, behaviors, speech, and thoughts. Rather than trying to convince an irritable, diagnosis-resistant manic (or hypomanic) or severely depressed client that they are out of control and need professional help, document the words and actions for presentation later when the individual is less irritable and is more receptive. Record dates of historic episodes with similar symptoms you have experienced or observed. Such records will help in the initial encounter with a therapist.

If in a crisis situation, take the person to an ED with an associated psychiatric inpatient unit. If available, use a university medical center. If the individual will not go voluntarily and is threatening or dangerous, call 911. First, make sure that the individual has no weapons and assure the authorities that the person is unarmed. Be certain to tell the police that the person has a mental disorder (Sects. 4.5 and 4.6).

This is an important step, because psychotic Bipolar clients are subject to getting shot in confrontations with law enforcement. Also give the therapist or admitting psychiatrist any available information about the individual's dangerous behavior.

Before concluding that a Bipolar Disorder is present, the influence of alcohol, illegal or prescription drug use/abuse, and other psychological or medical disorders must be considered and ruled out (Sects. 2.7, 3.6, and 3.7).

When convinced that a Bipolar Disorder is possible or likely, recognize that effective psychotherapy and medication depend on the correct diagnosis (Sect. 3.1). Getting the correct diagnosis depends on finding the right therapist and prescriber.

For the most effective treatment of Bipolar, two mental health professionals will be needed. The first is the psychotherapist who will be seen in 50-minute sessions weekly and will oversee care. This can be a PhD psychologist, a social worker, a nurse practitioner, or other psychotherapist. The second mental health professional will be a prescriber with an MD, a DO, or advanced RN degree. The MD or DO could be a psychiatrist or a primary care physician (PCP), and the nurse, a psychiatric nurse practitioner. Most therapists depend on their clients to find their own prescribers but some therapists may already have an established collaboration with a prescriber.

Vet potential therapists and prescribers alike for their knowledge in treating Bipolar. This may be evident in their bios, but their responses to e-mail or face-to-face questions about their frequency of diagnosing and treating Bipolar are important. Prescribers' frequent use of mood-stabilizing medications will be revealing of their knowledge of Bipolar.

Google available psychotherapists in your area. Research those therapists included in your insurance plan, or go out of network for a more qualified and experienced one. Out-of-network therapists may not cost much more than a therapist in network.

Initial sessions may be the client vetting the professional. Screening more than one therapist is advised since Bipolar has not traditionally been emphasized in the training of therapists. According to Barth (2014), "…you should judge your treatment provider according to how much effort he or she puts into determining what…if any…condition [diagnosis] you have."

Different therapists have different ideas about which symptoms are most important in making the diagnoses. For example, mental health workers have been taught that hallucinations and delusions mean "Schizophrenia," but this is not the case. Such psychotic symptoms are now recognized to be caused by *severe psychotic Mood Disorders*. There are other frequently diagnosed conditions with symptoms that overlap Bipolar, such as Major Depressive Disorder (MDD), ADHD, Borderline Personality Disorder (BPD), Antisocial Personality Disorder (APD), and others (Sects. 2.7 and 3.6). In children, the diagnoses of Oppositional Defiant Disorder (ODD), Intermittent Explosive Disorder (IED), and ADHD are prevalent (Sects. 2.7 and 3.6), but may not be correct.

The correct diagnosis matters because the diagnosis dictates the treatment plan (Chap. 6). Even with a correct diagnosis, different prescribers' and psychotherapists' treatment plans and preferred medicines can vary for the same diagnosis.

Once found, both the new therapist and prescriber will be helped in the initial interviews by the daily mood chart and a concise outline of one page or less describing any recent changes of mood.

Share your own ideas about your diagnosis with the therapist. Have your questions ready and request 10 minutes at the end of the initial session to ask them. Always include, at the top of the list of questions, one to confirm the therapist's diagnostic impressions regarding your diagnosis and the use of the diagnosis of Bipolar. Inquire about their drug preferences for Bipolar treatment. The most effective medications are the mood-stabilizing drugs (lithium, VPA/valproic acid [Depakene/Depakote], and lamotrigine [Lamictal]) rather than antidepressants and antipsychotics (Sect. 6.2).

In some cases, the Bipolar-knowledgeable psychotherapist will already have established a collaborative relationship with a Bipolar-knowledgeable prescriber. This will be of considerable benefit for the new Bipolar client.

5.2 Psychotherapists' Preparations for New Clients

The first challenge for psychotherapists is to gain knowledge and understanding of Bipolar in order to recognize Bipolar in both current and new clinic and client populations.

Some psychotherapy clients with Bipolar will also need medications. Learning about the several mood-stabilizing medications, their dosages, and side effects is easy and necessary in order to vet prescribers to ensure your client gets the most effective medications. The psychotherapist will collaborate closely with the client regarding finding a knowledgeable prescriber. "Knowledgeable" means that the prescriber frequently diagnoses Bipolar rather than "Schizophrenia," "Schizoaffective Disorder" (SAD), ADHD, and Personality Disorders (Sects. 2.7 and 3.6), because the symptoms of these disorders overlap with Bipolar and Bipolar is usually the diagnosis. Also critical for choosing the right prescriber is that they use the mood-stabilizing medications more often than the antipsychotic, antidepressant, and stimulant classes of drugs. Although these latter three drug classes may have some use in treating resistant Bipolar, they are fourth or fifth choices to be added in the case that the three mood stabilizers have failed (Sect. 6.2). Antipsychotics are needed initially along with three mood stabilizers in clients who are psychotic—but only as long as they remain psychotic, which is usually only for days to weeks.

Although most therapists leave it to their clients to find their own prescribers, it is recommended that the psychotherapist vet in advance a prescriber for referral of their clients for medications. This benefits clients, therapists, and prescribers. An ongoing collaboration with a Bipolar-knowledgeable prescriber includes cross-referrals and an agreement to prioritize attention to each other's calls and clients. The collaborating prescriber must agree to recognize the therapist's role as the primary caretaker for the client and must be willing to discuss diagnosis and treatment. Prescribers will be MD or DO psychiatrists, primary care physicians (PCPs), or psychiatric nurse practitioners who can prescribe.

Researching a prescriber knowledgeable about Bipolar and its treatment requires time, effort, and some expense that will pay rewards for both therapist and client. Some prescribers are not adequately knowledgeable about Bipolar or mood-stabilizing drugs, so gather as much data as possible about a prescriber's diagnostic and prescribing practices from their online CV. This research will narrow the field. Then contact several potential prescribers to meet to discuss a collaborative relationship. If necessary, it is worth paying for a lunch or even an interview session to discuss a collaboration and the prescriber's diagnostic and medication preferences for Bipolar and specifically the use of mood-stabilizing medications. Therapists may have to meet with several prescribers before finding one knowledgeable about Bipolar.

A therapist's established relationship with a prescriber is extremely beneficial for clients and for both professionals. The prescriber, who probably doesn't conduct psychotherapy, will appreciate having a known collaboration with a therapist for help in treating their Bipolar and other clients, since psychotherapy is mandatory for best care in Bipolar and other psychological conditions. Bipolar, mild to severe, is best treated with regular weekly psychotherapy as well as medications (Chap. 6). Recognize that, as a therapist, in addition to weekly psychotherapy, you also offer your client a vetted prescriber for medication management and suicide and psychotic symptom evaluations for inpatient placement.

Prescribers' understanding of therapists maintaining oversight for their Bipolar clients is important. Topics to agree upon are diagnostics, medication, cross-referral of clients, and prompt responses to inquiries.

5.3 The Initial Interview: Key Questions

Both moderate to severely depressed and manic clients can be difficult to interview because of their mood symptoms, which include disturbances in thoughts, emotions, and speech. Such deficits are diagnostic but can confuse client responses to questions asked. The depressed client may not spontaneously speak and the irritable manic can talk nonstop without the ability to focus on the questions asked, becoming irritated, if not angry, when interrupted with a question. Therapists can also feel frustrated and question continuing to work with such irritable clients. To increase therapist safety, consider asking new clients to come in with a significant other on the initial visit (Sects. 4.5 and 4.6).

Keep in mind that irritability and confusion are symptoms of a disorder you can treat and help the client with recovery to a productive life. In cases of acute mania with pressed speech and irritability, it may be best to allow the client to talk without interrupting to avoid a session-ending confrontation. Such behavior is consistent with mania and Bipolar, and clients will benefit with therapist input at a later point in the therapy about the negative impact of their manic behavior on their lives. If the client can be gently interrupted, ask if he or she will agree to stop talking and to focus on your question when you signal by raising your hand. Depending on the severity of the mania at the time, this may work. Once the client has become more stable, remind them about their disruptive speech and behavior during those past sessions and how without treatment it will interrupt their career and relationships.

Use judgement to determine when a manic client is stable enough to listen. If a delay is needed, give support, reschedule, and refer for mood-stabilizing medications.

In less obvious cases, an initial screening question for mania or hypomania is "Are you currently or have you ever experienced three or four days or more when you needed substantially less sleep than normal and yet had a considerable increase in energy and activities, felt wound-up, on top of the world, and experienced your thoughts as racing?" (Tables 5.1 and 5.2) Affirmative answers indicate mania and call for further exploration for a Bipolar diagnosis (Chaps. 2 and 3). A brief screening test is supportive to confirm Bipolar (Sect. 5.4).

Table 5.2 Detailed questions for psychotic or paranoid clients or their significant others

For mania
1. Have you needed less sleep over the past days to weeks? How many hours per night? How many nights with no sleep? Is this different from your baseline? Please explain further.
2. Describe your energy and activity levels during this time. What new activities have you begun?
3. Has your mind been going slower or faster than usual? Please explain.
4. Has anyone asked you to slow down or shut up?
5. Do you believe you possess special knowledge, powers, connections, or anything of substantial value? Please explain further.
6. Why are they after you? What do they want from you? Please explain further.
7. Have you been more irritable or more easily angered lately? How many physical or verbal altercations/fights have you been involved in lately? Is this typical for you? Give some examples.
8. What problems have you had with law enforcement?
9. Have you recently driven your car differently than is usual for you?
10. Who (what) presents a danger to you? Please explain.
For depression
1. Describe how you have been feeling in your mood or spirits over the past days to weeks. Have you been more tearful or felt like crying recently? Have you felt sad or empty? Is this different from your baseline? Please explain further.
2. Describe your energy and activity levels during this time. What activities have you given up?
3. Have you been enjoying usually pleasurable activities as much as usual? Please explain further and give examples.
4. Have you had feelings of guilt most days? Please describe in detail.
5. Have you felt worthless and that you deserved punishment for transgressions or sins in the past? Please explain in detail.
6. Have you stayed at home or in your room more than usual or not answered your telephone or door? Is this unusual for you? Please give details.
7. Have you experienced difficulty concentrating or focusing on a task? Help me understand how this is different from the normal you.
8. Have you had thoughts that life is not worth living? How have you thought about hurting yourself? What plans have you made? What is the closest you have come to hurting yourself? How close have you come to killing yourself in the past?

Continue to observe for and ask about *episodic* manic inflated self-esteem, grandiosity, irritable mood, quick anger, flight of ideas, racing thoughts, pressure to keep talking, and disabling distractibility (Chap. 3). Ask about similar past episodes and a family history of any blood kin with psychological or psychiatric contacts, suicidal behaviors, scripts for psychiatric medications, and psychiatric inpatient stays.

Continue to ask about past incidents of decreased need for sleep, poor judgement, reckless behavior, and spur-of-the-moment decisions often with painful consequences that lasted days to months; what was the most costly example? These symptoms are most severe in full mania defining Bipolar I and less severe in the hypomania of Bipolar II. Ask about the use of alcohol and other drugs that are frequently associated with Bipolar and must be addressed up front.

For Bipolar II with hypomania, ask about *episodes* of decreased hours of sleep, modest increases in energy, with productive goal-directed activities that associate with accomplishments, successes, and leadership roles but also with easy irritability and conflict (Sects. 3.2, 3.3, and 3.5; Tables 3.4 and 3.5). These episodes may last only three to four days or more, with the symptoms present 24/7. Such successes occur most often in Bipolar II and Cyclothymia but are also seen in Bipolar I clients before their mania becomes severe (Chap. 3; Table 1.1).

Successes in the lives of Bipolars can deter them from seeking or continuing treatment because they feel so invigorated and are often oblivious to the negative effects on others of their manic behavior. Therapists will be most successful in sustaining treatment contact when they discuss the potential of clients to terminate therapy, which can occur under various circumstances. One is when they feel so confident in mania/hypomania that they think they are cured or never had Bipolar. Emphasize that successes in hypomania are usually short-lived with either full destructive mania or depression to follow. Such cycling forecasts future increased cycling and increased severity. A second situation is when the manic client misperceives the therapist as rejecting. Therapists are encouraged to instruct their clients early in the therapy to confront the therapist with any concerns or disappointments they may have with the therapist.

When dealing with a grandiose manic client, recognize their grandiose thoughts and only gently challenge them. Document the delusions and manic behavior and address them later when the client is euthymic and more receptive to hearing such feedback.

Once hypomania and mania are surveyed, ask about depression. According to the Diagnostic and Statistical Manual (DSM), at least one Major Depressive Episode (MDE) is needed for a diagnosis of Bipolar Type II. There are usually multiple MDEs in both Bipolar I and II. Start with the depression screen first if the client presents with depression rather than mania.

If depression is established, ask about prior episodes of thoughts that life is not worth living. Assess risk for suicide here. If positive, go to a full screen for suicidality and homicidality (Sect. 6.6).

5.4 The Use of Brief Screening Instruments

There are many brief screening instruments that can supplement diagnostics and oral mental status questions. The screens noted here have been selected for their brevity and efficacy. Some are clinician administered; others are given to clients to complete in the waiting room. Clients can be given a packet of three to five self-administered screens to complete before their initial and follow-up interviews. The clinician can visually scan, if not score, the client's responses in a few minutes to gain valuable diagnostic data.

For example, the therapist-administered *Six-Item Cognitive Impairment Test* (6CIT-Kingshill Version 2000) takes only minutes. The *6CIT* requires no props, and the scoring system is on the one-page screen. If in the initial diagnostic interview, the client's responses do not seem rational, the 6CIT can identify cognitive problems. If the client's 6CIT responses are equivocal, initial focus must be on mental status. Has the client had complaints of memory and cognitive issues? If so, other mental status examinations that are more extensive may then be used. A referral to the PCP for a work-up and an MRI of the head is warranted.

For depression, the *Patient Health Questionnaire (PHQ-9)* can be client or clinician administered. The instructions for the interpretation of clients' responses are easy to understand. Another widely used rating scale for depression is the more extensive Hamilton Depression Scale (HAM-D).

The *Mood Disorders Questionnaire (MDQ)*, using only three questions, is an efficient *client-completed screen for mania*. The first question addresses specific symptoms of mania and consists of a 13-part "yes/no" checklist. The second question, also in a "yes/no" format, asks whether the symptoms from Question 1 occur at the same time. The third question asks about the severity of the impact of the symptoms on day-to-day life and is graded from "no problem" to "serious problem."

The very brief *Altman Self-Rating Scale for Mania (ASRM)* consists of five questions and clear instructions (Altman et al. 1997). Altman has also developed the more extensive and time-consuming Clinician-Administered Rating Scale for Mania (CARS-M) (Altman et al. 1994). The Young Mania Rating Scale (YMRS) is useful to evaluate manic symptoms at baseline and over time to assess changes in severity of mania (Young et al. 1978). It is clinician administered and requires 15–30 minutes to complete. The Mini Patient Health Survey (MPHS) can be clinician or client self-administered. It has four sections, all brief, that screen for Major Depression, Alcohol Use Disorder, and Panic and Social Anxiety Disorders.

Selecting three to five of these instruments and gaining confidence with their use should enhance Mood Disorder diagnostics.

References

6CIT-Kingshill Version. Swindon: The Kingshill Research Centre; 2000.

Altman EG, Hedeker D, Peterson JL, Davis JM. The Altman self-rating mania scale (ASRM). Biol Psychiatry. 1997;42:948–55.

Altman EG, Hedeker D, Janicak PG, Peterson JL, Davis JM. The clinician-administered rating scale for mania (CARS-M). Biol Psychiatry. 1994;36(2):124–34.

Barth FD. The importance of your diagnosis: why your diagnosis matters and how to get the right one. Psych Today May 9, 2014.

Young RC, Biggs JT, Ziegler E, Meyer DA. A rating scale for mania: Reliability, validity and sensitivity. Br J Psychiatry. 1978;133(5):429–35.

Chapter 6
Treatment

6.1 Psychotherapy

> "Bipolar-specific psychotherapy including psychoeducation, individual, family, and group is effective in combination with pharmacotherapy in delaying relapses, stabilizing episodes, and reducing episode length." (Swartz and Swanson 2014)

> "Psychotherapy is mandated for best care in treatment of Bipolar clients. Psychoeducation is a necessary component of all forms of psychotherapy. Needed is an information-oriented, didactic approach about Bipolar." (Miklowitz 2008)

Discussions of psychotherapy for Bipolar begin with a history of Cade's 1949 discovery of the magical efficacy of lithium in the treatment of Bipolar. This revelation of the effectiveness of lithium in stabilizing Bipolar clients discouraged the use of psychotherapy until the late twentieth century, when it was recognized that lithium and other mood-stabilizing medications gave *only partial relief. Pharmacologic interventions alone* have been associated with disappointingly *low rates of remission* and *high rates of recurrence*, *residual symptoms*, and *psychosocial impairment*. Current concepts consider Bipolar as a chronic disorder requiring a combination of pharmacotherapy and weekly psychotherapy for best management and results.

Bipolar causes a high degree of psychosocial impairment, low rates of compliance with appointments and medication, interpersonal dysfunction, and cognitive harm. These domains are effectively addressed by psychotherapeutic interventions in combination with pharmacotherapy. "*Bipolar-specific psychotherapy* is increasingly recommended as an essential component of illness management" (Swartz and Swanson 2014). Bipolar-specific psychotherapies use directive and symptom-focused strategies, such as *psychoeducation about the details of Bipolar*, *encouragement for appointment and medication compliance*, *involvement of family members*; development of *strategies for relapse prevention*; and exploration of the

C. R. Lake, *Bipolar for Psychotherapists and Their Clients*,
https://doi.org/10.1007/978-3-031-38750-0_6

reciprocal relationship between mood, cognition, interpersonal relationships, and a regular sleep-wake cycle.

Achieving remission in cases with active symptoms is no longer the only goal of treatment. *Preventing or delaying the next episode* after remission is essential for the successful lifetime management of Bipolar. Therapists must emphasize to clients and their families that a first step of effective treatment is to learn as much as possible about Bipolar Disorder. The goals of treatment and management of Bipolar are to reduce acute symptoms; to postpone or prevent recurrence; to minimize the severity of subsequent episodes, when they do occur; and to address clients' issues in their lives that can impact Bipolar episodes.

Building a therapeutic alliance is accomplished by eliciting clients' past and current issues, providing feedback, and conveying empathy, genuineness, and warmth. It is helpful to emphasize Bipolar as an illness of the brain and, to a degree, out of voluntary control. Still, psychotherapy can shift a negative view in life, often during depression, to a positive one—shifting a glass half empty to one half full.

Psychotic and nonpsychotic Mood Disorders are typically lifelong, episodic early in their course, and can be debilitating, especially with frequent episodes. Such conditions warrant major client and significant other involvement in care. The goal is to prevent these episodic disorders from becoming rapid cycling, chronic, persistent, and treatment-resistant disasters (Table 6.9).

Bipolar Disorders are severe diseases of the brain causing considerable morbidity and mortality from suicide and associated medical conditions. Continuous therapist-guided management is critical because many clients can remain symptomatic for more than half of their lives when untreated. Delayed treatment results from at least two factors: failure to recognize (Sect. 1.3, Chap. 3) and misdiagnosis as Major Depressive Disorder, Attention-Deficit Hyperactivity Disorder (ADHD), "Schizophrenia," "Schizoaffective Disorder," or others (Sects. 2.7 and 3.6). As clarified by the information provided previously and herein, these diagnoses are all likely to be psychotic Bipolar Disorders (Lake 2021).

Early onset of symptoms, delayed treatment, rapid cycling, and the number of previous psychotic and mixed episodes are potent risk factors for poor outcomes. Each episode of depression or mania is associated with *decrements in brain-derived neurotropic factor (BDNF)* and increases in oxidative stress markers, both of which endanger neurons and increase episodes. Bipolar gets worse and the next episode comes faster, so early accurate diagnosis and effective treatment are most important.

The correct diagnosis is critical to optimal treatment, and clients must accept some responsibility for receiving the right diagnosis. Substantial client effort is needed to accomplish this step for confidence in the right diagnosis (Sect. 1.3, Chap. 3). Potential clients can address this challenge by reading about Bipolar and Unipolar Disorders, learning among other things that even a single episode of mania or hypomania distinguishes a Bipolar from a Unipolar Disorder. Begin with Chaps. 2 and 3 of this book, the DSM-5-TR, and other sources such as textbooks, Wikipedia, and Google. The most comprehensive book about Bipolar Disorder is by Goodwin and Jamison 2007, *Manic-Depressive Illness*. The current book and the DSM-5-TR are good for the diagnostic criteria for mania and depression, which are summarized in Chap. 3. Productive questions for identifying Bipolar are found in Tables 3.3, 3.4, and 3.9.

Regular psychotherapy follow-up is recommended weekly to maximize the chances of client compliance, client understanding of their disease, the medications needed and their adverse effects (AEs), and recognition of early indications of recurrence, enabling a prophylactic increase in therapy and medication adjustment before a full-blown episode develops. The goal is prevention of episodes rather than the usual "catch up" treatment after a full relapse.

Therapy sessions must be a top priority in clients' lives and be seen as a lifeline to stability and functionality. If a rare priority overrides a scheduled session, it should be reset during the same week.

There are 12 steps therapists can teach their clients to help them manage their Bipolar. These reduce the risk for relapse and are as follows: (1) learn about Bipolar; (2) accept the diagnosis; (3) take the multiple medications; (4) insist on three mood stabilizers; (5) attend regular long-term psychotherapy; (6) avoid all alcohol and illegal drugs; (7) chart activities, mood, sleep, and medications daily (Fig. 6.3); (8) get regular exercise; (9) maintain a strict, consistent sleep-wake schedule; (10) recognize initial, subtle changes that herald an oncoming episode; (11) avoid kindling by identifying trigger factors known to start an attack; and (12) take charge of your treatment rejecting overconfidence even during long remissions (Table 6.9).

According to Miklowitz (2008), psychotherapy has been consistently recommended for Bipolar Disorder, and considerable efforts have investigated which interventions are effective for which clients. Psychotherapy is as important as pharmacotherapy in relapse prevention and episode stabilization and is associated with a 30–40% reduction in relapse rates over 12 to 30-month periods. Overall, psychotherapy enhances both the symptomatic and functional outcomes in Bipolar.

Untreated, up to 50% of Bipolar Type I clients do not recover from acute manic episodes within a year and only 25% gain full recovery of function. *With pharmacotherapy alone, rates of recurrence over 1 to 2 years are 40–60%.* Clients spend as much as 47% of their lives in symptomatic states, especially depression, despite taking their medicine. Clients who receive intensive psychosocial therapy have better functional outcomes than clients receiving routine pharmacological treatment alone over a one- to two-year period. Psychotherapy including individual, family, and group psychoeducation is effective in combination with pharmacotherapy in stabilizing episodes, delaying relapses, and reducing episode length.

6.1.1 Individual Psychoeducation (IPE)

Emphasis on early recognition of mood symptoms along with focus on interpersonal relationships, communication skills, and stress management is therapeutic. During individual psychoeducation (IPE), therapists collaborate with their clients in evaluating symptom changes, monitoring medication dosages and AEs, and developing relapse-prevention plans and illness-management strategies, such as a consistent sleep-wake cycle. Therapists and clients benefit from knowing the names, dosages, and AEs of their medications. Routine discussions of medications, their effects, and their AEs improve compliance and overall outcomes. Gaining an understanding of Bipolar, its history, biological basis, signs and symptoms, course, and relationship to successes may reduce stigma and enhance compliance. Such individual psychoeducation reduced the likelihood of manic recurrences from 57% to 27% (Perry et al. 1999). Swartz and Swanson (2014) reviewed 28 randomized trials of psychotherapy in Bipolar clients. In each of these studies, the psychotherapy was accompanied with pharmacotherapy.

Types of psychotherapy reviewed included Individual (IPE) and Group (GPE) Psychoeducation, Individual (ICBT) and Group (GCBT) Cognitive Behavioral Therapy (CBT), Family-focused Psychotherapy (FT), and Interpersonal and Social Rhythm Therapy (IPSRT).

IPE and GPE provide information about Bipolar causes, treatments, course and outcomes, and strategies to identify prodromal symptoms, early warning signs of relapse, and illness-coping strategies. Clients participating in IPE and GPE in general had prolonged time to manic relapse, fewer manic episodes over 18 months, lowered scores on the Hamilton Depression Scale, lower hospitalization rates, and improved symptoms over time.

6.1.2 Group Psychoeducation (GPE)

GPE can include lectures, handouts, and exercises to increase illness awareness, early detection with prodromal symptoms emphasized, and medication adjustments. Also considered are lifestyle changes such as avoiding abrupt late-night work or party events that cause alterations of sleep pattern that can trigger episodes (Sect. 2.5). GPE especially helps Bipolar clients with comorbid Substance Use Disorders.

6.1.3 Family Psychoeducation (FPE)

Family Psychoeducation (FPE) is effective in improving the course of Bipolar Disorder. Family-focused therapy emphasizes psychoeducation, communication-enhancement training, problem-solving, and strategies for regulating one's emotions. Clients in family-focused therapy had a greater likelihood of avoiding Bipolar relapse than clients in crisis-management treatment. "Family-focused therapy seemed more effective in preventing recurrence and rehospitalization compared to individual therapy" (Rea et al. 2003). The increased effectiveness of FPE may be due to the proximity of knowledgeable or invested family members for more hours per day than in IPE and GPE.

Family Therapy (FT) in general resulted in increased compliance with lithium; effective resolution of the index episode; longer delays to relapse; reductions in mood symptoms, especially depressive episodes; and fewer hospitalizations. FT hastened recovery and conferred protection against recurrence.

6.1.4 Cognitive Behavioral Therapy (CBT)

"CBT is a skills-based treatment that helps clients recognize and modify the link between maladaptive thoughts and mood. Through the use of *thought records*, *mood diaries*, and activity scheduling, clients learn to modify *automatic negative thoughts*, *remove distorted thinking*, and interrupt cycles of mania and depression" (Swartz and Swanson 2014). ICBT and GCBT lower the risk for relapse, improve scores on the Beck Depression Inventory (BDI), and result in significantly greater improvements in quality of life and fewer hospitalizations (Swartz and Swanson 2014).

Cognitive restructuring strategies address pessimistic explanatory styles in depression and overly optimistic biases in the manic or hypomanic phase (Johnson 2005). Other studies reviewed by Miklowitz (2008) show that clients in CBT and with pharmacotherapy fared better than those receiving pharmacotherapy and routine care. In general, clients receiving CBT and medication have *fewer hospitalizations*, *fewer days in the hospital*, *better social functioning*, *better medication adherence*, *lower depression* scores, and *fewer days of depressed mood* (Cochran 1984).

Results seem robust for one to two years; then effectiveness falls off, but this could be explained by CBT discontinuation. Nor did CBT appear as effective in severely ill Bipolars. CBT requires focus that is lost in moderate to severe mania. The effectiveness of CBT seems greater in depression than in moderate to severe mania; focus on medication compliance improves results.

6.1.5 Interpersonal and Social Rhythm Therapy (ISRT)

Poor interpersonal functioning is consistent with Bipolar, especially during depression. Interpersonal and Social Rhythm Therapy (ISRT) attempts to resolve interpersonal problems related to grief, role disputes, interpersonal conflicts, and interpersonal deficits. IPSRT addresses interpersonal problems and regulates and stabilizes Bipolar clients' social rhythms.

Social rhythms are those daily activities that help to set or disrupt underlying biological rhythms. Examples include sleep-wake schedules, mealtimes, work and school, and daily exercise (Frank 2005). IPSRT combines interpersonal psychotherapy (IPT) for depression with a behavioral strategy that sets daily routines (Social Rhythm Therapy) (SRT) and psychoeducation (PE) to increase compliance with medications. "IPSRT addresses 1) the identification and management of affective symptoms; 2) the link between mood and events; 3) the maintenance of regular daily rhythms…; 4) the identification and management of potential precipitants of rhythm dysregulation, with special attention to interpersonal triggers; 5) and the facilitation of mourning the lost healthy self" (Swartz and Swanson 2014). IPSRT is effective in both acute and maintenance treatments for Bipolar and has shown promise in monotherapy for Bipolar II depression.

Sleep-wake cycle changes can trigger manic episodes. Daily use of the *mood tracker* or other form is critical to record sleep/wake cycles, as well as mood (Fig. 6.3). These records are a weekly source for discussion in therapy sessions.

Clients treated with ISRT have *longer well intervals* (Frank 2005). ISRT appeared effective in *delaying recurrences*, especially of depression, in the maintenance phase when clients were able to stabilize their social rhythms.

Although no particular psychotherapeutic modality is superior to others, research results suggest that the different techniques operate through different change mechanisms and in turn effect different outcome variables. Therapists are encouraged to use psychotherapy techniques they are used to, with emphasis on education of clients about details of Bipolar. This requires therapists to know about Bipolar. The next priority is stressing the importance of compliance with weekly attendance, charting, and medication.

Psychotherapy plus medication have consistently demonstrated superiority over medication only. Bipolar-specific psychotherapy plus mood-stabilizing medications hasten recovery from depressive episodes, reduce new mood episodes, and improve daily functioning and quality of life.

Psychotherapy is mandated for best care in treatment of Bipolar clients. Psychoeducation is a necessary component of all forms of psychotherapy for Bipolar clients. An information-oriented, didactic approach about Bipolar is needed.

Assume that compliance will become an issue for all clients at some point and create an atmosphere in which ambivalence and obstacles can be anticipated, discussed, and simple behavioral techniques introduced (such as pairing medication taking with routine activity) to facilitate adherence (Scott 1995).

6.2 Medications

"Given the risk for a life-devastating course from a recurrent or persistent psychotic Mood Disorder, the benefit-to-risk ratio for these drugs, especially the mood stabilizers, is large. A missed diagnosis usually eliminates chances for such benefit." (Post 2007)

"In rational polypharmacy, conventional doses and blood level targets are not the primary goal. Rather, maximizing therapeutic efficacy and minimizing adverse effects (AEs) of the entire regimen is the aim." (Post 2007)

"In the absence of AEs data support maintaining full doses of each agent in the entire regimen that resulted in the acute improvement into the continuation and long-term prophylactic phases…stay the course." (Post 2007)

"Because these [second-generation antipsychotic] drugs [SGAs] have safety issues, physicians should prescribe them only when they are sure patients will get substantial benefits." (Alexander et al. 2011)

> "These new drugs [SGAs] accounted for more than $10 billion in U. S. retail pharmacy prescription drug costs in 2008, representing the largest expenditure for any single drug class…" (Grohol 2011)

> "[Because the second-generation antipsychotics(SGAs)] worsen long-term outcomes…continual medication therapy [with SGA drugs]…does more harm than good." (Whitaker 2004)

> "If a patient with … atypical 'Schizophrenia' … has suffered one or more manic symptoms at index admission…*great care should be taken in diagnosing 'Schizophrenia' in [such] a patient who also has manic symptoms* [because] … when they actually have a Bipolar Affective Disorder [they] will not have an opportunity to benefit from this [lithium] treatment." (Tsuang et al. 1976)

Psychotherapy training programs do not teach about medications. For Bipolar, the number of drugs is limited and important to know. Even though therapists usually do not prescribe, they will benefit their clients and themselves by knowing about the drugs for Bipolar. By learning about the drugs, their dosages, and AEs, therapists can teach their clients and consult with their clients' prescribers. Prescribers must be notified with medication data that warrant changes. In this way, therapists become managers of Bipolar cases.

Polypharmacy, the use of several drugs at once, has been the treatment of choice for many medical diseases, such as cancers, heart disease, AIDS, tuberculosis, and rheumatoid arthritis, and is now considered standard of care for the treatment of Mood Disorders (Fig. 6.1).

Compliance with therapy and medications is absolutely necessary to manage risk for relapse. *Some 50% of Mood-Disordered clients* do not regularly take their prescribed medications; many drop out of therapy and are lost to follow-up.

There are studies that address ways to improve compliance. Some of these focus on Bipolar, where adherence rates are as low as *35%* (Torem 2013). Psychotherapists must invest themselves in urging client compliance by discussing it in each session. In an attempt to counter compliance failure, encourage clients to participate in their treatment decisions, even to take charge of the management of their Bipolar. When possible, working with their families in their medication titration schedules under therapist and doctor guidelines is a benefit. Emphasize that Bipolar, its treatment, including several medications and psychotherapy, and other life changes are for life…analogous to diabetes. Discuss *clients' opinions of what their treatment outcome goals are*, and encourage them to express their ideas about how to reach such outcomes. "Understanding the client's expectations of how treatment is carried out will allow therapists to provide them with a rational view of treatment and *establish a partnership based on realistic expectations*" (Torem 2013). It is recommended that *clients engage in choosing their medications within the mood-stabilizer class*, setting *their treatment goals* and *targeting symptoms to be relieved*. The times and frequency of medication administration can be mutually addressed with the goal of choosing the best time to enhance remembering. Use of a daily medicine reminder container helps with compliance and prevents double dosing. Some of the anti-seizure mood stabilizers sedate, so are best taken at bedtime. Lithium is best taken with food to decrease the chance of nausea.

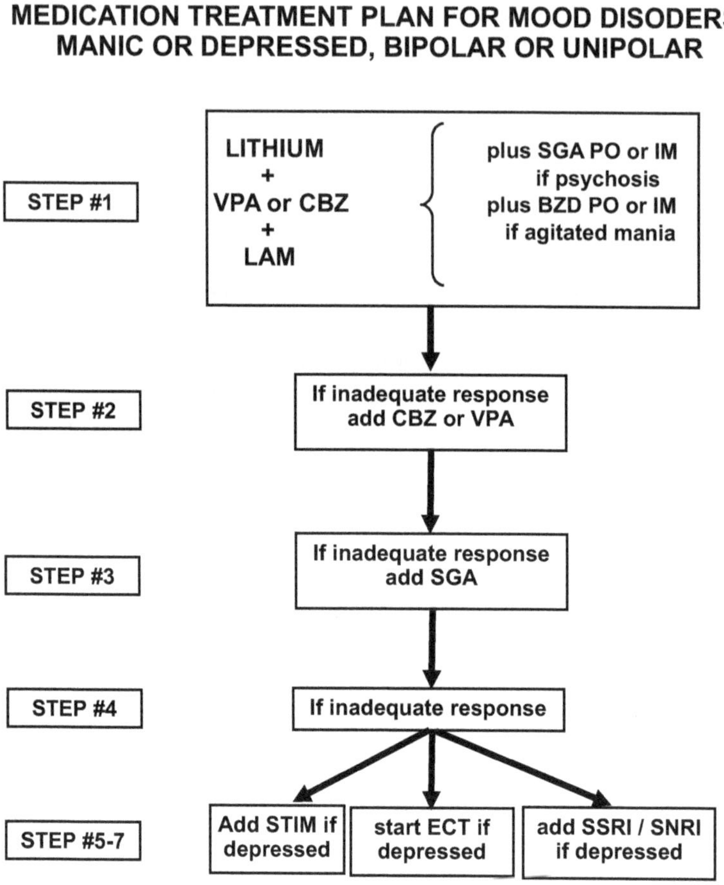

Fig. 6.1 Medication treatment plan for Mood Disorders, manic or depressed, Bipolar or Unipolar

The treatment for Mood Disorders is the same whether manic or depressed and whether Unipolar or Bipolar. *If not psychotic*, begin with three mood-stabilizing medications. Recommended are Lithium, VPA (or CBZ) and LAM. Starting dosages are 300–600 mg/day of lithium with food, 250 mg of VPA usually qhs and 25 mg/day of LAM. Lithium and VPA can be titrated up as tolerated. LAM is limited to increases of 25 mg/week because of the danger of Stephens-Johnson Syndrome (a severe rash) (Fig. 6.2). Discuss medications with your clients and work for consensus on drugs and dosages. If the prescriber has not given the medications in the dosages deemed necessary, contact him/her. Getting blood levels of lithium and VPA can be considered on daily dosages of 600–900 mg and 500–1000 mg, respectively. If the response is inadequate on therapeutic levels, Step 2 is to add another mood stabilizer or a low dose of an SGA. NOTE: VPA, CBZ, and SGAs are sedative, should be given qhs, and can cause dose-limiting daytime sedation.

If response remains inadequate, discuss Steps 5, 6, and 7: only if client is depressed consider a stimulant, ECT or an SSRI/SNRI. Some recommend ECT even before an SGA in non-psychotic severely depressed individuals (Swartz and Shorter 2007).

For agitation, a BZD can help.

Abbreviations: qhs Give at bedtime, *LAM* lamotrigine (Lamictal), *SSRI* selective serotonin reuptake inhibitor (Table 6.3), *STIM* stimulants (Table 6.5), *SNRI* serotonin norepinephrine reuptake inhibitor (Table 6.3), *ECT* electroconvulsive therapy, *CBZ* carbamazepine (Tegretol), *BZD* benzodiazepine, *VPA* valproic acid (Depakote), *SGA* second-generation anti-schizophrenia drug.

It is important to *encourage clients (and families) to self-monitor* mood changes, sleep, anger episodes, and symptoms identified as early signs of an oncoming episode. Trigger situations and specific individuals who trigger are identified. Sometimes such known triggers can be gradually approached in an attempt to desensitize reactivity rather than using a trigger-avoidance strategy (Sect. 6.4).

Give clients the ability to hold at a given dose rather than continue to increase if there are mild to moderate AEs. Recommend clients avoid stopping a drug altogether unless side effects are severe. Rather, it is suggested that the dose be taken down one step to see if adverse effects diminish or go away. An exception is a rash, especially while taking lamotrigine (Lamictal), when the medication(s) must be discontinued immediately and the client must go to the ED (Fig. 6.2). Clients should recognize that there are a limited number of drugs in each class, especially in the mood stabilizers group (Table 6.1).

Continue to *warn of overconfidence* during extended euthymic episodes when there is a strong tendency to conclude that the diagnosis is a mistake and no treatment is needed. Case examples of this resistance to accept the Bipolar diagnosis are found in Sects. 4.2, 4.3, and 4.4. One example is Mr. S. M., a brilliant tax lawyer, who withdrew from treatment during euthymia on five occasions and relapsed after six months to a year each time. He finally said, "Never again" and has reduced his cycle rate with consistent therapy and medication compliance (Sect. 4.2, Case 4.3).

Polypharmacy for Mood Disorders consists of two or three *mood-stabilizing drugs at once*; SGAs should be used only in cases of psychosis or multiple concomitant mood-stabilizer resistance. *SGAs are never used alone in Bipolar* but only in combination with several mood-stabilizing medications.

There are some exciting alternative treatments for depression, either Bipolar or Unipolar. These include ketamine, aggressive high-dose thyroid replacement therapy, and transcranial magnetic stimulation (TMS). Electroconvulsive therapy (ECT) continues to be an effective treatment for medication-resistant depression. The benefit-to-risk profile for ECT exceeds that of the SGAs (Sect. 6.5).

Rapid-cycling Bipolar is disappointingly resistant to treatment. Nor is rapid cycling rare, with some reporting that almost *40% of inpatient Bipolars* suffer four episodes a year. This is despite polypharmacy, with an average of three medications plus psychotherapy. Studies show that only 12.5% of rapid-cycling Bipolar clients are acutely stabilized with lithium or valproic acid/divalproex (Depakene/Depakote) separately; *25% are stabilized on the combination*. One disappointing study reported only 50% of Bipolar clients respond to a year of polypharmacy plus psychotherapy.

Modafinil (Provigil), a stimulant, may help in residual depression and low energy in Bipolar depressed clients but poses a risk for a switch to mania. *Triiodothyronine (T_3) or levothyroxine (Synthroid, T_4) augmentation* is helpful in difficult-to-stabilize depressed Bipolar and Unipolar clients. The positive effects are independent of abnormalities in the thyroid axis (Sect. 6.5).

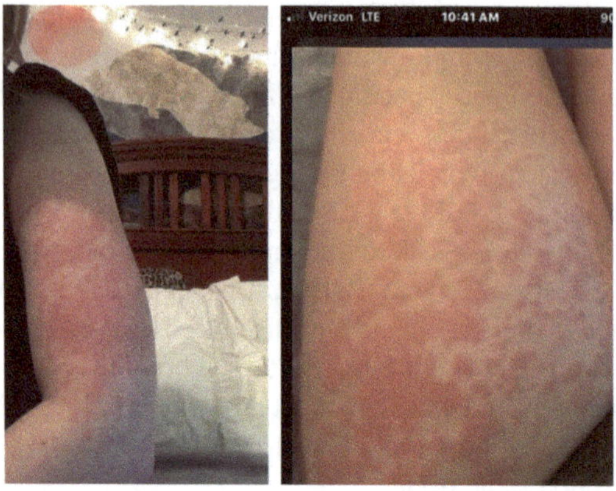

Fig. 6.2 Lamotrigine (Lamictal) potential rash

Figure 6.2 shows the rash caused by lamotrigine (Lamictal), which typically occurs within weeks of starting this medication. In contrast to the manufacturer's indications of a 1% incidence, the current author experienced at least a 10% incidence or higher in women. Patients were started on 25 mg per day, with increases of 25 mg weekly, building to a total daily dose of between 200 and 400 mg per day, less if valproic acid/divalproex (Depakene/Depakote) was prescribed concomitantly. The rash, as depicted here, usually appeared within a few weeks, sometimes within hours to days of beginning the drug and the upward titration.

The rash usually appeared on the upper thighs, arms, and chest. This rash can substantially worsen to Stevens-Johnson Syndrome, which can be fatal if the drug is continued. None of the author's patients' rashes progressed to Stevens-Johnson Syndrome.

All patients prescribed lamotrigine (Lamictal) were told to stop the drug immediately at the appearance of any rash, and these orders were followed. Several patients went to the ED, were reassured since they had stopped the drug, and some were given diphenhydramine (Benadryl). In general, the rash resolved over one to three weeks. The most detrimental sequela was that the patient could no longer take a very useful mood-stabilizing drug. There are too few effective mood-stabilizing drugs available. In one case a female patient who suffered the rash on 25 mg/day insisted on trying it again a year later, having cycled into a severe manic episode. She restarted at 5 mg/day and did not have a recurrent rash despite slow upward titration.

Table 6.1 Examples of mood-stabilizing medications

Name	
Generic // trade	Maint/max dosage (mg/day[a])
lithium carbonate, citrate[b] // Eskalith, Lithobid, Lithane	600–1500/1800
Valproic acid, divalproex sodium[c] // Depakene, Depakote	250–2000/3000
Carbamazepine[c] // Tegretol	200–1200/1200
Oxcarbazepine[c] //Trileptal	600–1200/1200
Lamotrigine[b,c] // Lamictal	100–400/400[b,d]
Topiramate[c,e] // Topamax	200–400/600
Gabapentin[c,e] // Neurontin	900–1800/1800
Levetiracetam[c,e] // Keppra	1000–3000/3000
Zonisamide[c,e] // Zonegran	200–800/800

[a]These dosages are broad estimates
[b]Especially effective in treating depression
[c]Antiepileptic drugs
[d]Half the dose if also taking Depakote
[e]Data less convincing of efficacy in Bipolar

6.2.1 Mood-Stabilizing Medications

Clients newly faced with taking long-term maintenance medications for Bipolar must evaluate benefits versus AEs with their therapists. The benefit-to-risk ratio of the mood-stabilizing agents surpasses that of the other four groups of drugs used in Bipolar. It is the effectiveness of the mood stabilizers that stands out as superior to the others in stabilizing mood. Another major advantage of the mood stabilizers is that plasma levels of lithium, valproic acid/divalproex (Depakene/Depakote), carbamazepine (Tegretol), and oxcarbazepine (Trileptal) can be measured to help determine if the client is taking the right dose to reach the known therapeutic blood level; also revealed is whether clients are taking their medicine at all. Therapeutic blood levels are used as guidelines (Post 2007). Plasma levels for lamotrigine (Lamictal) are not available. *Blood levels* are recommended every three to six months for a year and then every six to 12 months indefinitely. Dose changes may warrant additional measurements. Therapists can oversee AEs, suggesting that their Bipolar clients get blood levels measured, and making recommendations to the prescriber to change dosages.

The *mood-stabilizing medications* are a small group of effective drugs with a high benefit-to-risk ratio, but they are not prescribed as often as their effectiveness warrants (Table 6.1). There are only five; lithium is an element, while carbamazepine (Tegretol), oxcarbazepine (Trileptal), lamotrigine (Lamictal), and valproic acid/divalproex (Depakene/ Depakote) are anti-seizure medications as well as mood stabilizers.

For moderate to severe manic and depressed clients *without psychotic features*, the current author suggests starting *three mood stabilizers at once*. The literature is clear that *lithium is the most effective antidepressant, anti-suicide* medication, and its anti-manic and mood-stabilizing properties have been documented since the 1950s. Valproic acid/divalproex (Depakene/Depakote) and carbamapezine (Tegretol) also have a long-established record of efficacy in stabilizing mood. Their side effect of sedation is useful in mania, and particularly to initiate sleep toward normalizing to a healthy sleep cycle.

Lamotrigine (Lamictal) is especially useful in depression as well as in overall mood stabilization. It has a low side-effect profile, except for a 1% chance of Stevens-Johnson Syndrome, a rash that can be brutally fatal (Fig. 6.2). In this author's experience, the incidence of rash is higher than 1%, especially in women (10%), but there have been no deaths or near deaths in his practice. Risk of rash seems to be diminished with slow titration, but this substantially prolongs reaching an effective dose and is no assurance of no rash. In order to minimize the risk of a severe rash (*Stevens-Johnson Syndrome*), a starting dose of 25 mg per day is recommended, to be increased by 25 mg every week until a daily dose of 300–400 mg a day is reached. This takes about three months, so it is not a drug to give alone in acute cases. Valproic acid/divalproex (Depakene/ Depakote) inhibits the catabolism of lamotrigine (Lamictal) and effectively doubles the plasma level, so when giving both, lower the target lamotrigine (Lamictal) daily dose to 200 mg.

Anxiety may be present in as many as 40% of Bipolar clients. *Gabapentin (Neurontin)*, an anticonvulsant also used for pain relief, can be useful in alleviating anxiety, although the anxiety associated with Bipolar generally improves with mood stabilization. *Topiramate (Topamax)*, another anti-epileptic drug, has a benefit in reducing intake and craving for alcohol and may offset weight gain stimulated by some of the mood-stabilizing medications. Both of these anticonvulsant drugs may have some mood stabilization properties in some clients.

A Bipolar Disorder can present in psychotic or nonpsychotic depression or mania, and the current pharmacological management is surprisingly similar if not identical despite the marked differences in mood and behavior (Table 6.1; Fig. 6.1). Presentations to therapists during depression are more common than during mania and frequently occur postpartum. Presumptive Unipolar Depression can be effectively medicated the same as Bipolar with mood stabilizers, *not antidepressants*, especially if some of the nonmanic Bipolar factors suggesting Bipolar depression are present (Sect. 3.5) (Table 3.11). In psychotic mania, Unipolar or Bipolar Depression, immediate short-term *use of an SGA drug is appropriate*, started simultaneously with three of the first-line mood-stabilizing medications (Fig. 6.1).

Bipolar is viewed as a neuroprogressive degenerative disorder, and there is evidence that lithium is neuroprotective, although it may cause "cognitive dulling" (Nunes et al. 2013; Gray and McEwen 2013a, b; Mauer et al. 2014; Koek 2015; Schou 1979a). Lithium is among the oldest of effective treatments (Alda 2015). The modern history of lithium in the treatment of Bipolar began in Australia with Cade's (1949) accidental discovery of the effectiveness of lithium for manic-like symptoms in rats.

6.2.2 Lithium

After nearly 70 years, the data are overwhelming that lithium is one of the most, if not *the most, effective medication for acute and prophylactic treatment of MDD and Bipolar*. To date, lithium represents the standard of long-term Bipolar treatment against which other medications are compared. Lithium is standard of care in a polypharmaceutical cocktail of three mood-stabilizing drugs in psychotic or nonpsychotic Mood Disorders, depression, or mania. Further, lithium produces a *fivefold decrease in suicide risk* compared to placebo and other active treatments (Schou 1967, 1968, 1979a, b; Wehr and Goodwin 1987; Goodwin 1989; Calabrese et al. 2001). By reducing the high medical morbidity and mortality, lithium lowers the cost of Bipolar. The potential savings are estimated at $8 billion in the US alone (Koek 2015).

Although the efficacy of lithium is unsurpassed, only about 30% of Bipolar clients are full responders. The predictors of response include a family history of

Bipolar, a classic presentation with an episodic course with remissions, low rates of comorbidity, intermediate age of onset, the absence of rapid cycling, positive social support, good compliance, employment, and a low number of life stressors. There is a wide variability in time for response to lithium from a *few days to weeks.*

One reason clients fail to respond to lithium is failure to take it. As many as *47% of Bipolar clients discontinue their lithium* on at least one occasion and 34% on two or more. Side effects of lithium, such as nausea, tremor, and weight gain, often cause client discontinuation.

When lithium is prescribed, it is reasonable to begin with 300 mg once or twice a day with food and to titrate this dosage up by 300 mg *as tolerated* over a week or two to as much as 600 mg twice a day if tolerated. At one to three months, it is appropriate to measure the level of lithium in the blood. One should not have taken a dose of lithium within eight hours of having blood drawn. Depending on the individual client's metabolism, between *600 and 1800 mg per day* may be tolerated to yield a therapeutic plasma level of between *0.6 and 1.2 meq/L* for clients younger than 60 years of age; for clients between 60 and 80, aim for serum level of 0.4–0.8 meq/L. For those aged 80 and over, the best serum level is between 0.4 and 0.7 meq/L (Shulman et al. 2019). It is reasonable for therapists to involve themselves in their clients' labs and blood levels in order to evaluate the need to discuss medication changes with clients and their prescribers. For standard of care, psychotherapists will need to know these levels.

6.2.3 Anti-seizure Mood-Stabilizing Medications

Simultaneously with lithium, valproic acid/divalproex (Depakene/Depakote) or carbamazepine (Tegretol) should be started at 250 mg or 200 mg, respectively, at bedtime. If no AEs occur and severe mania or depression continues, the dose should be increased by 250 mg or 200 mg, respectively, every two or three nights up to 500–1500 mg or 400–1600 mg per night, respectively, *as tolerated* and their *levels obtained after one to three months along with lithium levels*, a CBC, and a chemistry panel. *A thyroid screen* is also useful to rule out a hypothyroid contribution to depression (Sect. 6.5). Sedation can be a limiting factor in dose increases for both valproic acid/divalproex (Depakene/Depakote) and carbamazepine (Tegretol). Their sedative side effects make them good choices in agitated mania or mixed manic depressions with initial insomnia.

A third mood stabilizer, such as lamotrigine (Lamictal), is also recommended to be started day one, but its titration is more gradual than the other mood stabilizers because of the risk of a serious rash that usually occurs during the upward titration, especially if rapid. Warn your therapy clients to be vigilant about the danger of a rash, and document your warnings in the chart. Calabrese et al. (2001) report efficacy of lamotrigine (Lamictal) in Bipolar I even when used alone and in rapid cycling Bipolar II. Lamotrigine (Lamictal) is not advised alone because of the extended time to reach a therapeutic dose.

In severe depression, after two or three weeks of three mood-stabilizing medications at therapeutic levels without an adequate response, discuss with the client how to approach the prescriber, or if collaborative relationship is established, make the contact directly to recommend adding a low dose of an SGA. Other options are an antidepressant, a stimulant, or a fourth mood-stabilizing medication, ketamine, or ECT (Fig. 6.1). In addition to ketamine, there are additional, more recent treatments that seem to have potential for efficacy in treatment-resistant cases (Sect. 6.5). Once psychotic symptoms resolve, expect or suggest that the client request that the prescriber titrate down and discontinue the SGA (Calabrese et al. 2001; Whitaker 2004).

In clients presenting with psychotic mania or depression, an SGA drug plus three mood-stabilizing drugs are recommended by many psychopharmacologists. Disruptive, dangerous manic clients may need hospitalization and the use of four mood-stabilizing drugs. Such clients may also warrant an IM plus oral SGA, titrated up to maximum tolerated followed by the addition of a PRN IM benzodiazepine, if needed. Since upward titration can be more rapid in the inpatient setting, hospitalization in severely psychotic cases is recommended. ECT should be available for severe depression. As Dick Cavett said, "ECT is [my] game changer."

For depression, several psychopharmacologists first prescribe lithium and other mood stabilizers, even when there are no hints of a Bipolar Disorder and even if all of the points in Table 3.11 are negative and the diagnosis is a Major Depressive Disorder (MDD) or Postpartum Depressive Disorder (PPD) (Fig. 6.1). Antidepressants are not recommended for Bipolar depression or even for MDD because some data suggest the antidepressants increase cycling in Unipolar Depression as well as in Bipolar (Schou 1967, 1968, 1979b; Wehr and Goodwin 1987; Goodwin 1989; Calabrese et al. 2001). Moreover, some 50% of MDD-diagnosed clients actually have Bipolar depression, never MDD. If one or more of the items in Table 3.11 are positive, the choice of mood stabilizers, especially lithium, and the avoidance of antidepressants are supported. Valproic acid/divalproex (Depakene/Depakote) and lamotrigine (Lamictal) are also recommended in addition to lithium from the start in moderate to severe depression, Bipolar or Unipolar. Certainly there are psychopharmacologists who recommend one of the selective serotonin reuptake inhibitors (SSRI) or serotonin norepinephrine reuptake inhibitors (SNRIs) as the first drugs in presentations of depression, but the current author's read of the literature is that this strategy is counterproductive.

The benefit-to-risk ratio for ECT in the treatment of severe Major Depression is superior to that for an SGA drug, according to Swartz and Shorter (2007). *Ketamine* may be a major breakthrough in the treatment of depression, and if the current optimism holds, ketamine may become a back-up second choice in drug-resistant depression, Bipolar or Unipolar. In depressed clients, if the TSH is higher than 1.5 μIU/L, it is appropriate to supplement with *high-dose thyroid hormone* (Kelly 2018).

The mood-stabilizing drugs have been on the market for so long that all are available in generic form, are inexpensive, and not a major income source for the manufacturers. Thus, pharmaceutical companies do not invest in marketing these drugs to doctors or directly to the public in media advertisements. This lack of advertisement compared to that for the SGAs is a disservice to Bipolar clients because the mood stabilizers are more effective in long-term prevention and are also important in acute episodes.

Furthermore, the pharmaceutical industry has not developed new mood-stabilizing drugs, the class most effective in Bipolar since 2003; profit has overridden client welfare. Lamotrigine (Lamictal), the most recent mood stabilizer, was Federal Drug Administration (FDA) approved for treatment of Bipolar in 2003 and earned $1.27 billion in 2008. Now available generically, it is inexpensive. Pharmaceutical efforts have focused on other, more profitable psychiatric drug classes, the SGAs, antidepressants, and stimulants. For example, olanzapine (Zyprexa) and quetiapine (Seroquel), both antipsychotics, *earned revenues of $4.70 and $4.45 billion* in 2008 for Eli Lilly and AstraZeneca respectively.

6.2.4 Antipsychotic Medications (SGAs)

The *second-generation antipsychotics (SGAs)* have been widely recommended in the media by the pharmaceutical manufacturers and some investigators for the treatment of nonpsychotic Bipolar Disorders, especially depression. Consensus considers it critical to use SGAs simultaneously with mood stabilizers in *psychotic* Bipolar clients, either manic or depressed. The SGAs are used sparingly and primarily for psychotic symptoms by the current author, as discussed below. Some *discourage all use of SGAs* because of their AEs (Whitaker 2004).

Some of the newer "atypical" or *second-generation antipsychotics (SGAs)* are not yet available generically, expensive to purchase, a significant source of profit for their manufacturers, and heavily marketed by pharmaceutical sales representatives and on television (Tables 6.2 and 6.9). Samples are given to doctors to pass on to their clients along with data generated by drug companies about the advantages of their drugs. Some PCPs and psychiatrists are not attentive to the bias of media and drug representatives' presentations.

Aripiprazole (Abilify) and cariprazine (Vraylar) are examples of atypical SGA drugs that are FDA approved for depression and/or mania and are advertised on television. Prime-time TV advertisements are expensive and effective in selling more product, but they are misleading. In the TV ad, aripiprazole (Abilify) is said to be doctor-recommended as a first-line back-up choice to be added to an initial antidepressant to treat what is advertised as unresponsive depression. Cariprazine (Vraylar) is advertised as an effective treatment for mania and depression. The cartoon ad for aripiprazole (Abilify) implies that its addition causes the client's depression to vanish. A cartoon ad for iloperidone (Fanap) implies that the drug treats "Schizophrenia" with symptoms of hallucinations and paranoia. This ad promotes the diagnosis of "Schizophrenia" when these symptoms are instead diagnostic of a psychotic Mood Disorder. The advertisements for these SGAs are misleading and are examples of attempts by the pharmaceutical industry to influence clinical decisions by encouraging clients to ask for aripiprazole (Abilify), cariprazine (Vraylar), and iloperidone (Fanap) and doctors to prescribe them.

Table 6.2 Examples of antipsychotic medications[a]; typical vs atypical

First generation or typical				Second generation or atypical			
Generic name	Trade name	Maint/max dose (mg/day[b])	Half-life (hrs)	Generic name	Trade name	Maint/max dose (mg/day[(2)])	Half-life (hrs)
Chlorpromazine	Thorazine	200–600/2000	20–40	Aripiprazole	Abilify	10–20/30	75–146
Chlorprothixene	Taractan	50–400/600	8–12	Clozapine	Clozaril	300–450/900	6–26
Fluphenazine decanoate	Prolixin Decanoate	12.5–50 IM every 1–4 weeks	4–9 days	Iloperidone	Fanapt	12–24/24	16–31
Haloperidol	Haldol	1–30/30	20	Lurasidone	Latuda	40–80/160	20–40
Haloperidol decanoate	Haldol Decanoate	25–250 IM every 2–4 weeks	21 days	Olanzapine	Zyprexa	10–20/20	32–52
Loxapine	Loxitane	60–100/250	4–12	Paliperidone	Invega	3–12/12	23
Perphenazine	Trilafon	16–32/64	8–20	Quetiapine	Seroquel	300–800/800	7–12
Pimozide (for Tourette's)	Orap	2–4/10	55	Risperidone	Risperdal	2–8/16	2–4
Thioridazine	Mellaril	200–800/800	5–26	Risperidone depot	Risperdal depot	25 IM every 2 weeks	4–6 days
Thiothixene	Navane	20–30/60	10–20	Ziprasidone	Geodon	40–60/200	7
Trifluoperazine	Stelazine	15–20/40	22	Asenapine	Saphris	10–20/20	24
				Brexpiprazole	Rexulti	2/3	91
				Cariprazine	Vraylar	1.5–6/6	2–7

[a]Note: Most recent data suggest that the benefit-to-risk ratio is unacceptable in moderate to long-term use, i.e., over four weeks and that there are no appreciable differences in AEs between the typical versus the atypical antipsychotic drugs (Whitaker 2004; Zarate Jr and Tohen 2004; Tyler and Kendall 2009)

[b]These dosages are broad estimates

One significant flaw to such advertisements is the incorrect assumption that an antidepressant should be used first in Mood Disorders with depression. Moreover, the side effect profile of the SGAs is not adequately explained. Although some of the SGAs have won FDA approval for treating mania and depression, they are not second- or even third-line choices in nonpsychotic clients. These drugs are designed and developed to treat psychotic symptoms and are effective in acutely psychotic mania and depression, but their long-term mood-stabilizing effects are not adequately tested when compared to the long-term trials conducted over multi-decades of the first-line mood stabilizers, especially lithium, valproic acid/divalproex (Depakene/Depakote), and carbamazepine (Tegretol). An SGA can be therapeutic in nonpsychotic Bipolar clients resistant to three mood stabilizers. Any pharmacologic treatment plan is subject to failure because of poor compliance.

The seriously mentally ill are often not compliant with medications, so some psychiatrists use weekly or monthly IM SGAs in these circumstances. Such chronic administration of IM SGAs is not advised, with very few, if any, exceptions because of the SGA AE profile (Tables 6.7 and 6.8). Weekly psychotherapy can usually eliminate the need for IM SGAs.

6.2.5 Antidepressant Medications

The *antidepressants* have a long history in the treatment of depression. This group of drugs is large like the SGAs; over five times as many antidepressant and antipsychotic drugs have been developed and marketed compared to mood-stabilizing drugs. Like the antipsychotics, the antidepressants have been profitable so pharma has invested in developing more of them compared to the mood stabilizers (Table 6.3).

At one time, antidepressants were prescribed widely for any type of depression and anxiety. It is true that Bipolar depressed clients and those with MDD or PPD all have the same neurovegetative symptoms, but more recently, this widespread use of antidepressants has been restricted based on the drugs' propensity to switch clients from depression into mania (Aiken 2017c). The antidepressants given alone to Bipolar depressed clients can cause 10% to switch to mania and thus increase the rate of cycling, making the condition worse (Carlson and Goodwin 1973; Wehr and Goodwin 1987; Goodwin 1989). Other data suggest the antidepressants also *increase the rate of cycling of depressive episodes* in recurrent MDD (Goodwin 1989; Prien et al. 1984). The recognition of the spectrum versus the established all-or-none concept of Bipolar and Unipolar has further reduced the advisability of using antidepressants (Table 3.11). Some now rarely, if ever, prescribe them.

The rate of switching is greater in youths than in adults. A switch to mania increases the risk for violence, homicide, and suicide (Chap. 4). Since data suggest that as many as 50% of clients initially diagnosed with MDD actually have Bipolar Disorder, many psychiatrists now recommend using lithium and other mood stabilizers, avoiding antidepressants. Data suggest lithium is as effective in Unipolar depression as in Bipolar depression (Carlson and Goodwin 1973; Wehr and Goodwin 1987; Schou 1979a, b; Goodwin 1989; Goodwin and Jamison 1990, 2007; Calabrese et al. 2001).

The nonmanic Bipolar factors encourage the diagnosis of Bipolar depression in depressed clients and the use of mood-stabilizing drugs without antidepressant drugs (Phelps 2018a, b). An argument can be made for the use of an SSRI or an SNRI in severe depression, Unipolar or even Bipolar, when the client is resistant to three mood-stabilizing drugs and an SGA, all at once and at therapeutic levels or doses. *ECT and ketamine are alternatives or actually preferred* treatments (Sect. 6.5).

Table 6.3 Examples of antidepressant medications

First generation				Second generation			
Name			Dosage	Name			Dosage
generic	Trade/brand	Class	maint/max/(mg) day[a]	generic	Trade/brand	Class	maint/max/(mg) day
Phenelzine	Nardil	MAO-I[b]	15–30/90	Fluoxetine	Prozac, Sarafem, Symbyax	SSRI[c] (the first)	40–60/120
Tranylcypromine	Parnate	MAO-I	20–30/40	Sertraline	Zoloft	SSRI	25–200/200
Selegiline (patch)	Emsam	MAO-I	6 mg/day patch	Citalopram	Celexa	SSRI	20–40/40
Amitriptyline	Elavil, Endep	TCA[d]	50–150/300	Fluvoxanime	Luvox	SSRI	100–300/300
Imipramine	Tofranil	TCA	50–200/300	Escitalopram	Lexapro	SSRI	10–20/40
Nortriptyline	Aventyl, Pamelor	TCA	75–100/150	Paroxetine	Paxil, Pexeva	SNRI[e]	10–50/60
Clomipramine	Anafranil	TCA	25–100/250	Venlafaxine (IR)[f]	Effexor	SNRI	75–375/375
Protriptyline	Vivactil	TCA	15–40/60	Venlafaxine (ER, XR)[g]	Effexor	SNRI	75–225/225
Desipramine	Norpramin	TCA	75–200/300	Duloxetine	Cymbalta	SNRI	40–60/120
Amoxapine	Asendin	TCA	200–300/600	Bupropion	Wellbutrin	dopaminergic	300–450/450
Doxepin	Sinquan, Sinequan	TCA	75–150/300	Desvenlafaxine	Pristiq	SNRI	50–200/400
Mirtazapine	Remeron	Tetra-cyclic	15–45/45				
Trazodone	Desyrel	non-TCA SARI[h]	150–200/1,000				

[a]These dosages are broad estimates
[b]Monoamine Oxidase Inhibitor
[c]Serotonin Specific Reuptake Inhibitor
[d]Trycyclic Antidepressant
[e]Serotonin Norepinephrine Reuptake Inhibitor
[f]Immediate Release
[g]Extended Release
[h]Serotonin Antagonist and Reuptake Inhibitor

6.2.6 Benzodiazepines (BZDs)

The *benzodiazepines (BZDs)* are a very useful class of drugs. They replaced the dangerous barbiturate drug class typified by phenobarbital. The therapeutic index (TI) of the BZDs is very safe compared to the barbiturates, lithium, and the SGAs. The BZDs are also referred to as the *antianxiety class of drugs* as they are the short-term treatment of choice for Generalized Anxiety, Social Anxiety, and Panic Disorders. They are used for other conditions, both psychiatric and medical, such as PTSD, acute muscle cramps, alcohol withdrawal, seizures, and for inducing sedation. Some of the BZDs are available in injection form (IM) and are extremely valuable in acutely psychotic, agitated, and threatening manic clients. They can be given in addition to an IM SGA. Although the BZDs are therapeutic, they should be used daily only short-term, for days to weeks, because they produce tolerance and are highly addictive. They are best given only when needed and only *three or four times a week* rather than daily. Examples of BZDs are Chlordiazepoxide (Librium), flurazepam (Dalmane), clorazepate (Tranxene), *alprazolam (Xanax), clonazepam (Klonopin), lorazepam (Ativan), and temazepam (Restoril). Triazolam (Halcion)* is a short half-life BZD, most commonly used to treat insomnia. New, non-BZD analog drugs with ultra-short half-lives of less than six hours include *zolpidem (Ambien), eszopiclone (Lunesta), and zaleplon (Sonata)* and are designed for sleep. The FDA has recently approved a sublingual preparation of zolpidem (Ambien) called Intermezzo that aims to manage middle-of-the-night awakenings accompanied by difficulty falling back to sleep (Table 6.4).

The BZDs are useful in Bipolar in only a few circumstances. Severe, acute, agitated mania with or without psychosis warrants sedation usually with the combination of an SGA and a BZD. Intramuscular preparations of both SGAs and BZDs are available. In addition, since the regulation of sleep is a major issue in Bipolar (Sect. 2.5), the BZDs can help in reestablishing a regular sleep pattern. The BZDs, which have no mood-stabilizing effects, can be life-saving in agitated, acutely suicidal clients. However, the sedative mood stabilizers do not produce tolerance and do have potent mood-stabilizing effects.

6.2.7 Stimulants

The *stimulants* are almost never warranted for use in Bipolar. The rare exception would be an extremely depressed client who has not responded to the simultaneous administration of at least three mood-stabilizing medications and one SGA. In such a case, a stimulant could be added short term before going to ECT (Table 6.5). Psychotherapists can be prepared to recommend ECT to such severe clients and their prescribers.

Table 6.4 Examples of benzodiazepine medications

Name				
Generic // trade	Average/max dosage (mg/day)[a]	Onset of action (min)	Peak onset (hrs)	Duration of action (hrs)
Chlordiazepoxide // Librium	5–75/100	15–30	2–4	24–48
Diazepam // Valium	5–50/50	15	1	20–50
Alprazolam // Xanax	0.25–4/4	15–30	0.7–1.6	6–20
Clonazepam // Klonopin	0.5–3/20	15–30	1–4	18–39
Lorazepam // Ativan, Temesta	0.5–4/4	15–30	1–1.5	10–20
Temazepam // Normison, Restoril	7.5–30/30	30–60	0.75–1.5	10–20
Triazolam // Halcion	0.125–12.5/12.5	15–30	0.75–2	1.6–5.5
Clorazepate // Tranxene	10–50/100	Variable	Variable	32–152
Oxazepam // Serax	10–120/120	30–60	2–3	3–21
Flurazepam // Dalmane	15–30/30	15	0.5–2	4–6

[a]These dosages are broad estimates; often taken in divided dosages

Table 6.5 Examples of stimulant medications

Name		
Generic // trade	Average dosage (mg/day[a])	Duration of action (hrs)
Amphetamine sulfate // Evekeo; Dyanavel	5–40/40	6–12
Dextroamphetamine // Dexedrine Spansule	5–60/60	6–8
Dextroamphetamine and amphetamine // Adderall XR[b]; Mydayis	5–60/60	8–12
Dexmethylphenidate ER[c] // Focalin XR	10–40/40	6–10
Lisdexamfetamine // Vyvanse	50–70/70	10–12
Methylphenidate // Ritalin LA[d]; Ritalin SR[e]	18–36/36	4–12
Methylphenidate // Concerta	18–36/36	8–10
Modafinil // Provigil	100–200/200	8

[a]These dosages are broad estimates
[b]XR - extended release
[c]ER - extended release
[d]LA - long acting
[e]SR - sustained release

Another relationship of the stimulants to Bipolar involves misdiagnosed ADHD in unrecognized Bipolar clients (Sects. 2.7 and 3.6). When seeing a new client who is taking a stimulant prescribed for their ADHD diagnosis, a critical reevaluation of the diagnosis is appropriate (Sects. 2.7 and 3.6). After discussion of the issue with the ADHD misdiagnosed client, the prescriber must be contacted and the appropriate changes recommended. A change in prescriber may be warranted.

As with the BZDs, tolerance occurs rapidly and withdrawal is troublesome. The most commonly prescribed *stimulants for ADHD are dextroamphetamine/amphetamine (Adderall), methylphenidate (Concerta, Ritalin, and Methylin), dextroamphetamine (Dexedrine, Mydayis)*, *atomoxetine* (*Stratera*), *lisdexamfetamine (Vivanse)*, and *modafinil (Provigil)*. When the diagnosis is more likely Bipolar, not ADHD, the stimulants must be tapered and discontinued while the mood stabilizers are added simultaneously and titrated up to effective therapeutic doses.

Although strikingly different in symptom presentation, mania and depression, both Bipolar and Unipolar, are most effectively treated with the same drugs: three mood stabilizers plus an SGA in cases of psychosis or a two-month response resistance to the three mood stabilizers. An antidepressant and/or a stimulant can be a fifth add-on to three mood stabilizers and an SGA in resistant depressions before going to ECT. The stimulant will show benefits within a day; an antidepressant could take weeks.

6.3 Adverse Effects (AEs) of the Medications

Compliance with their medications is a major goal of the psychotherapy that will directly benefit clients (Sect. 6.4). Clients are at risk of stopping their medications when they incur adverse effects (AEs). Therapists' knowledge about the Bipolar medications and their side effects forms a critical part of the psychoeducation therapy that can support compliance. Substantial therapy time is well spent discussing medications and their AEs.

6.3.1 Lithium AEs

Lithium and the four anti-epileptic mood stabilizers have significant AEs (Table 6.6). All associate with some weight gain.

At therapeutic levels, lithium may be associated with *thirst*, *polydipsia*, a *fine tremor* typically observed in the hands and fingers, a metallic taste, *weight gain*, anorexia, *acne*, and *nausea*. Nausea should be countered by taking lithium with food, in divided dosages, with dinner, and in the extended-release preparation. Clients should be asked about their AEs at each session. When these AEs are mild, clients are encouraged to tolerate them; if the AEs worsen to the extent that clients are distressed, suggest clients contact the prescriber to reduce the dose a minimal amount to attain the highest dose tolerated by a client. Clients must realize that they have the best chance to avoid another episode when they have the highest circulating blood level that they can tolerate.

At toxic levels, most of the AEs listed above worsen and confusion, gait instability, seizures, coma, and death are possible. Note that if the person who achieves a therapeutic plasma level of lithium on 600 mg per day takes more than triple this amount, they are likely to become toxic and possibly need hospitalization. The *therapeutic index (TI) for lithium is low at three*. This means that the *toxic dose is only three times the therapeutic dose*. If in an overdose toxic levels are surpassed, treatment is available since lithium is *dialyzable* out of the body.

Table 6.6 Examples of adverse effects of the first-line mood-stabilizing medications

Medication name	Common, mild to moderate side effects	Rare, severe to life-threatening side effects or with OD	Comments
Lithium	Thirst; frequent urination; fine tremor in the hands; dehydration; mild nausea; headache; weight gain; symptoms of hypothyroidism; metallic taste; acne	Renal diabetes insipidus due to renal impairment; coarse tremor; irregular heartbeat; visual changes; rash; swelling of the eyes, face, lips, tongue, throat, hands, feet, ankles or lower legs; ataxia; dysarthria; nystagmus; confusion; seizures; coma; death	Lithium inhibits anti-diuretic hormone, thereby inhibiting the ability of the kidney to reabsorb water from the urine, i.e., an inability to concentrate urine leading to loss of body water and thirst. Thiazide diuretics are contra-indicated with lithium. Must monitor plasma lithium levels and thyroid and kidney function on a regular basis. Lithium is a teratogen causing birth defects. Lithium inhibits thyroid hormone causing symptoms of hypothyroidism
Anti-seizure mood-stabilizing medications (carbamazepine, valproic acid, lamotragine, oxcarbazepine)	Sedation; dizziness; decreased coordination; nausea; headaches; double vision; insomnia; anxiety; vivid dreams; missed or painful menstrual periods; cough; dry mouth; constipation; diarrhea; weight gain; hair loss (valproic acid)	Cardiac arrhythmias; aplastic anemia; agranulocytosis; syndrome of inappropriate anti-diuretic hormone (carbamazepine); cognitive anomalies; rash in the form of *Stevens-Johnson syndrome* or toxic epidermal necrolysis (*especially lamotragine*); vomiting; fever; dark urine; jaundice; liver damage; blood in the urine; hallucinations; drug eruptions; drug reaction with eosinophylia and systemic symptoms (DRESS syndrome) (especially lamotragine); seizures, coma and death possible in overdose	Carbamazepine (Tegretol) is a CYP450 inducer increasing clearance (decreasing blood level and effectiveness) of warfarin (Coumadin), phenytoin (Dilantin), theophylline and valproic acid (Depakote). Drugs increasing the level of carbamazepine include erythromycin, cimetidine (Tagamet), propoxyphene (Darvon) and calcium channel blockers. Valproic acid inhibits the catabolism of carbamazepine and lamotragine and increases their activity. Lamotragine (Lamictal) has relatively few side effects but does rarely cause a potentially fatal rash called Stephens-Johnson syndrome. Blood monitoring is not avalible. Valproic acid and carbamazepine do require blood level and liver function monitoring

Lithium is excreted by the kidneys and must be used with care in clients with impaired renal function, in those taking diuretics, and those over 60 years old. Long-term use can adversely affect kidney and thyroid function (Table 6.6). Chronic lithium use over years to decades can impair urinary concentrating capacity, causing nephrogenic diabetes insipidus and nephropathy. Lithium-induced *nephrogenic diabetes insipidus* is usually self-limiting and not clinically dangerous. Renal impairment can be estimated by following glomerular filtration rate (GFR) and *creatinine levels greater than 1.5 mg/dL* and at worst can progress to dialysis and kidney transplantation. Nephropathy generally occurs only after decades of maintenance exposure. Most recommend using a lower lithium-plasma target for long-term maintenance in order to reduce the risk of nephrotoxicity. Some clients with severe Bipolar may require continuation of their lithium treatment despite increases in creatinine (Azab et al. 2015). There are cases of clients who value their lithium so much that they are willing to undergo dialysis and a renal transplant in order to keep using it.

Lithium impacts *thyroid function* more commonly than the other mood stabilizers. Lithium maintenance causes *hypothyroidism in 30% of Bipolar clients* and as many as 50% of these have goiters detectable by ultrasonography compared to 20% of non-Bipolars. *Women* are at higher risk for *hypothyroidism*. Hypothyroidism is not a contraindication to lithium. Some recommend monitoring thyroid-stimulating hormone (TSH) every three months during the first six to 12 months of lithium therapy and *every six to 12 months indefinitely*. Also recommended is *lowering of the cut-off for high TSH from 5 to between 1 and 2 μIU/mL* or even less. Consider hypothyroidism-induced depression in Bipolar clients maintained on lithium as hypothyroidism is a common cause of organic or secondary depression. Lithium can also induce hyperthyroidism that can present as mania. A TSH of 2 or more requires thyroid replacement which is a benign process and can reverse depression. Psychiatrists, PCPs, and nurse practitioners can manage low thyroid function with high-dose supplemental levothyroxine (Sect. 6.5).

Lithium can cause *hypercalcemia and hyperparathyroidism* by its direct effect on parathyroid calcium sensitivity. One study reports 8.6% of lithium-maintained Bipolar clients have hyperparathyroidism. *Check calcium levels* on clients' chemistry panels. This AE can include benign parathyroid adenomas.

Lithium is in the FDA Category D regarding safety in pregnancy because of the Epstein and other cardiovascular anomalies in the fetus associated with first trimester exposure. There is a *20% greater risk of complications during pregnancy* in women maintaining their lithium. Lithium poses a risk to breast feeding as it is in *high concentrations in breast milk*.

There is a *risk of relapse to depression or mania upon discontinuation of lithium* including after long-term remission. Even a gradual discontinuation of lithium can cause recurrence of mania or depression and an increased risk for suicidality. Abrupt, as compared to gradual, *discontinuation substantially increases relapse and suicide risk. After discontinuation of lithium, some clients are refractory to its benefits when restarting it* (Post 2012).

6.3.2 *Anti-seizure Mood-Stabilizing Drug AEs*

Although the list of adverse reactions of the *anti-seizure mood stabilizers* is long, lethal side effects are rare. All are metabolized in the liver, have drug-drug interactions, and must be used with care in clients with impaired liver function. Nonlethal adverse effects of the anti-epileptic mood stabilizers include sedation, hair loss, weight gain, nausea, dizziness, headache, and occasional activation with lamotrigine (Lamictal). See Table 6.6 for additional AEs. Clinical experience with the mood-stabilizing drugs is extensive over the past 50 years with the exception of lamotrigine (Lamictal) that has been in use for just over a decade.

Lamotrigine (Lamictal) can cause a fatal rash called *Stevens-Johnson Syndrome* in about 1% of recipients. This author finds a higher percentage, possibly as high as a 10% incidence in women, despite a slow upward titration. None of his clients required hospitalization as the rashes were caught early, the drug was stopped, and the rash resolved over days to a week. The rash usually occurs when titrating the dose upward (Fig. 6.2).

The anti-seizure mood-stabilizing drugs can suppress bone marrow production of blood cells leading to *aplastic anemia* and especially *agranulocytosis*, a reduction in white blood cells, which predisposes to infections and possible death. At toxic levels, seizures, coma, and death are possible. All of these are rare.

Carbamazepine (Tegretol) has several pharmacokinetic interactions because it induces cytochrome P-450 3A4 especially in the liver. Estrogen levels such as with birth control pills are lowered by carbamazepine (Tegretol), so birth control medication is less effective. Erythromycin and calcium channel blockers markedly increase carbamazepine (Tegretol) levels. Oxcarbazepine (Trileptal) is considerably less potent as an enzyme inducer than carbamazepine (Tegretol), so there is less risk for hematological toxicity but it can cause hyponatremia (low sodium levels).

Decreased cognitive function is both a feature in Bipolar Disorders, especially depression, and a potential side effect of drugs that treat Bipolar; thus, it is important to inform clients of this phenomenon of depression so that medications are not blamed and discontinued. Cognitive function may not recover as quickly as mood symptoms resolve during treatment (Goodwin and Jamison 2007; Aiken 2017a). Techniques to address this issue are recommended during psychotherapy. Mood-stabilizing and SGA medications can also impair cognitive function depending on dosages. The most likely offending drug should be titrated down slowly. Elicit the client's help in judging the source of the cognitive impairment. Use of the 6CIT may be helpful (Sect. 5.4).

Lithium and lamotrigine (Lamictal) may improve some areas of cognition. Some evidence indicates that the reputation of lithium's poor cognitive profile is inaccurate. One study finds no clear evidence of lithium's having a negative cognitive impact and another study suggests that *lithium improves verbal fluency* (Nunes et al. 2013). Impaired cognition in clients taking lithium could be due to depression or subclinical hypothyroidism. In any case, cognitive side effects are generally worse from the anti-epileptic mood stabilizers and the SGAs than from lithium. The goal in psychotherapy is to educate clients about these issues and to emphasize the lifestyle changes recommended below (Aiken 2017a, b).

6.3.3 Antipsychotic Drug AEs

The second-generation antipsychotic drugs (SGAs) are widely advertised for the treatment of Bipolar and Major Depression. They have a poor benefit-to-risk ratio compared to any of the other drug classes used in the treatment of Bipolar (Whitaker 2004; Lake 2021). SGAs are prescribed in larger, usually escalating dosages over the lifetime of clients misdiagnosed with "Schizophrenia." One reason has been the universal misunderstanding that for "Schizophrenia," the SGAs are necessary for life in order to prevent psychotic relapse. With compliance, the SGAs do acutely reduce hallucinations and delusions, but "… they [the SGAs] have not enhanced functional recovery (for example, employment)…" (Insel 2010). Across Europe, less than 20% of clients treated chronically with SGAs are employed. Sustained recovery of only about 15% is recorded by two groups of researchers. Other studies report nearly 20% of such clients were homeless at one-year follow-up and had a high rate of incarceration (Insel 2010). These outcomes may be iatrogenic, caused by the AEs of the SGAs prescribed long-term (Table 6.7).

If these data derive from Mood-Disordered clients misdiagnosed with "Schizophrenia," it is possible that these dismal statistics might improve with the correct diagnosis, the addition of mood-stabilizing medications long-term, and only temporary use of the SGA drugs.

Data reviewed by Whitaker (2004) suggest that the SGA drugs "…*worsen long-term outcomes*…and that 40% or more of all … patients [treated with SGAs] would fare better if they were not so medicated…The preponderance of evidence shows that the current standard of care – continual medication therapy [with SGA drugs] for all patients … does more harm than good…The real-world *first-year relapse rate for clients maintained on neuroleptics [SGAs] is understood to be 40%*."

Manic clients maintained on SGA drugs "… were more likely to have a shorter time to depressive relapse, discontinue the study, and have increased rates of dysphoria, depressive symptoms, and extrapyramidal symptoms. … There were no short-term benefits with the continued use of atypical antipsychotics [SGAs] after achieving remission from an episode of acute mania. In fact, its *[SGA] continued use was associated with detrimental effects*" (Zarate Jr and Tohen 2004). According to some, the SGA medications themselves prevent full remissions or may cause relapses into psychotic episodes as seen in *tardive psychosis*, which occurs months to years after taking an SGA (Swartz 1995; Whitaker 2004).

Severe AEs of the SGA medications involve disfiguring movement disorders as well as other life-threatening reactions (Tables 6.7 and 6.8) . Symptoms of tardive dyskinesia can last for years; these are highly disfiguring and life-altering, often leading to the loss of employment and dysfunction. Another name for tardive dyskinesia is the *bucco-facial-lingual syndrome* because the abnormal movements involve repetitive lip pursing, facial grimacing, and tongue protrusions on a fairly constant waking basis, worsened by anxiety (Table 6.8). Tardive dyskinesia has been difficult to treat. The treatment of choice is to discontinue the SGA, not to add another drug to try to counter the symptoms.

Table 6.7 Examples of adverse effects of antipsychotic medications

Common, mild to moderate side effects	Rare, severe to life-threatening side effects	Comments
Sedation; slurred speech; dry mouth; diarrhea; glucose intolerance; rash; skin pigmentations especially in regions exposed to sunlight; hyperprolactinemia leading to breast swelling or discharge and amenorrhea, ovarian cycle dysfunction, loss of libido, hirsutism, false positive pregnancy tests, risk of osteoporosis in women, in men, impotence and loss of libido; contact dermatitis; decreased night vision, tunnel vision, increased sensitivity to light; akathisia (restlessness); dry mouth; dizziness; irritability; insomnia; constipation; urinary retention; fatigue; orthostatic hypotension; increased appetite and weight gain [ziprasidone (Geodon) may cause less weight gain]; missed periods; apathy; lack of emotion; hyperglycemia and diabetes mellitus; brain zaps; dental problems and discoloration of teeth; impaired erectile function; increased salivation; lowered seizure threshold; stuffy nose; movement disorders (Table 6.8)	Tardive dyskinesia; tardive psychosis; neuroleptic malignant syndrome; acute dystonic reaction; metabolic syndrome with substantial weight gain and diabetes mellitus; risk of death in elderly patients with dementia-related psychosis; torsades de pointes and other arrhythmias; severe Parkinson's syndrome; stroke; allergic reaction with swelling in the mouth and throat, itching and rash; liver damage; inflammation of the pancreas; body temperature dysregulation; aplastic anemia; agranulocytosis; cognitive and motor impairment; priapism; ocular tissue deposits; blindness in overdose, seizures, coma, and death	About 20 million people world-wide have taken olanzapine (Zyprexa). Quetiapine (Seroquel) had annual world-wide sales of $5.7 billion and $2.9 billion in the U.S. Eli Lilly, maker of olanzapine (Zyprexa), agreed to pay up to $1.2 billion to settle lawsuits from people who claim they developed diabetes or other injuries. Pfizer makes ziprasidone (Geodon) and pleaded guilty to misbranding "with the intent to fraud or mislead" agreeing to pay $2.3 billion in settlement for promotion of its drug for use in conditions that have not been approved by the FDA. Several of these atypical anti-schizophrenic drugs have received FDA approval for use in psychotic Mood Disorders

Note: Most recent data suggest that the benefit-to-risk ratio is unacceptable in moderate to long-term use, i.e., over four weeks and that there are no appreciable differences in AEs between the typical versus the atypical antipsychotic drugs (Whitaker 2004; Zarate Jr and Tohen 2004; Tyler and Kendall 2009)

Table 6.8 Movement disorders caused by the antipsychotic medications

Movement disorder	Time to onset of symptoms[a]	Symptoms of movement disorder	Treatment
Akathisia	Hours to days	Restlessness; inability to sit still; agitation	Benzodiazepines; discontinue SGAs STAT
Acute dystonic reaction (ADR)	Minutes to days; 50% within two days; 90% within five days	Sudden onset of frightening, painful muscle cramps; dramatic presentation sometimes confused with a seizure or stroke; muscles affected are neck, face and eyes; torticollis with neck twisted or head drawn back and fixed to one side; oculogyric crisis causes the eyes to be turned upward and/or to one side	Discontinue SGAs STAT; STAT IV push of diphenhydramine (Benadryl), 25-50mgs or benztropine mesylate (Cogentin) 1–2 mg PO/IM/IV; prophylactic anticholinergic agent such as benztropine mesylate (Cogentin) recommended for first five days (Boyer et al. 1987)
Parkinson's syndrome	Days to a few weeks	Rigidity; instability; resting tremor; shuffling gait; masked facies; urinary retention; depression	Discontinue SGAs STAT; anticholinergic and/or dopaminergic agents
Tardive dyskinesia (TD)	Months to years	Bucco-facial-lingual syndrome with repetitive lip pursing, grimacing and tongue protrusions	Discontinue SGAs STAT, despite ads of other drugs to treat
Neuroleptic malignant syndrome	Weeks	Life-threatening neurological side effect of the SGAs presenting with high fever, sweating, unstable blood pressure and heart rate, muscular rigidity, autonomic dysfunction, stupor, coma, and death	Discontinue SGAs STAT

[a]Approximate time from starting a course of an antipsychotic drug

The other SGA-induced movement disorders are also disfiguring, disturbing, and life-altering. *Akathisia* can begin within a few hours to days of starting an SGA drug. This movement disorder is described as a very uncomfortable sensation of an inability to sit still or relax. Clients are driven into nongoal-directed movement and agitation. At least one client described the sensation as having "ants in my pants." The benzodiazepine class of anti-anxiety drugs, such as alprazolam (Xanax) and clonazepam (Klonopin), can give partial relief but produce tolerance and sedation. Akathisia usually goes away within days to a week or two after discontinuing the SGA. The challenge is the recognition of akathisia as an SGA side effect rather than an individual client's idiosyncratic or worsening psychotic behavior.

Acute dystonic reactions are acute in onset, dramatic, painful, frightening, and due to muscle contractures typically in muscles of the neck, face, and eyes, called *torticollis* and *oculogyric crisis*. These movements involve locking of the head at an angle because of twisting of the neck, facial muscle spasms, and a fixed upward gaze of the eyes. Onset typically occurs within a few hours to days of beginning a course of an SGA drug. An SGA drug-induced acute dystonic reaction is considered a *medical emergency* and in the ED warrants a *STAT IV push of diphenhydramine (Benadryl), 25–50 mg*. Prophylactic anticholinergic drugs, for example, benztropine (Cogentin) have been recommended in parallel with starting an antipsychotic drug, especially in younger, muscular male clients (Boyer et al. 1987). The addition of such drugs adds to the side effect profile of the treatment. The correct treatment is the discontinuation of the SGA.

SGA drug-induced Parkinsonian movements can begin within days to weeks of starting the drug (Table 6.8). These abnormal and disfiguring movements are basically the same as those seen in idiopathic Parkinson's disease. They include loss of balance, a shuffling gait, propensity to fall, limb rigidity, a resting tremor, masked face, and flat affect (an inability to show emotions in the facial muscles). *Depression is likely*. These side effects usually resolve within weeks of discontinuing the SGA drug, but, as with akathisia, other drugs, in this case, the anticholinergic drugs, have often been added to try to counter these Parkinsonian side effects in order to continue the SGA drug. These added anticholinergic drugs have adverse effects of their own, and the SGA should be discontinued. In some cases, the drug-induced Parkinson's syndrome does not resolve after discontinuing the offending SGA drug (Jimenez-Jimenez et al. 1997).

Other adverse effects of the antipsychotic medications are considered by severity and frequency, shown in Table 6.7. Life-threatening but rare effects include sudden cardiac death, bone marrow suppression with aplastic anemia or agranulocytosis, *Neuroleptic Malignant Syndrome (NMS)* and *Serotonin Syndrome*. Common but generally nonlife-threatening, adverse effects are *sedation*, often severe; *weight gain*, often substantial; nausea; constipation or diarrhea; dizziness upon standing (orthostatic hypotension [OH]); fainting; blurred vision; rapid heartbeat; sensitivity to the sun; cognitive dulling, and others (Table 6.7). Abnormal shifts in sleep patterns with extreme fatigue and weakness can occur. The fatigue can cause avolition, amotivation, dysfunctionality, and a stuporous state.

The SGAs seem to cause depression in some cases. Sexual side effects include a reduction in sexual interest, impaired sexual performance, with failure to ejaculate in males and abnormal menstrual cycles and infertility in females. Both sexes are subject to *breast enlargement* and lactation. Since 2003 the FDA has required all manufacturers of the SGAs to include a warning about the risks of hyperglycemia, hyperlipidemia, and diabetes. This common group of side effects includes *substantial weight gain and diabetes*, which have been called the *metabolic syndrome*. One reference cited the prevalence of the metabolic syndrome in clients treated with the SGA drugs to be about *40%* (McEvoy et al. 2005). McIntyre et al. (2012) calls the SGA weight gain a "deal breaker" for their use. Obesity in Bipolar "increases the risk of depression and…reduces the likelihood of…recovery from a manic episode." McIntyre states that SGA weight gain is a "brain hazard…because it may also change the underlying brain structure and function." The newer SGAs cause all of the AEs of the older typicals including the life-threatening NMS and serotonin syndrome.

The term "atypical antipsychotics" or SGAs is criticized as a marketing strategy, and any substantial differences from the typicals are questioned. Tyler and Kendall (2009) state that "… the second-generation drugs *[SGAs] have no special atypical characteristics that separate them from the typical*, or first-generation, antipsychotics. As a group they are no more efficacious, do not improve specific symptoms, *have no clearly different side-effect profiles* than the first-generation antipsychotics, and are less cost effective. The spurious invention of the atypicals can now be regarded as invention only, cleverly *manipulated by the drug industry for marketing purposes* and only now being exposed."

6.3.4 Antidepressant Adverse Effects (AEs)

Overall, the AEs of the antidepressants as a class are minimal compared to those of the SGAs. The therapeutic index (TI), which measures the effective dose relative to the toxic dose, is much safer as compared to the TI of lithium at three. The concern for antidepressants is not primarily about an initial antidepressant-induced switch to mania or hypomania but the danger that the switch associates with the *kindling-induced onset of rapid cycling and mixed features*. The course of the disease may be worsened. Some argue that an antidepressant is more acceptable in Bipolar II depression, but the danger here is a switch to Bipolar I. Ninety-four per cent of psychiatrists are concerned about prescribing antidepressants alone to Bipolar II depressed clients; 56% feel antidepressants can be helpful only with mood stabilizers; 39% generally avoid antidepressants in Bipolar Disorders. Although switches into hypomania from depression are desired by clients, this hypomania likely leads to more depressive episodes, mixed states, emotional instability, and "painful life consequences" (Aiken 2019).

The other AEs of the antidepressants depend upon which neurotransmitter system is most affected, norepinephrine, serotonin, or dopamine. The SSRI and SNRI antidepressants are thought to have their effects by blocking the reuptake inactivation of these neurotransmitters at their pre- and post-synaptic membranes. This enhances the effective half-lives of these neurotransmitters, giving them longer access to and increased activation of their pre- and postsynaptic receptors, magnifying their physiological effects.

There are other classes of antidepressants. Use of the *monoamine oxidase inhibitors (MAOIs)* began in the 1950s, and *they are effective*. These drugs gain their antidepressant effects by inhibiting monoamine oxidase, an enzyme that breaks down and inactivates the monoamine neurotransmitters noted above. Although effective, the MAOIs are less used today because of early dietary restrictions. More recent findings show that the diet initially required eliminating tyramine-containing foods because of the fear of a hypertensive crisis. That diet was overly strict. Examples of such foods include aged cheeses and meats, beer and wine, smoked fish, and other aged foods.

The two most common MAOIs are *tranylcypromine (Parnate) and phenelzine (Nardil)*. A transdermal delivery system called *selegiline (Ensam)* is reported to have fewer side effects. Meperidine (Demerol) is dangerous when used in combination with an MAOI; the SSRIs and SNRIs are also contraindicated with the MAOIs because of the danger of a serotonin syndrome episode.

The *tricyclic antidepressants (TCAs)* were also developed in the 1950s when an antipsychotic drug prototype was found to have antidepressant properties. For the names of MAOIs and TCAs, see Table 6.3. The TCAs are effective antidepressants, but their side effect profile is substantial. Like the antipsychotic drugs from which they were derived, they cause the anticholinergic AEs of dry mouth, constipation, urinary retention, blurred vision, and confusion and in overdose, seizures, coma, and possibly death. Orthostatic hypotension (OH), sedation, dizziness, fainting, tachycardia, *weight gain*, and *sexual dysfunction* are common.

The first *Selective Serotonin Reuptake Inhibitor (SSRI)*, *fluoxetine (Prozac)*, was released in 1988 and considered a miracle drug at the time. In two years, it was the number one prescribed drug in the United States. Its financial success prompted the pharmaceutical industry to focus considerable efforts at developing additional drugs in this class. The two most profitable drug classes have been the antidepressants and the antipsychotics.

All of the antidepressants may have withdrawal symptoms after months to years of use, and especially if abruptly discontinued. Initially, these drugs were thought not to cause the tolerance of more addictive drugs, such as the stimulants and benzodiazepines. The main advantage of the SSRIs over the TCAs and the MAOIs is not efficacy in treating depression but rather a higher TI meaning that they are considerably *safer in overdose* with fewer AEs in general. The common, mild side effects of the SSRIs include palpitations, nausea, anxiety, sedation, insomnia, hypersomnia, *sexual and erectile dysfunction,* and *weight gain*, as much as *eight pounds a year*. The SSRIs are more risky in the elderly because they cause cognitive decline, OH, dizziness, and falls. Falls lead to fractures that associate with overall decline in function and death often within six months after a fracture.

The SSRIs primarily block the reuptake inactivation of serotonin. Newer antidepressants have been developed that also block norepinephrine and dopamine reuptake inactivation. These are called atypical serotonin and norepinephrine reuptake inhibitors (SNRIs). The side effects of the SNRIs are similar to the SSRIs, but in addition, the SNRIs are more likely to cause hypertension, anxiety, *stimulation*, and *insomnia*.

Bupropion (Wellbutrin) is an example of an atypical antidepressant which has the same side effect possibilities as the SSRIs and the SNRIs with the addition of an increased risk for seizure. It may be more likely to cause anxiety and insomnia but may be less likely to switch Bipolar depression to mania. Another significant AE is the *serotonin syndrome*, which causes fever, sweating, cardiovascular instability, tachycardia, hypertension, muscular twitching, and rigidity, confusion, coma, and possibly death. According to Aiken (2017c), all of these classes of the newer antidepressants can switch Bipolar depression to mania.

6.3.5 *Benzodiazepine (BZD) Adverse Effects (AEs)*

The AEs of the BZDs are less life-threatening with a safer TI than the SGAs or lithium. They cause sedation, and with overuse or overdose, there can be oversedation, decreased cognitive function, slurred speech, an unsteady gait, and risk of falls, especially in the elderly. In a massive overdose, seizures, coma, and death are possible. They cause tolerance and addiction. They share receptors with alcohol so that the effects of combining BZDs and alcohol may be more than additive and more dangerous to life.

BZSs are used to treat and prevent life-threatening *alcohol withdrawal seizures*. After long-term use, *BZDs can cause anxiety*, the very symptom they are supposed to treat. As the BZD blood level falls several hours after ingestion, anxiety is generated. BZDs seem to degrade sleep quality over time. Again, BZDs should not be prescribed daily for more than days to weeks with a few exceptions such as end of life and some chronic medical disorders. Taking only 0.5 mg three or four times a week is safe, except for the propensity to increase this dose.

Non-BZDs, used as sleep aids, eszopiclone (Lunesta), zaleplon (Sonata), and zolpidem (Ambien), are advertised to cause less dependence and cognitive impairment than the BZDs. Non-BZDs interfere less with rapid eye movement as well as Stage III and IV delta sleep. The short-acting sleep aid zolpidem (Ambien) is now linked to *sleep walking*, *sleep eating*, and *sleep driving* in some users. According to Wegmann (2015), there is often no memory for these bizarre physical behaviors. There are now FDA warnings for them.

Withdrawal from chronic BZD use is difficult and can be approached in two ways. Some prefer an inpatient, rapid detox over three or four days, while others recommend a very slow tapering over months to a year. The withdrawal symptoms of the BZDs include generalized discomfort, flu-like symptoms, electric shock sensations in the extremities, BZD craving, anxiety, muscle cramps, decreased ability to concentrate, headache, loss of appetite, and, most significant, seizures are possible if the withdrawal is too acute.

6.3.6 *Stimulant Adverse Effects (AEs)*

The stimulants produce tolerance and are *very addictive*. Taken chronically in increasing dosages, the stimulants cause psychotic reactions. They were commonly taken for weight loss and were available over the counter until the Bureau of

Narcotics and Dangerous Drugs (BNDD), the forerunner of today's Drug Enforcement Administration (DEA), recognized their potential for psychosis and addiction and classified them as *Category II* drugs in 1970 and 1971.

The stimulants' major relevance to Bipolar involves Bipolar clients misdiagnosed with ADHD and prescribed stimulants that make their Bipolar Disorder cycle faster, induce rapid cycling and mixed episodes, and may associate with mood-stabilizer treatment resistance. These clients are unaware of these AEs. As stated above, the challenge regarding the stimulants used in newly referred Bipolar clients misdiagnosed with ADHD is correcting the diagnosis and discontinuing the stimulant. Trust must be gained before suggesting this type of change.

6.4 Life Changes

> "As someone who suffers chronic… mental illness, this app is perfect to find trends in what is making me ill." (Caldeira et al. 2017)

> "I have a Mood Disorder and the graphs make a great visual aid for sharing mood fluctuations with my doctor." (Caldeira et al. 2017)

Weekly psychotherapy is a major *risk reducer* as are several life-change behaviors. These include *daily mood charting* and avoiding all alcohol, illegal drugs, and prescription and over-the-counter stimulants, including caffeine. Additional risk-reducing behaviors are the addition of a *daily exercise program*, the identification of episode triggers, and the stringent avoidance of overconfidence when life is going well. Intensely involving family will reduce relapse risk (Table 6.9).

Table 6.9 A survey of steps to manage your Bipolar

1. Learn about Bipolar.
2. Accept/embrace your diagnosis of Bipolar.
3. Expect multiple drugs, at least three (3), likely for life.
4. Insist on three (3) mood stabilizers, such as: lithium, Depakote, Lamictal
5. Commit to weekly long-term psychotherapy.
6. Avoid alcohol, street drugs, prescription steroids, and stimulants; minimize caffeine.
7. Chart mood, sleep, energy, and meds daily for life.
8. Adopt a daily exercise routine.
9. Establish a consistent daily sleep-wake schedule.
10. Identify early subtle symptoms that precede a major episode.
11. Identify triggers that are likely to initiate an episode.
12. Take charge of your treatment; know your medications, dosages, plasma levels, and side effects.

6.4.1 Chart Mood, Sleep, Energy, and Medications Daily for Life

An initial high-priority life change is daily charting of mood and sleep. Although charting takes less than about five minutes a day, it is a challenge for clients; therapists generally do not insist enough. However, charting is essential for understanding the soul of each client's Bipolar. Lifetime daily charting reveals the pattern of recurrence and facilitates detection of early symptoms that herald onset of an episode of either mania or depression.

For clients, begin charting by journaling retrospectively the date of the first lifetime episode, the lifetime total number of episodes, how often they occur, how long they last, whether the episodes are generally the same or whether one or more have been noticeably different. How are they different? Clients can also record the level of dysfunctionality caused by the episodes.

From there, therapists should encourage clients to journal on a daily basis their mood on, for example, a 1–100 scale, the total hours of sleep, their energy level, and medications. Therapists can ask relatives to help clients rate mood and energy levels.

In your journal, on a 100-point scale, make 0–10 signify severe, likely *psychotic depression*, *suicidal thoughts*, and hospitalization needed; 90–100, out of control, dangerous, psychotic *mania* with super energy, and hospitalization needed. A score of 45–55 is *baseline mood* and energy or *euthymia*. Clients must record the number of hours of sleep and medication dosages taken daily when changes occur. Additional optional items for clients to *journal* are appetite, level of enjoyment of day-to-day activities, level of irritability, rate of speech, activity level, crying spells, and sociability/isolation level. Recording delusional thoughts, typically involving grandiosity, guilt, suspiciousness, paranoia, and fear of harm is also helpful (Sects. 3.9, Chap. 4).

There are convenient paper and digital forms already set up for this, and Fig. 6.3 is a flow sheet to offer to clients to record such data every day over each month. The use of paper and pencil charts allows clients to make a copy for the therapist to examine with them in every session. Such paper charts have been superseded by the use of digital apps available on I-Phones that are carried on one's person during waking hours. With the ready availability of digital devices, refining methods for frequent, at least daily mood monitoring in Bipolar is easier and can identify relapse signatures between episodes of mania and depression (Malik et al. 2012). Paper copies of these online charts can be made for therapy sessions. Reviews in the literature detail the advantages of different apps that are available to monitor and record mood (Malik et al. 2012; Caldeira et al. 2017). Some apps allow the quantification of client reactivity to specific stressful life events, a gauge for judging the likelihood of onset of mania and for recognizing triggers.

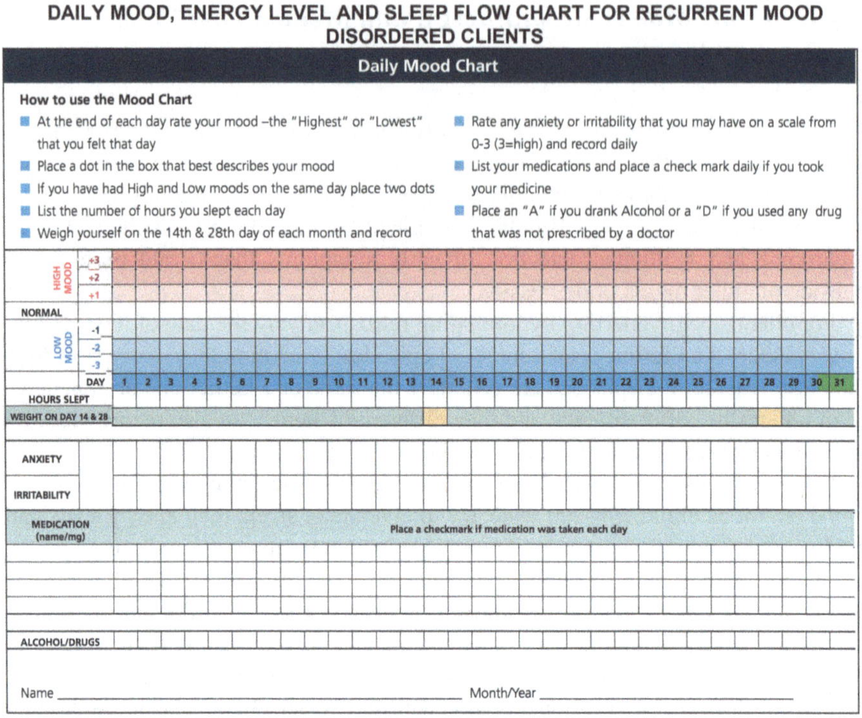
DAILY MOOD, ENERGY LEVEL AND SLEEP FLOW CHART FOR RECURRENT MOOD DISORDERED CLIENTS

Daily Mood Chart

How to use the Mood Chart

- At the end of each day rate your mood –the "Highest" or "Lowest" that you felt that day
- Place a dot in the box that best describes your mood
- If you have had High and Low moods on the same day place two dots
- List the number of hours you slept each day
- Weigh yourself on the 14th & 28th day of each month and record
- Rate any anxiety or irritability that you may have on a scale from 0-3 (3=high) and record daily
- List your medications and place a check mark daily if you took your medicine
- Place an "A" if you drank Alcohol or a "D" if you used any drug that was not prescribed by a doctor

HIGH MOOD +3 +2 +1

NORMAL

LOW MOOD -1 -2 -3

DAY 1 2 3 4 5 6 7 8 9 10 11 12 13 14 15 16 17 18 19 20 21 22 23 24 25 26 27 28 29 30 31

HOURS SLEPT

WEIGHT ON DAY 14 & 28

ANXIETY

IRRITABILITY

MEDICATION (name/mg) — Place a checkmark if medication was taken each day

ALCOHOL/DRUGS

Name ______ Month/Year ______

Fig. 6.3 Daily mood, energy level, sleep flow chart for recurrent Mood-Disordered clients
This form is to be used daily by clients with recurrent Mood Disorders, either Bipolar or Unipolar. Begin each month by printing your name, the month and the year on the new sheet at the bottom of the form. Next, add the names of your medications and the number of milligrams in each tablet also at the bottom of the form. See instructions at the top for rating daily mood, anxiety, irritability, and hours slept. Try to rate at approximately the same time every day. Abbreviate life events on another form and rate the impact of each between a −3 and +3 depending upon negative or positive impact upon one's mood. Note the hours of sleep for the night before. Women are asked to circle days of their menstrual period. Medication side effects can be noted under life events or in one of the rows available for medications at the bottom of the form. Target sleep time is one's average hours of sleep per night when euthymic.
Several online apps are available for accomplishing daily mood and sleep ratings. Your doctor may ask you to print your ratings for the month before each appointment.
Bring this form or a print of your online ratings with you to your appointments with your therapist and psychiatrist.

Different apps use different methods to record and rate mood. For example, MOBIMOOD and eMOODS use colors to designate mood. Aurora and IMoodJournal support self-tracking with users' photos to judge their moods by their photos. Medisafe enables convenient tracking of medication. MoodLog provides for mood tracking as well as related symptoms such as headache, nausea, panic, and menstrual pain. MOODZOOM permits Bipolar clients to rate anxiety, elation, sadness, anger, irritability, and energy on a 1–7-point Likert Scale ("not at all" through "very much"). Other apps use emojis.

A "short message service" system has been developed at Oxford University, Oxford, England. Clients are signaled by their phones to respond to a specific question, and the answer is recorded. This system allows for charting of mood and other variables such as sleep, also on a 1–7 Likert Scale. Instructions for this procedure require 15 minutes of orientation and an instruction card is credit-card sized. This system offers the opportunity for recording of mood changes in relationship to environment, such as the identification of environmental triggers (Chap. 6.4). Mobile phone monitoring of mood improves upon paper charting by increased convenience, assurance against loss, and reliability as the time of data entry is automatically recorded. The use of such mood-rating apps has grown exponentially in recent years (Caldeira et al. 2017). They benefit users by helping to increase awareness of their mood patterns that can be shared with their health care providers and family members to enhance management. Episodes can be anticipated.

Charting is most informative for documenting a hypomanic episode that can be overlooked without charting. This charting effort is for life and will form an invaluable data base that can yield a pattern of episodes that is critical for ideal management and can give the best chance for the prevention of rapid cycling and treatment resistance. After a very few days of scores above 70 or below 30, an extra trip to the therapist, the psychiatrist, the ED, or the hospital is warranted.

6.4.2 Avoid Kindling, Alcohol, and Illegal Drugs

Bipolar and Substance Use Disorders have a close and complex relationship, existing together more often than one might anticipate. The relationship between Mood and Substance Use Disorders has been observed for more than 2,000 years (Goodwin and Jamison 2007). Approximately 43–60% of Bipolar clients also develop Alcohol Use Disorder during their lifetimes. Bipolar individuals self-medicate with drugs and alcohol in an effort to numb the painful symptoms of their Bipolar. As a CNS sedative, *alcohol temporarily alleviates social anxiety* and makes interacting in groups more comfortable. Alcohol can blunt manic symptoms, and its use increases more during mania than during depression. Specific symptoms of mania that alcohol can moderate include excessive energy, hyperactivity, and decreased need for sleep. Alcohol sounds like a perfect drug for treating mania, but it is not. First, it can induce a switch from mania or euthymia to depression. Intoxication more likely increases poor decisions in mania, such as sexual indiscretions and conflict and contact with law enforcement. The literature is conclusive that *alcohol increases the negative effects of Bipolar* at both poles, mania and depression. *Alcohol destabilizes Bipolar Disorder.* Drinking while taking Bipolar medications increases the chances of adverse effects. It is said that some clients choose alcohol over medications because of a medication's side effects. The answer here is for clients to report to their therapists and then for the therapists to report the side effects to the prescriber and suggest a reduction of the doses of the offending medications, to avoid clients resorting to alcohol or illegal drugs. The prognosis is worse when Bipolar precedes the development of a Substance Use Disorder.

Alcohol Use and Bipolar Disorders must be treated concurrently as a *dual diagnosis* to have the best chance for a good outcome. An integrated treatment approach with a team of professionals who work together to address issues associated with both disorders maximizes effectiveness. After discharge, such dual diagnosis clients must continue psychotherapy and are usually expected to attend Substance Use Disorder therapy, which includes group therapy and social support groups that would include other dual diagnosis clients. One common and inexpensive social support group is *Alcoholics Anonymous (AA)*. Therapeutic approaches in individual psychotherapy include Cognitive Behavioral Therapy (CBT) and individual and group psychoeducation therapy. Other treatments include vocational rehabilitation, job training, childcare, and parenting instruction. Ongoing case management is useful. A common goal is to identify triggers and risk factors that can lead to relapse. Alcohol or drug detox can be accomplished on an inpatient basis. Medications for Bipolar are continued throughout this entire program, including the acute detox.

There are several useful medications for the treatment of Alcohol Use Disorder. These are only given to clients who have stopped drinking. *Disulfram (Antabuse)* was the first medicine approved for the treatment of Alcohol Use Disorder. It causes nausea and vomiting in most people who drink while taking it. A doctor's warning that there have been fatalities after drinking while taking disulfram (Antabuse) usually deters clients from a spur-of-the-moment drink. One must discontinue disulfram (Antabuse) for *at least three days* before it is safe to drink. This is very useful in blocking an acute desire to drink. *Naltrexone (Revia, Depade, and Vivitrol* in IM weekly form) works by changing tastes to bitter and by blocking other positive feelings from the brain that people experience when they drink alcohol or take opioids or cocaine. When combined with psychotherapy, Naltrexone reduces alcohol and drug cravings and decreases relapse rates. *Acamprosate (Campral)* is the medication most recently approved for the treatment of Alcohol Use Disorder. It reduces the discomfort, both physical and emotional, during withdrawal.

Young men with Bipolar are more likely to develop a Substance Use Disorder than females or older men and to take dangerous risks, including self-destructive behaviors. *Drug Use Disorders occur in some 41% of clients with Bipolar I.* Approximately 5% of Bipolar clients have a Cocaine Use Disorder, with more Bipolar Type I than Type II individuals involved. Cocaine use seems to be more common when manic than when depressed. One study reports 25% of their manic clients and 20% of their depressed Bipolar clients also suffer with Opiate Use Disorder. Another study finds only 5% of their manic clients use opiates.

The amphetamine analogs, once available over the counter but now controlled, can also precipitate psychoses, more likely in predisposed Bipolar clients. Ecstasy or *methylenedioxymethamphetamine (MDMA)* is a popular party stimulant known by several names. It is both a stimulant and a psychedelic street drug. Like the stimulants, it produces tolerance, which means it is addictive, at least psychologically. MDMA use in Bipolar risks the onset of a manic episode with rapid cycling, mixed features, and treatment resistance.

Marijuana Use Disorder is more prevalent among the Bipolar than the non-Bipolar population. There is a wide range of marijuana use (15–65%) reported in different studies in Bipolar Disorder. Chronic use leads to *reduced motivation, lethargy, depression*, anxiety, paranoia, and possibly memory loss. *Acute intoxication with marijuana* associates with anxiety, agitation, euphoria, grandiosity, paranoia, and *psychotic paranoid manic episodes* (Sects. 4.4 and 4.5; Cases 4.27, 4.30, and 4.31).

Alcohol and drug use make Bipolar worse. A first manic episode in a vulnerable individual (and no one knows who is subject to it) can be triggered by a stimulant such as cocaine or methamphetamine, marijuana, or a hallucinogen such as LSD or PCP. These drugs can also cause psychoses in Bipolar clients. Alcohol and Drug Use Disorders in Bipolar lead to higher rates of treatment resistance, rapid cycling, mixed states, impulsivity, aggression, destabilization of both mood and sleep, and poor outcome. Time to recovery from Bipolar episodes is slowed by Alcohol and Drug Use Disorders. Drug and alcohol use also increases the probability of non-compliance with treatment for Bipolar and decreases the effectiveness of Bipolar medications; chances of suicide increase. When confronted, Bipolar clients who drink or use drugs usually want to "cut back" their use but this rarely works. As AA says, "The easiest drink to refuse is the first."

Prescription drugs can also be abused by Bipolar clients. The most common classes are the benzodiazepines (BZDs), the stimulants, and steroids. The first two of these classes produce tolerance and are sought after by some with Bipolar Disorders. BZDs are used for sleep and to take the edge off mania and anxiety. Steroids, both prescribed and those used for body building, kindle mood episodes. None are mood-stabilizing, and the BZDs can increase anxiety with overuse as blood levels fall. The prescription stimulants do have mood-elevating properties but are dangerous because of their propensity for addiction, their ability to switch depression into mania, to increase the rate of cycling, and cause rapid cycling, mixed states and treatment resistance. The most likely circumstance for Bipolar clients to receive scripts for stimulants is when they are misdiagnosed with ADHD. The stimulants are the treatment of choice for ADHD, but ADHD is often unrecognized Bipolar (Sect. 2.7). These two classes of drugs, the BZDs and the stimulants, should be prescribed rarely and avoided by Bipolar clients.

Over-the-counter stimulants such as ephedrine and pseudoephedrine, as well as caffeine, are also best minimized or avoided altogether in Bipolar. These drugs are also capable of initiating a manic episode. Caffeine-containing beverages such as Red Bull contain substantial amounts of caffeine as does strong coffee. There are risks to indulging in the benefits of caffeine's stimulant effects. Abstinence from alcohol and illicit or nonprescribed medications is important to lower the risk of a poor outcome in Bipolar. Prescribed or online steroids for various medical/surgical disorders or anabolic steroids for body building are of concern in Bipolar clients as they can cause the onset of an episode of mania or depression (Sect. 3.7).

6.4.3 Daily Exercise and a Consistent Sleep-Wake Schedule

A sedentary lifestyle is common among those with mental illness, especially depression. Physical activity is recommended for the prevention and treatment of depression. Melo et al. (2016) review the effects of exercise in Bipolar clients, concluding that "*Physical activity is associated with less depressive symptoms*, better quality of life, and increased functioning."

Bipolar has a high comorbidity with obesity, diabetes, hypertension, and cardiovascular disease, all of which respond positively to exercise. The anti-inflammatory properties of frequent exercise are considered especially beneficial. Several groups recommend exercise as a healthy, nonpharmacological addition to depression treatment. Other authors show that exercise training reduces depressive symptoms. Physical activity seems to increase hippocampal brain-derived neurotrophic factor (BDNF) levels and to stimulate neurogenesis, which is associated with good mental health.

Disturbances in sleep and Bipolar are intimately linked (Sect. 2.5). Substantial data support the conclusion that Bipolar is related to *circadian rhythm disruptions,* such as changes in one's sleep pattern. The onset of a change in sleep routine often indicates, even predicts, a Bipolar episode. Mood regulation depends on consistent sleep regulation. Shift work, all-night partying and "all nighters" for exams, and meeting other deadlines risk a switch from euthymia into mania or depression. The degree of sleep disturbance affects the overall course of Bipolar, the effectiveness of its treatment, and the client's quality of life. A regular and *consistent six- to eight-hour sleep pattern* lowers the risk of mood episodes.

Bipolar episodes associate with *changes in the seasons*, more specifically, changes in hours of daylight (Sect. 2.5, Case 2.2). Seasonal Affective Disorder (SAD) is a type of Mood Disorder in which depression begins in the late summer and fall into the winter and mania begins in the late winter and spring and into the summer. The regulating factor is the number of daylight hours; these are exaggerated at extreme latitudes (Sect. 2.5).

6.4.4 Identify Triggers

Classic Bipolar Disorder is usually a chronically cycling lifelong disease. The primary goal in managing Bipolar is to postpone or prevent the next episode of mania or depression. Such mood episodes seem random and uncontrollable, but they *often occur in a pattern*, unique in each case. Episodes are frequently preceded by identifiable phenomena and can be triggered by specific factors. The identification of these triggers and the early, subtle prodromal symptoms is worth the effort. Some of these differ from one client to another, but others are common to most Bipolar clients. There is a body of literature on prodromal symptoms and triggers (Vann 2017; Kvarnstrom 2018; Nowak 2018). Identifying them empowers Bipolar clients to recognize and better manage their transitional symptoms. Usually no blame is due for a relapse; Bipolar is a brain disease generally out of the client's control, yet individuals can make the choice to avoid common triggers, such as drinking alcohol, smoking weed, and studying or partying all night.

As discussed above in Sect. 6.4, charting mood, hours of sleep, and environmental factors related to mood change can identify for each individual Bipolar client their specific prodromal symptoms and triggers. Both alcohol and recreational drug use can trigger mania, hypomania, and depression. Heavy, long-term use of alcohol and/or marijuana substantially increases the risk for a poor outcome in Bipolar. Even casual and occasional use of alcohol or drugs, such as Mr. V. N.'s weed, can trigger a major psychotic episode (Sect. 4.4; Case 4.31).

Common prodromal warning signs for an oncoming manic episode include a decreased need for sleep and clear increases in energy, irritability, rate of thoughts, rate of speech, self-confidence, intrusiveness, speeding, excessive buying, poor judgement, increased interest in sex, and in the use of substances, including alcohol.

The early signs for the onset of an episode of depression involve an increase in wanting to stay in bed, social withdrawal, procrastination or failure to complete things, negative opinions, forgetfulness, and cognitive decline; there are decreases in enjoyment, motivation, interest in usually pleasurable activities, energy, and ability to concentrate. There can be weight gain or loss and a change of at least 5% over a month is suggestive; there is no enjoyment in food.

The consideration of triggering in Bipolar clients is an important factor in gaining stability and preventing damaging interpersonal conflict. Some of the triggers for Bipolar clients are more individualized and personal compared to these general lists of early warning signs. Examples would include contact with a specific relative, such as one's mother-in-law in the case of Mr. H. S. (Sect. 4.4; Case 4.28). Others are triggered by anniversaries of painful events and current negative life events, such as separation, divorce, relationship break-ups, financial or job losses, conflicts with friends and family, and holidays. Crowds, loud parties, perceived disrespect, arguments, and fights can trigger a manic or depressive episode. Once triggers are identified, it is the responsibility of clients to avoid them. Alternatively, exclusive of substance use, one can reduce and eliminate reactivity or triggering by controlled exposure, as in desensitization.

Clients will invariably blame their manic, angry outbursts on someone or something "triggering" them. Examples are: "My mother-in-law always triggers me when my wife and I go over for a visit," "I am triggered by crowds and loud noise," "Just a couple of beers triggers me every time," "When something goes wrong at the office, I am triggered when I get home."

Helping clients understand the flaw in the logic of these blame statements will enable them to better stabilize and avoid crises. Help clients understand that we have control of how we respond to triggers. Most often we unknowingly indulge ourselves in "getting triggered," but that is a choice we do not have to make. The better choice is to avoid allowing ourselves to become triggered despite being confronted by triggers. How do we do this?

The initial step is to help clients recognize that they can be in control and do not have to succumb to getting triggered. Instant recognition is key. Once it is recognized that one can choose to maintain control of one's angry emotions, one can refuse to indulge oneself in one's usual out-of-control rage episodes. Mr. H.S. (Sect. 4.4; Case 4.28) can desensitize himself to his angry episodes when he goes to his mother-in-law's by determining to recognize his rising anger but choosing to remain calm.

The next step is to help clients identify the early thoughts and feelings when in a typically stressful or triggering situation. This is a relatively easy step when triggering situations are known beforehand. New and unknown triggering situations require more effort. Clients are encouraged to journal their thoughts and feelings in these kinds of situations. The "Notes" on a cell phone is a convenient means for journaling. Journaling episodes of irritability and anger on a daily basis is helpful if not mandatory to make progress. Support clients' efforts and expect failures. Reward successes.

Another trigger in women is the reproductive cycle, which can bring on depression premenstrually, as in Premenstrual Dysphoric Disorder (PDD). Sixty-eight per cent of women may have a menstrual cycle mood change, usually depression. Pregnancy and the post-partum period also impact mood, triggering depression in otherwise stable clients or initiating the first episode of Bipolar depression. Rarely a negative life event can trigger mania. More often positive events and goal attainment trigger mania. Examples would be winning an award, getting a promotion, falling in love, or going on vacation.

Sleep change can be both an early warning symptom and also a trigger.

Bipolar clients, when in remission and euthymic, must remain vigilant to early symptoms of an oncoming episode and avoid triggers identified above or unique to each individual. This strategy gives the best chance to maintain stability.

6.5 Other Treatments

6.5.1 Ketamine

Sometimes effective treatments derive from unexpected sources. One example has been ketamine, which was developed as an anesthetic agent in the 1960s, then became an illegal street drug, and is now FDA approved for severe depression. Although it was ideal as an anesthetic agent in not causing respiratory depression or hypertension, some clients awoke psychotic and its use in humans was discontinued. It is still widely used in veterinary anesthesia. Then, due to its hallucinatory properties, ketamine became known as a party drug or "Special K."

More recent studies of its effects in *treatment-resistant depression* have been exciting. According to Miller et al. (2019), there is optimism for its effectiveness in *treatment-resistant depression*, Bipolar as well as Unipolar. Research and development of *esketamine (Spravato)* as an antidepressant by Janssen has spanned the last nine years and involved over 1,700 clients with resistant depression. *Brain-derived neurotropic factor (BDNF)*, associated with mood stabilization, is increased by ketamine. Neuroimaging studies find increased *global brain connectivity or synaptogenesis,* especially in the hippocampus and prefrontal cortex, *within hours* to days of a single dose. These effects are associated with improvement in mood. "Remarkably, the *brain's structure appears to rewire in hours after a single dose of ketamine…*" (Miller et al. 2019). In 2000, *intravenous (IV) ketamine* showed a *significant antidepressant effect within 72 hours* after the first treatment and without significant adverse effects. Certified clinics are established around the country where esketamine (Spravato) is administered either *IV or intranasally*. Clients must remain in the clinic for two hours post-nasal or IV infusion. AEs include sedation, disassociation, and increased blood pressure. Dosages demonstrating efficacy have been 56 mg and 84 mg. Still unknown is the propensity of ketamine to switch Bipolar depressed clients into mania. In March of 2019, the FDA approved *esketamine (Spravato)* as an intranasal spray to treat resistant depression in combination with traditional mood stabilizers.

6.5.2 High-Dose Thyroid Replacement Therapy

High-dose thyroid replacement therapy (HDT) is another effective treatment for Bipolar and MDD. Hypothyroidism associates with depression. *Thyroid-stimulating hormone* (TSH) is an *inverse index of thyroid gland activity* and is measurable in the blood. The higher the TSH, the lower the thyroid gland output of thyroid hormone. *High TSH means hypothyroidism* or low levels of thyroid hormones. TSH is secreted by the anterior pituitary gland so it is high when the hypothalamus in the brain measures too little circulating thyroid hormone. TSH stimulates the thyroid gland to produce more thyroid hormones, triiodothyronine (T3) and thyroxine (T4). High TSH is also common in depression, so more thyroid hormone may help depression. Thyroid hormone is available in oral preparations.

Phelps (2018a, b) has recently reviewed the efficacy of thyroid hormone replacement in Bipolar depression. The relationship between hypothyroidism and severe, refractory rapid cycling is established since 1990 (Bauer et al. 2003; Bauer and Whybrow 2012). TSH levels between 2.5 and 4.0 milli International units per liter (mlU/L) associate with more severe symptoms and treatment-resistant MDEs, both Unipolar and Bipolar. The strategy in treating depression with thyroid replacement hormone therapy is to give enough thyroid hormone to reduce easily measurable *TSH levels to low values, around 1 mlU/L.*

The AEs of endogenous hyperthyroidism are an increased risk for atrial fibrillation, decreased bone density, and congestive heart failure. Exogenous levothyroxine does not seem to carry these same risks. Kelly (2018) has published a book on HDT for the treatment of Bipolar depression. He recommends considering levothyroxine augmentation in Bipolar depressed clients with a TSH level greater than 1.5; start with at least 50 μg/day and with a *target to reduce the TSH level down to around 1.0 m/U/L*. Phelps (2018a, b) recommends starting at *75 μg/day with a range of 50–100 μg a day*.

In Bipolar high-dose thyroid replacement (HDT) may decrease cognitive decline and may also decrease the considerable medical morbidity and mortality (Kelly 2018). HDT has been an effective treatment for mood disorders since Kraepelin taught about the use of desiccated sheep thyroid (Kraepelin 1899). Despite this, HDT treatment for Bipolar has not been widely embraced. It is effective in combination with mood stabilizers and not as monotherapy. When combined with carbamazepine (Tegretol), higher doses of thyroid hormone are required. *HDT is especially useful in treatment resistance and rapid cycling cases*.

6.5.3 Simvastin (Zocor)

Another old drug with a new use in psychiatry is *simvastatin (Zocor)*. It crosses the blood-brain barrier more easily than other statins and has anti-inflammatory effects, inhibiting cytokines IL-1 and TNF-alpha (tumor necrosis factor), among other effects. These may link simvastatin (Zocor) to efficacy in depression. This drug was initially associated with antidepressant effects in rats but more recently in humans as well (Phelps 2018a, b). It is superior to placebo as an adjunct to fluoxetine (Prozac) and reduces negative (depressive) symptoms.

6.5.4 Tamoxifen (Nolvadex)

Tamoxifen (Nolvadex) is a selective estrogen receptor modulator used in breast cancer treatment. It inhibits protein kinase C (PKC), an effect similar to valproic acid/divalproex (Depakene/Depakote) and lithium. Because of this similarity of mechanism with established effective drugs in Bipolar, Tamoxifen has been tried, with mixed results. British investigators found Tamoxifen to be promising in the treatment of mania (Palacios 2019). It was superior to placebo in lowering mania scale scores when used in monotherapy. Other results have been disappointing (Zarate et al. 2007).

6.5.5 AXS-05 (Alzforum)

On June 26, 2020, the FDA granted "Breakthrough Therapy Designation" to *AXS-05* for the treatment of MDD and Alzheimer's. AXS-05 is made up of *dextromethorphan*, a noncompetitive N-methyl-D aspartate (NMDA) receptor antagonist, and *buproprion (Wellbutrin)*, a norepinephrine and dopamine reuptake inhibitor that also increases the bioavailability of dextromethorphan. AXS-05 is said to have led to substantial, rapid, and statistically significant reductions in depressive symptoms when compared to buproprion (Wellbutrin) alone. AEs included nausea, dizziness, dry mouth, decreased appetite, and anxiety.

6.5.6 Electroconvulsive Therapy (ECT)

According to Wikipedia, agents producing seizures were used to treat psychotic psychological conditions as early as the sixteenth century. In 1785, *seizure induction* was documented as therapeutic in psychotic clients in the *London Medical Journal*. In 1934, the Hungarian neuropsychiatrist Meduna believed that "Schizophrenia" (psychotic depression) and epilepsy were antagonistic disorders. He therefore successfully used convulsive therapy to treat psychotic clients at that time. To induce seizures, he initially used camphor and later metrazol. Metrazol convulsive therapy was used worldwide by 1937 when the first international meeting on convulsive therapy was held in Switzerland. In 1938, the Italians *Cerletti and Bini* used electricity (*electroconvulsive therapy, ECT*) as a substitute for metrazol to more safely produce seizures in clients. For this they were nominated, but did not win the Nobel Prize. By 1940, ECT was introduced in both the United Kingdom and the United States, and through the 1940s and 1950s, the use of ECT became widespread. The widespread negative portrayal of ECT in the popular media, such as Ken Kesey's novel and movie *One Flew Over the Cuckoo's Nest*, where ECT was used as an instrument of punishment and terror, has reduced the acceptance of this effective treatment.

ECT is a very effective short-term treatment for severe depression, Bipolar or Unipolar, despite its negative reputation. The procedure passes an electric current through the scalp and skull to cause a generalized seizure. The entire procedure takes about 30 minutes; *the actual shock treatment lasts seconds*. Short-acting anesthesia is used. Its beneficial effects are rapid, usually after three to five treatments. ECT is called for when mood or psychotic symptoms are unresponsive to several concomitant medicines or when symptoms are so severe that it may be unsafe to wait until drugs take effect. It may be the treatment of choice for severe depressive episodes during pregnancy.

It is generally given three times a week, usually for two to three weeks. Maintenance treatments can continue weekly or monthly supplemented with psychotherapy and mood-stabilizing medications. A course of ECT is effective in about *50% of cases* with treatment-resistant major depression, either Bipolar or Unipolar. ECT is generally one of the *safest treatments*, with risks relating to the anesthesia *Short-term memory loss is common*, occurring in some 33% of clients. *It is not permanent*. Other side effects are headache, jaw pain, muscle aches, nausea, and confusion, and these effects may last from hours to days.

6.5.7 *Light Therapy*

According to Wikipedia, the use of *light therapy* has a long history, dating from many ancient cultures, such as the Greeks, Egyptians, Romans, Inca, Assyrians, and Germans. Medical literature from India dating from 1500 BCE as well as Buddhist (200 CE) and Chinese (900 CE) sources recommended natural sunlight for treatment of various disorders.

Niels Finsen is credited as the father of modern light therapy. He developed the first artificial light source and received the *Nobel Prize in Physiology and Medicine* in 1903. Light therapy is also known as phototherapy or heliotherapy and consists of exposure to light of specific wavelengths. The use of light therapy in the treatment of Seasonal Affective Disorder (SAD) is linked to the artificial light making up for lost hours of sunlight during the fall and winter seasons. Morning exposure has provided the best results.

There are data questioning the effectiveness of light therapy but these are in a minority of studies overall. A review in 2008 concluded that "overall, bright light therapy is an excellent candidate for inclusion into the therapeutic inventory available for the treatment of…depression…" (Even et al. 2008).

Light therapy uses a light box which emits up to 10,000 lux of light at a specific distance (Aiken 2017b). Precise wavelengths of light are used from the blue (460 nm) to the green (525 nm) areas of the visible spectrum. Green light therapy has been shown to suppress melatonin. Side effects can include rash or skin irritation, headache, eye irritation, and nausea.

6.5.8 *Transcranial Magnetic Stimulation (TMS)*

Transcranial magnetic stimulation (TMS) is used in adult clients with *depression*, Unipolar and Bipolar, who have failed to respond to medications. There are a few studies indicating success in manic clients as well. There are several theories of the mechanisms of action of TMS. The AEs of TMS are minimal and include headache, pain at the site of stimulation, a low risk of TMS-induced seizures or memory impairment, and conflicting reports regarding TMS-induced mania in depressed clients. There is no post-procedure recovery and no anesthesia is used.

6.5.9 *Opioid Systems*

The *opioid* system has become a therapeutic target for treatment-resistant depression. Opioid receptors populate cortical and subcortical brain areas involved in stress and emotional responsivity. Blockage of kappa opioid receptors is reported to have antidepressant effects; their activation causes dysphoria. Ketamine binds to kappa receptors and this may explain its benefits. Buprenorphine, a partial agonist at mu receptors and an antagonist at delta receptors, also binds at kappa receptors where it is a strong antagonist. Twelve studies find benefit of low doses of buprenorphine augmentation (2 mg) in depression (Stanciu et al. 2017).

There are other pharmacological and physical treatments for Bipolar.

6.6 Suicide/Homicide Evaluations for Therapists, Clients, and Their Families

Suicide, the tenth leading cause of death in the United States, is the most tragic consequence of depression, and its prevention is a critical responsibility of mental health professionals. Worldwide, about a million people die by suicide yearly, and the suicide rate in Bipolar depression is about 15–25%. Suicide occurs predominantly in severely, usually psychotic, depressed clients with a few exceptions, such as end-of-life decisions. Suicidal ideations occur in about 4% of the US population annually; this equals 13 million people who think of killing themselves in a year. Most of these individuals are depressed. There are about *36,000* suicides per year in the United States, of which over 14% occur in people over 65. Rates are said to be soaring among middle-aged Americans with a rise of 28% over the last decade (Wendling 2013).

Males are four times more likely to succeed than females but females attempt suicide three times more often than males. Among suicides in people younger than 24 and older than 65, about *85% are male*. Caucasians and Native Americans have the highest rate among all races (Freeman 2012). The ratio of attempted to completed suicide is 100–200 to one in individuals 15–24 but four to one in those over 65. *Guns* are the most common method for completed suicide. According to the Centers for Disease Control and Prevention, nearly 20,000 of the 30,000 deaths annually from guns in the United States in 2010 were suicides. Suicidal acts with guns are fatal in 85% of cases versus just 2% in overdose cases (Desilver 2013).

The first step to suicide prevention is the *recognition of depression* because suicide predominantly occurs during severe depression. Depressed clients may not volunteer symptoms of depression or their suicidal ideations or even recognize that they are depressed. *About 50%* of clients who killed themselves saw their primary care physician (PCP) within four weeks of their suicide and about a *third within two weeks*. In other studies, 35% of physicians did not diagnose depression or did not recognize a risk for suicide in 54% of their clients who subsequently took their own lives.

To uncover suicide risk, the initial focus must be on a brief screen for depression. There are a number of screening instruments for suicide such as the APA Practice Guideline, the Chronological Assessment of Suicide Events (CASE), Columbia-Suicide Severity Rating Scale (C-SSRS) and the *four-question, 90-second screen* discussed below. If these are incorporated into every client encounter, more depressed clients should be identified and their risk for suicide better appreciated (Table 6.10).

Table 6.10 Screening questions for suicidal risk assessment

A. *Four-Part Screen for Suicidal Risk*:
When one or more of the four-questions of the "90-second depression screen," especially question 4 (Table 5.1), are positive or there are other indications of depression or suicidality (SI), the following screen for SI is one of several available. Emphasis is on the order and wording of questions and eliciting exquisite detail. Since the four questions focus the client on the emotional symptoms of depression, the following sequence appropriately follows the four questions. In this format there are four parts to the screen for suicidal risk. Assessments of low, moderate and high risk remain subjective.
Part I: Thoughts, Plans, Actions *during the H.P.I. or recently*
1. "Have you had thoughts about hurting yourself?" If negative, go to Parts II, III and IV. If positive, proceed with question #2.
2. "Tell me about these thoughts." Get detail. If only passive SI, such as, "I wouldn't care if I didn't wake up in the morning" or "I wouldn't care if the airplane crashed," proceed to Parts II, III, and IV. If active SI, proceed to question #3.
3. "Tell me about the plans you have made to hurt yourself." Get detail. If negative, consider asking Question #2 again or going to Parts II, III, and IV. If positive proceed to question #4.
4. "What actions have you taken?" Proceed to question #5 regardless of positive or negative response.
5. Ask detail of plan and/or actions depending on the client's response in questions #3 and #4. For example:
If the plan involves overdose, ask "What pills?" "How many?" "Where did you get them?" "Have you stock-piled?" "Where do you keep the pills?" "Do you hide them?" "Have you gotten the pills out in your hand?" "What is the closest you have come to swallowing them?" "Have you researched the lethal dose?"
If by hanging, ask, "What preparations have you made?" "Have you bought a rope or selected one at home?" "Describe where you would do it." "Have you put the rope around you neck?" "What is the closest you have come?"
If with a gun, ask, "Do you own a gun or have you decided where to buy one?" "How long have you owned the gun?" "Did you recently buy it?" "Have you taken the gun out and loaded it with the thought of shooting yourself?" "Have you put it to your head?" If a revolver, "Have you played Russian roulette?" "What is the closest you have come?"
If by carbon monoxide, "What preparations have you made?" "Have you selected or bought a hose?" "Do you have or have you bought duct tape?" "Have you sealed the garage?" "Have you put the hose in the tailpipe and sat in the car?" "With the car running?" "For how long?" "Describe the closest you have come."
If by cutting, ask "With what?" "Have you taken the razor blades or knife out?" "Describe your plan; hot bath? direction of cut?" "What is the closest you have come?"
If by jumping, ask, "Have you picked a spot?" "Have you gone there?" "What prevented you from jumping?"
6. "What thoughts have you had about avoiding rescue?" "What would you do to avoid rescue?"
7. "What thoughts, ideas, and activities have prevented you from hurting yourself?"
8. "Have you made or altered your will lately? Given things away? Bought a plot...all in preparation for killing yourself?"
Part II: Thoughts, Plans, Actions, *Ever*
1. Ask when thoughts of suicide have occurred in the past. If negative, i.e., no thoughts in the past and Part I was negative, may stop the suicide screen here. If positive, proceed to question #2.

(continued)

Table 6.10 (continued)

2. "What actions to hurt yourself have you taken in the past?" "Please describe." If negative and Part I was negative, it may be appropriate to stop the screen here. If positive, proceed to question #3.
3. "What is the closest you have come to killing yourself in the past?" Focus on one or two of the most severe episodes. Proceed to question # 4.
4. As in Part I, require detail. For example, "Was medical attention sought?" "If so, what happened?" "How close did you come to dying?" "How many stitches?" "Units of blood?" "Loss of consciousness?" "Ventilator?" "Days on the ICU?" "Admitted directly to Inpatient Psychiatry?" "Discharged from the Emergency Dept. to home?" "Band-Aid?"
Part III: Models
1. "Who do you know that has killed themselves or attempted suicide?" If positive, proceed to question #2.
2. "Who? How? When? Relationship to you? How close of a relationship?"
Part IV: Thoughts, Plans, and Actions, *Now* and in the *Future*
1. Follow the questions in Part I.
2. "What are your thoughts (and plans) about hurting yourself in the future?"
B. Summary of Some Predictive Factors for Suicide
1. Severe depression, especially in a mixed Bipolar episode
2. Increasing anxiety and agitation
3. Long current episode of severe depression getting worse
4. Access to lethal means
5. Has a detailed plan for suicide
6. Recent loss or separation
7. Alcohol or Substance Use Disorder, severe
8. Age (for males, the older, the higher the risk; for women, between 55 and 65 years old)
9. Older, unmarried male
10. Recent bona-fide attempt; lethal, premeditated prior behavior
11. Refusal of help and/or a plan to avoid rescue
12. Psychosis; especially voices/thoughts saying "die" or "kill yourself"
13. Caucasian or Native American
14. Recent suicide by a friend or fellow student
15. Giving away personal belongings

The first question of the four-question screen is a combination of the two DSM diagnostic criteria required for a diagnosis of Major Depression. Question 1 is "Over the past few weeks (or months) have you been getting less enjoyment out of your life and/or feeling more down in the dumps, sad, or blue?" The second question is "Out of the blue have you felt weepy or like crying more than is usual for you?" Questions 3 and 4 may be unnecessary if the answers to Questions 1 and 2 are negative. If answers to either 1 or 2 are positive, determine whether the symptoms have lasted for at least *two weeks* and been *present 24/7*. Next, proceed to Questions 3 and 4, which evaluate risk for suicide. Question 3: "How often do you awake in the morning wishing you had not woken up?" Question 4 asks, "How often have you been thinking that your life is not worth living?" If the answers to these questions above are negative, the risk for suicide is low. If the answers to the four questions are positive, however, a more thorough line of questions to determine risk for suicide will be needed (Table 6.10).

This pursuit for suicide risk will be more productive with a focus on creating a safe emotional environment in which the client is comfortable being vulnerable about their thoughts and intentions. Remain calm and *listen more than you speak, maintain eye contact*, use open body language, ask and act with confidence. Reassurance must be conveyed by the interviewer that suicidal ideation is common and that the therapist is comfortable talking about suicide. At first, listening without reassurances is recommended (Weinberg 2016). Once trust is established, "Curiosity is your best tool, and it will guide your questions" (Jha 2013). Ask for details such as how the client experiences suicidal thoughts, what time of day, more in the morning or more in the evening. Identify triggers such as specific events. Explain that suicidal thoughts come and go and that they will subside at least for a time if they are not acted upon. Asking does not increase risk; not asking is worse and *discussion can reduce risk.*

Additional questions focus on thoughts, plans, and actions taken (Table 6.10). Determining methods considered and actions taken reveals an index of commitment. Examples of actions include preparations such as buying a gun, rope, or hose for the car's exhaust, or stockpiling medicine. Risk factors are known: *extreme psychic anxiety*, *agitation*, *active psychosis*, anhedonia, decreased ability to concentrate, insomnia, panic attacks, hopelessness, a history of suicide attempts, positive family history of suicide, active alcohol or substance abuse, anger, rage, risk-taking, *reckless and erratic behaviors*, lacking purpose, experiencing a loss, and a *recent suicide by a friend or fellow student. Giving away possessions*, being older, unmarried, male, and Caucasian or Native American, having *access to lethal means,* and *having a detailed plan* for suicide are also high risk factors (Freeman 2012). Busch and Fawcett (2004) find that 79% of clients who suicided had extreme *psychic anxiety* and *agitation* and 54% were actively *psychotic*.

Other treatment considerations include an attempt to understand the individual's strengths, weaknesses, and relationships. Most clients are ambivalent about killing themselves, so explore that ambivalence with regard to why the client *wants to live.* "Considering all of your difficulties, what has kept you alive? What is important to you now?" "Look for the attachment to someone or something positive and reinforce that" (Jha 2013).

Protective factors can be assessed using the "Reasons for Living" inventory (Lineham et al. 1983). Prevention focuses on factors that can serve as obstacles to clients killing themselves. Restrict access to lethal means and *forcefully follow up.* Hospitalization is the best means for ensuring safety in high-risk suicidal clients.

Useful medications for suicidal clients include the *benzodiazepines for agitation* in an acutely suicidal client. The data are persuasive that lithium can reduce the mortality rate from suicide for clients with Mood Disorders and that this effect persists (Baldessarini et al. 2006; Tondo and Hennen 2003). *Lithium is remarkable* in the consistency of reports of its efficacy in *reducing suicidal acts and attempts by over 90%*; another study finds that this drug reduces suicide completions by 82% (Müller-Oerlinghausen et al. 2003). A drawback is that lithium is toxic at only three times its therapeutic dose and does not work instantly but may take days to a week or two to be effective. That means that the therapist could consider monitoring a suicidal client's lithium for distribution in sessions that are increased to daily or every other day. Consider allowing only enough for a few days.

Electroconvulsive Therapy (ECT) can *reduce suicidal thoughts and acts* by 38% after one week and 80% overall. One report finds amelioration of suicidal thoughts after just one treatment of ECT (Kobeissi et al. 2011). Therapists should not hesitate to refer acutely suicidal clients for inpatient care and ECT.

There are situations when risk of suicide is not clear, generating a dilemma regarding hospitalization. Some factors to consider follow. Hospitalization is the best choice (1) if there is no family or significant other to observe and care for the client; (2) when Alcohol or Substance Use Disorders are comorbid factors; (3) when there has been a recent bona-fide suicide attempt; or (4) when the client is extremely anxious, agitated, psychotic, hostile and/or angry. In such cases, commitment must be considered (Sect. 6.7).

Questions and epidemiology to assess *homicidal risk* are given in Table 6.11. Begin by asking if the client has any thoughts about hurting anyone else. A negative answer usually ends the screen. When there is not a denial, further exploration is recommended.

Saxton et al. prefer the use of actuarial tools in assessing risk for homicide (Saxton et al. 2018). A structured tool such as the *Classification of Violence Risk* can be helpful. *Past violence is the best predictor* of future violence because violence risk increases with each violent episode. *Prior arrest for any crime*, especially in one's teens, increases future risk. Being *young*, *male* and of *low socioeconomic status* are risk factors. Fifteen- to 24-year-old males are most likely to perpetrate violence. Other risk factors include *mental illness*, *psychosis*, *unstable employment*, *less education*, *low intelligence*, a history of *head trauma*, *childhood abuse*, *witnessing violence in the home*, *parental loss*, early disruptive behavior, a predisposition to *anger and hatred*, hostile attributional biases, *violent fantasies*, *poor anger control*, *impulsivity*, *substance abuse*, and *availability of weapons*.

Targeted violence is defined as a "predatory act of violence intentionally committed against a preselected person, group of people, or place." Targeted violence was responsible for the *Tarasoff case* in which a client discussed killing an individual during a therapy session and later followed through; the therapist was prevented from reporting the situation based on client confidentiality. The resultant ruling mandates therapists to override client confidentiality and warn the potential victim and law enforcement in such cases. To assess seriousness of intent to harm, Saxton et al. (2018) recommend asking the following: "How likely are you to carry out this act of violence? Do you have a plan? Have you taken any steps toward this plan? Do you see other, non-violent solutions to this problem? What do you hope that we can do for you to help with this problem?" The authors recommend that it may be prudent to get a second opinion.

Table 6.11 Screening questions and epidemiology for homicidal risk assessment

A. Screening questions:
1. Have you had some thoughts about hurting anyone? (if negative, the screen can usually end; if a "yes," proceed with the questions below to determine likelihood for violence.)
2. Who do you plan to hurt?
3. What do you plan to do?
4. Do you plan to kill this person?
5. How are you planning on carrying out the attack?
6. Where are you planning on attacking?
7. How likely are you to carry out your plan?
8. What steps have you taken toward your plan?
9. Could there be other, nonviolent, solutions to this conflict?
10. How can we work together in therapy to prevent such a drastic, life-changing action for both of you?[a]
B. Epidemiology; factors that increase risk for homicide:
1. Past violence
2. Prior arrest for any crime
3. Male 15–24 years old
4. Mental illness
5. Availability of weapons
6. Low socioeconomic status
7. Low intelligence
8. Unstable employment
9. Less education
10. Childhood abuse
11. Witnessing violence growing up
12. Parental loss or absence
13. Early disruptive behavior
14. Predisposition to hatred and anger
15. Violent fantasies
16. Poor anger control
17. Impulsivity
18. Substance abuse

[a]Based on the Tarasoff case, when there is a threat of violence, the therapist is obligated to override patient confidentiality and inform both the intended victim and law enforcement.

6.7 Commitment Issues: Outpatient Rescheduling Versus Hospitalization

"Early onset of symptoms, delayed treatment, rapid cycling and the number of previous psychotic and mixed episodes are potent risk factors for poor outcomes." (Goodwin and Jamison 2007)

"Each episode of depression or mania is associated with a worsening of the Bipolar so that the next episode comes faster, is more severe, and can become treatment resistant." (Goodwin and Jamison 2007)

> "Achieving remission in cases with active symptoms is no longer the only goal of treatment. Preventing or delaying the next episode after remission is essential for the successful lifetime management of Bipolar." (Post 2007)

> "Regular psychotherapy follow-up is recommended weekly to maximize the chances of client compliance, patient understanding of their disease, the medications needed and recognition of early indications of recurrence, enabling a prophylactic increase in therapy and medication adjustment before a full-blown episode develops. The goal is prevention of episodes rather than the usual "catch-up" treatment after a full relapse." (Lake 2021)

A treatment dilemma arises in severe cases of clients presenting in danger of harm. When such clients are unwilling to voluntarily hospitalize themselves, forced commitment must be considered if not mandated. Civil commitment means the forced hospitalization of clients with severe mental illness. Aspects of civil commitment are discussed below.

A potentially life-saving aspect of mental health treatment is civil or involuntary commitment. The decision to recommend forcibly holding a client versus releasing them falls to the evaluating therapist and then usually the ED. For clients unwilling to voluntarily go to the ED, the options include warning law enforcement. If there is a significant other, they could be notified that the client could present some danger (Chap. 4; Case 4.60).

Law enforcement is empowered to transport psychotic clients in need of commitment to the ED. This process to detain a person in a psychotic crisis without a court order for two or three days in the hospital to evaluate need for commitment is consistent across the states, but it is up to the ED doctor whether to hospitalize.

Once in the ED, most are declined admission. At this time, commitment guidelines warranting forced admission are too strictly interpreted. Clients are often released when it is judged that they are not in *imminent or immediate danger* of hurting themselves or anyone else but many of these clients are still at risk for life-threatening decisions based on the dysfunction caused by their mental illness. Needed reforms are hindered by the cost, effort, and time required.

In severely mentally ill clients who may present imminent danger and need but refuse hospitalization, a treatment dilemma arises between involuntary commitment to the hospital and release to the care of family with scheduled outpatient follow-up. Mr. Fertuck (Sect. 4.6, Case 4.60) is an example of a dangerous individual whose therapist warned his parents not to keep him in the house. He was not committed by his parents or psychiatrist and he killed his parents before suiciding.

In at least four cases reviewed in Sects. 4.5 and 4.6, families either notified the police, asked the psychiatrist to hospitalize their relative, or the client was brought to the mental health center, but warnings were not heeded and the client murdered or attempted murder (Sect. 4.5, Mr. Cho, Case 4.36; Mr. Bedell, Case 4.37; Mr. Hinckley, Case 4.38; Mr. Loughner, Case 4.41).

The Treatment Advocacy Center is a national nonprofit organization "dedicated exclusively to eliminating barriers to the timely and effective treatment of severe mental illness" (Torrey et al. 2014). This center's report published in February, 2014, surveying mental health commitment laws finds that "…every Western nation, and every US state has established civil commitment laws and criteria that govern when the condition of an individual with acute or chronic psychological symptoms warrants a court order to mandate mental health treatment in a hospital or, where enabling statutes exist, as a condition of living in the community." This less restrictive option of court-ordered community treatment is called *Assisted Outpatient Treatment or AOT*. However, in the "vast majority of states the quality of civil commitment laws is far below what is necessary to provide a readily accessible path to treatment and recovery for severely mentally ill clients who are unable to seek care for themselves [but are not imminently suicidal or homicidal]."

> The tragic consequences of ignoring the needs of individuals with the most severe mental illnesses who are unable or unwilling to seek treatment are on vivid display nationwide: on our streets, where an estimated *quarter million people with untreated psychological illness roam homeless; in our jails and prisons* which now house ten times as many people with severe mental illness as do our psychiatric hospitals; *in our suicide and victimization statistics, where individuals with psychotic disorders are grossly over-represented*; and *in our local news* which reports daily *on violent acts committed by individuals whose families struggled vainly to get them into treatment* (Torrey et al. 2014) (Chap. 4).

Responsibility for these tragedies falls to state and local governments, who are *failing to adequately fund* their mental health systems to meet the needs for hospital beds (at least *50 beds per 100,000 population* are needed), medications, community-based services, and intensive case management. Some *$1.6 billion was cut from state funds* for mental health services between 2009 and 2011, according to a report by the National Alliance on Mental Illness (NAMI).

Criteria for commitment vary from state to state. Before the 1960s, obtaining involuntary commitment was straightforward: all that was needed was the determination that a person required care for their mental health issues. However, commitments were allowed to be continued indefinitely without ongoing judicial oversight. These laws were reformed in the 1960s. The 1975 US Supreme Court ruling in O'Connor v Donaldson, in which Kenneth Donaldson sought release from 15 years of hospital confinement without treatment, effectively restricted the ability to commit.

The understanding of the meaning of "a danger to self or others" became exceedingly narrow. To be involuntarily committed, it was understood that the person had to be at imminent risk of suicide or homicide. This strict interpretation saved state and local governments millions of dollars as they were able to close many state hospitals and lay off thousands of mental health workers. The deinstitutionalization moved mentally ill clients out of hospitals and into community mental health center treatment, the streets, and prisons, if not to early deaths.

The standards of "*grave disability*" and "*need for treatment*" as bases for commitment are much more liberal but not widely applied. "Grave disability" includes individuals that pose a physical threat to themselves because they are unable to provide for their basic necessities for human survival, but are not necessarily suicidal. This standard allows for the commitment of persons whose untreated mental illness has led them to living on the streets and foraging in dumpsters to eat. The "need for treatment" standard enables the commitment of mentally ill clients who suffer a deterioration of general health, psychological damage, and loss of the ability to function independently. These people are unable to seek help on a voluntary basis because of their mental illness and if not treated, there will be severe suffering and harm to their mental and physical health.

These standards are not often followed because of the prevailing idea that the individual must present an *imminent* threat to self or others. Commitment should be available below the imminent threat bar when mental illness causes persistent and acute disability, meaning that if not treated, there is a "substantial probability of the person continuing to suffer severe and abnormal mental, emotional, or physical harm that significantly impairs judgement, reason, behavior, or capacity to recognize reality."

There are several blocks to needed commitments. First is the misinterpretation of the necessity of imminent danger to self or others. Admitting ED doctors and psychiatrists who screen potential clients in the ED may be motivated to interpret imminent danger more stringently in order to reduce the number of people who qualify for a bed and their own client work-up time that will be required if they admit.

In cases where mental health professionals justifiably commit one of their own long-term clients, client feelings of betrayal and anger can permanently break the therapeutic bond. Psychotic clients needing commitment may spend days, if not weeks, in the ED because there are no beds available on the psychiatric unit. Another block to commitment is the reluctance by psychologists and psychiatrists to give time required for expert testimony to have a client committed. This testimony, usually in front of a judge, is time-consuming and typically goes uncompensated.

There have been worthwhile suggestions of allowing private persons such as family or significant others to petition the court for commitment. Empowering private individuals to petition for evaluation gives voice to the observers most likely to recognize [psychotic behavior] and frees families from being forced to wait for the individual to exhibit the sort of violent behavior that tends to draw police attention… The more broadly this right is extended, the better.

Assisted Outpatient Treatment (AOT) is a practice of the court, ordering a mentally ill client who meets certain legal criteria to adhere to a specific program of outpatient treatment as a condition of remaining in the community. AOT significantly reduces a number of negative outcomes such as hospitalization, incarceration, suicide, violence, and crime. AOT saves money as well. AOT laws are active in all but a very few states.

Although there have been improvements, "The quality of *civil commitment laws* in the vast majority of states *remains far below what is necessary* to provide a readily accessible path to treatment and recovery for individuals with the most severe mental illnesses who are unable to seek care for themselves" (Torrey et al. 2014).

References

Aiken C. The year in bipolar: seven practice-changing papers from 2017. 2017a Psychiatr Times. 8 Dec 2017a. On line.

Aiken C. How to use light therapy in bipolar disorder. Psychiatric Times. 12 Oct 2017b. On line.

Aiken C. Who gets worse on an antidepressant? Psychiatric Times. 10 Nov 2017c. On line.

Aiken C. Antidepressants in Bipolar disorder. Psych. Times 2019;36(5):np On line.

Alda M. Lithium in the treatment of bipolar disorder: pharmacology and pharmacogenetics. Mol Psychiatry. 2015;20(6):661–70.

Alexander GC, Gallaher SA, Mascola A, Moloney RM, Stafford RS. Increasing off-label use of antipsychotic medications in the United States, 1995–2008. Pharmacoepidemiol Drug Saf. 2011;20:177–84.

Azab AN, Schnaider A, Osher Y, Wang D, Bersudsky Y, Belmaker RH. Lithium nephrotoxicity. Int J Bipolar Disorders. 2015;3(1):28.

Baldessarini RJ, Tondo L, Davis P, Pompili M, Goodwin FK, Hennen J. Decreased risk of suicides and attempts during long-term lithium treatment: a meta-analytic review. Bipolar Disord. 2006;8(5 pt 2):625–39.

Bauer M, Whybrow PC. Impact of sunlight on the age of onset of bipolar disorder. Bipolar Disord. 2012;14(6):654–63.

Bauer M, Mazda A, Bschor T, Heinz A, Rasgon N, Frye M, Grunze H, et al. Clinical applications of levothyroxine in refractory mood disorders. Clin Appr Bipolar Disord. 2003;2:49–56.

Boyer WF, Bakalar NH, Lake CR. Anticholinergic prophylaxis of acute haloperidol-induced acute dystonic reactions. J Clin Psychopharmacol. 1987;7:164–6.

Busch KA, Fawcett J. A fine-grained study of patients who commit suicide. Psychiatr Ann. 2004;34(5):357–64.

Cade JFJ. Lithium salts in the treatment of psychotic excitement. Med J Aust. 1949;36:349–52.

Calabrese JR, Shelton MD, Bowden CL, Rapport DJ, Suppes T, Shirley ER, Kimmel SE, et al. Bipolar rapid cycling: focus on depression as its hallmark. J Clin Psychiatry. 2001;62(Suppl 14):34–41.

Caldeira C, Chen Y, Chan L, Pham V, Chen Y, Zheng K. Mobile apps for mood tracking: an analysis of features and user reviews. AMIA Annu Symp Proc. 2017:495–504.

Carlson GA, Goodwin FK. The stages of mania: a longitudinal analysis of the manic episode. Arch Gen Psychiatry. 1973;28:221–8.

Cerletti U, Bini L. L'elletroshock. Archivio Générale di Neurologia. Psichiatria et Psicoanalisi. 1938;19:266–8.

Cochran S. Preventing medical non-compliance in the outpatient treatment of bipolar affective disorder. J Consult Clin Psychol. 1984;52(5):873–8.

Desilver D. Suicides account for most gun deaths. Pew Research Center. May 24, 2013. On line.

Even C, Schroder CM, Friedman S, Rouillon F. Efficacy of light therapy in nonseasonal depression: a systematic review. J Affect Disord. 2008;108(1–2):11–23.

Frank E. Treating bipolar disorder: a clinician's guide to interpersonal and social rhythm therapy. New York: Guilford Press; 2005.

Frank E, Thase ME, Mallinger AG, Kupfer DJ, et al. Two-year outcomes for interpersonal and social rhythm therapy in individuals with bipolar disorder. Arch Gen Psychiatry. 2005;62:996–1004.

Freeman S. Targeting acute risk factors: focus on time-sensitive factors that may respond to treatment. Curr Psychiatr Ther. 2012;11(1):53–6.

Goodwin FK. The biology of recurrence: new directions for the pharmacologic bridge. J Clin Psychiatry. 1989;50:40–4.

Goodwin FK, Jamison KR. Manic-depressive illness: bipolar disorders and recurrent depression. 1st ed. Oxford: Oxford University Press; 1990.

Goodwin FK, Jamison KR. Manic-depressive illness: bipolar disorders and recurrent depression. 2nd ed. Oxford: Oxford University Press; 2007.

Gray JD, McEwen BS. Dynamic plasticity: the role of glutocorticoids, brain-derived neurotrophic factor and other trophic factors. Neuroscience. 2013a;239:214–27.

Gray JD, McEwen BS. Lithium's role in neural plasticity and its implications for mood disorders. Acta Psychiatr Scand. 2013b;128:347–61.

Grohol JM. Evidence for atypical antipsychotic drugs called into question. Psych Central News. 8 January 2011. http://psychcentral.com/news/2011/01/07/atypical-antipsychotic-medication-evidence-called-into-question/22419

Insel TR. Rethinking schizophrenia. Nature. 2010;468:187–93.

Jha A. Community technical assistance center. Suicide prevention training. 2013. www.ctacny.com/.../ctac_suicide_prevention_training_-_aruna_jha-_7-17-13_1.pdf

Jimenez-Jimenez FJ, Garcia-Ruiz PJ, Molina JA. Drug-induced movement disorders. Drug Saf. 1997;16:180–204.

Johnson SL. Life events in bipolar disorder: towards more specific models. Clin Psychol Rev. 2005;25:1008–27.

Kelly T. The art and science of thyroid supplementation for the treatment of bipolar depression. Scotts Valley: CreateSpace; 2018.
Kobeissi J, Aloysi A, Tobias K, Popeo D, Kellner CH. Resolution of severe suicidality with a single electroconvulsive therapy. J ECT. 2011;27(1):86–8.
Koek RJ. Tips, cautions and successes in treating bipolar patients with lithium. Psychiatr Times. 2015;32(4):np On line.
Kraepelin E. Psychiatrie. Ein lehrbuch fur studierende und arzte, 6 Auflage, 1. Band, Barth, Leipzig. 1899.
Kvarnstrom E. Understanding bipolar disorder triggers and how to prevent them. 24 Apr 2018; Bridges to Recovery On line.
Lake CR. Bipolar. London: Elsevier; 2021.
Lineham G, et al. Reasons for staying alive when you're thinking of killing yourself: the reasons for living inventory. J Consult Clin Psychol. 1983;51(2):276–86.
Malik A, Goodwin GM, Homes EA. Contemporary approaches to frequent mood monitoring in bipolar disorder. J Exp Psychopathol. 2012;3(4):572–81.
Mauer S, Vergne D, Ghaemi SN. Standard and trace-dose lithium: a systematic review of dementia prevention and other behavioral benefits. Aust N Z J Psychiatry. 2014;48:809–18.
McEvoy JP, Meyer JM, Goff DC, Nasrallah HA, Davis SM, Sullivan L, Meltzer H, et al. Prevalence of the metabolic syndrome in patients with schizophrenia: baseline results from the Clinical Antipsychotic Trials of Intervention Effectiveness (CATIE) schizophrenia trial and comparison with national estimates from NHANESIII. Schizophr Res. 2005;80:19–32.
McIntyre RS, Taylor VH, Sharma A. Beyond pharmacotherapy: understanding links between obesity and chronic mental illness. Can J Psychiatr. 2012;57(1):5.
Melo MC, Daher EF, Albuquerque SG, de Bruin VM. Exercise in bipolar patients: a systematic review. J Affect Disord. 2016;198:32–8.
Miklowitz DJ. Adjunctive psychotherapy for bipolar disorder. Am J Psychiatry. 2008;165(11):1408–19.
Miller OH, Moran JT, Hall BJ, Basel C, Hoffmann F. Two cellular hypotheses explaining the initiation of ketamine's antidepressant actions: direct inhibition and disinhibition. Neuropharmacology. 2019;100:17–26. https://doi.org/10.1016/j.neuropharm.2015.07.028.
Müller-Oerlinghausen B, Berghofer A, Ahrens B. The anti-suicidal and mortality-reducing effect of lithium prophylaxis: consequences for guidelines in clinical psychiatry. Can J Psychiatr. 2003;48(7):433–9.
Nowak L. The signs and triggers of a bipolar relapse – what can you do? BrightQuest 21 Sept 2018 On line.
Nunes MA, Viel TA, Buck HS. Microdose lithium treatment stabilized cognitive impairment in patients with Alzheimer's disease. Curr Alzheimer Res. 2013;10:104–7.
Palacios J. Tamoxifen for bipolar disorder: systematic review and meta-analysis. J Psychopharmacol. 2019;33:177.
Perry A, Tarrier N, Morriss R, McCarthy E, et al. Randomised controlled trial of efficacy of teaching patients with bipolar disorder to identify early symptoms of relapse and obtain treatment. Br Med J. 1999;318:149–53.
Phelps J. A new treatment for bipolar depression: part 1. Psychiatr Times. 2018a;35(9):np On line.
Phelps J. A new treatment for bipolar depression: part 2. Psychiatr Times. 2018b;35(10) On line
Post RM. The case for polypharmacy in the treatment of bipolar disorder. Psychiatr Times. 2007;24:1–4.
Post RM. The sorry state of treatment research in bipolar disorder: an ongoing but preventable catastrophe. J Nerv Ment Dis. 2012;200(11):924–7.
Prien RF, Kupfer DJ, Mansky PA, Small JG, Tuason VB, Voss CB, Johnson WE. Drug therapy in the prevention of recurrences in unipolar and bipolar affective disorders: report of the NIMH Collaborative Study Group comparing lithium carbonate, imipramine, and a lithium carbonate-imipramine combination. Arch Gen Psychiatry. 1984;41:1096–104.
Rea MM, Thompson M, Miklowitz DJ, Goldstein MJ, et al. Family focused treatment vs individual treatment for bipolar disorder: results of a randomized clinical trial. J Consult Clin Psychol. 2003;71:482–92.

Saxton A, Resnick P, Noffsinger S. Chief complaint: homicidal: assessing violence risk. Curr Psychol. 2018;17(5):27–34.
Schou M. Therapeutic and prophylactic action of lithium. Act Nerv Super. 1967;9:440.
Schou M. Special review: lithium in psychiatric therapy and prophylaxis. J Psychiatr Res. 1968;6:67–95.
Schou M. Artistic productivity and lithium prophylaxis in manic-depressive illness. Br J Psychiatry. 1979a;135:97–103.
Schou M. Lithium as a prophylactic agent in unipolar affective illness: comparison with cyclic antidepressants. Arch Gen Psychiatry. 1979b;36:849–51.
Scott J. Psychotherapy for bipolar disorder. Br J Psychiatr. 1995;167:581–8.
Shulman K, Almeida O, Herrman N, Schaffer A, Strejilevich S, Paternoster C, Amodeo S, Dols A, et al. Delphi survey of maintenance lithium treatment in older adults with bipolar disorder: an ISBD task force report. Bipolar Disord. 2019;21(2):117–23; epub 2018 Nov 16.
Stanciu CN, Glass OM, Penders MT. Use of buprenorphine in treatment of refractory depression – a review of current literature. Asian J Psychiatr. 2017;26:94–8.
Swartz CM. Tardive psychopathology. Neuropsychobiology. 1995;32:115–9.
Swartz CM, Shorter E. Psychotic depression. New York: Cambridge University Press; 2007.
Swartz HA, Swanson J. Psychotherapy for bipolar disorder in adults: a review of the evidence. Am Psychiatr Publ. 2014;Sum 12:251–66.
Tondo L, Hennen J. Lithium treatment and suicide risk in major affective disorders: update and new findings. J Clin Psychiatry. 2003;64 Suppl 5:44–52.
Torem MS. Participatory pharmacotherapy: 10 strategies for enhancing adherence. Curr Psychiatr Ther. 2013;12(7):21–5.
Torrey EF, Zdanowicz MT, Kennard AD, Lamb HR, Eslinger DF, Biascotti MV, Fuller DA. The treatment of persons with mental illness in prisons and jails: a state survey. 8 Apr 2014.
Tsuang MT, Dempsey GM, Rauscher F. A study of "atypical schizophrenia": a comparison with schizophrenia and affective disorder by sex, age of admission, precipitant, outcome, and family history. Arch Gen Psychiatry. 1976;33:1157–60.
Tyler P, Kendall T. The spurious advance of antipsychotic drug therapy. Lancet. 2009;373:1007.
Vann MR. 9 Most common triggers for bipolar mood episodes. Everyday Health. 9/18/2017:62.
Wegmann J. Psychopharmacology: straight talk on mental health medications. 3rd ed. Eau Claire: PESI Inc; 2015.
Wehr TA, Goodwin FK. Can antidepressants cause mania and worsen the course of affective illness? Am J Psychiatry. 1987;144(11):1403–11.
Weinberg I. Psychiatry advisor. Is this patient suicidal? Tips for effective assessment. http://www.Psychiatryadvisor.com/suicide-and-self-harm. 8/17/2016.
Wendling P. Suicide rates soaring among middle-aged adults. Clin Psychiatry News. 2 May 2013.
Whitaker R. The case against antipsychotic drugs: a 50-year record of doing more harm than good. Med Hypotheses. 2004;62:5–13.
Zarate CA Jr, Tohen M. Double-blind comparison of the continued use of antipsychotic treatment versus its discontinuation in remitted manic patients. Am J Psychiatry. 2004;161:169–71.
Zarate CA, Singh JB, Carlson PJ, et al. Efficacy of a protein kinase C inhibitor (Tamoxifen) in the treatment of acute mania: a pilot study. Bipolar Disord. 2007;9:561–70.

Chapter 7
Future Changes in the World of Bipolar

7.1 Bipolar Will Be More Openly Accepted and Understood with Less Stigma

The number of publications about Bipolar has increased substantially over the past 10 years. As there are more publications about Bipolar, both academic and lay, more people will read about, accept, and understand Bipolar as a medical disorder of the brain that often associates with success. This increase in the Bipolar literature will lead to increased recognition and understanding in the general population by potential Bipolar clients and by psychotherapists.

Training programs in psychotherapy, social work, and psychology will recognize the need for preparing more mental health professionals to meet the need for treatment of this growing population. As more individuals are identified with Bipolar, the greater its acceptance will be. Additional academic focus on Bipolar will substantially raise the knowledge level of Bipolar and further increase the number of identified Bipolar clients (Sect. 7.2). Bipolar-knowledgeable mental health professionals will both benefit from this increase in the identified Bipolar population and help to alleviate suffering of Bipolar clients.

The number of famous advocates for Bipolar should also increase in this process and they will reinforce recognition and acceptance of Bipolar more than any other group. Twelve case summaries of famous Bipolar people are included in Sect. 4.3, some of whom have widely advocated for the personal acceptance of Bipolar; others did not. Recognition and acceptance, especially by the famous, reduce stigma and shame.

C. R. Lake, *Bipolar for Psychotherapists and Their Clients*,
https://doi.org/10.1007/978-3-031-38750-0_7

7.2 Psychotherapy Training Programs Will Emphasize Bipolar Disorders

For 25 years it has been reported that less than 50% of Mood-Disordered clients are appropriately recognized, diagnosed, and treated. Considering that some 16 million people in the United States have Bipolar, recognized or not, there is a large number of underserved clients. There are many more psychotherapists than psychiatrists, but the majority of non-MD mental health workers are not adequately trained to identify and manage Bipolar clients. When more therapists are trained, many more Bipolars will be diagnosed and better treated earlier in their lives. This will reduce the cost of their Bipolar morbidity and mortality, now an average of nine years shorter lifespan, and the potential disastrous chaos in their lives as well as that in their significant others' lives.

Depression is the fourth highest cause of disability in the United States and around the world, and because suicides occur during depression, usually Bipolar depression, its recognition and management are critical as the first steps in preventing suicide (Prestidge and Lake 1987; Pignone et al. 2002) (Sects. 3.4 and 6.6).

Academic psychology and schools of social work and psychotherapy may have some responsibility for more effective education of their students so that, as future mental health professionals, they will better identify Bipolar depression, other Mood Disorders, and risk for suicide among their clients. The heads of psychotherapy programs will recognize that there is a large population of unrecognized or inadequately managed Bipolar clients and that their graduates will be able to manage them best. Courses about Bipolar will be integrated into the teaching programs for psychotherapists. Exposure to Bipolar will include didactic and clinical sessions. Students will have the opportunity to interview new Bipolar clients under supervision.

Therapists will learn about Bipolar, its signs and symptoms, and they will be better able to recognize, diagnose, and manage the cycles, coordinate the needed medication changes with prescribers, and advise about their side effects (Sects. 3.2, 6.2, and 6.3).

Such training programs might consider consulting with chairs of Academic Departments of Psychiatry to contract a psychopharmacologist to teach a three-hour course on Bipolar during the first year of training. An upper-level clinical exposure to a Bipolar or mood clinic would be important in this project of helping these future psychotherapists gain confidence in their ability to manage Bipolar clients. Therapists' education about Bipolar will benefit many Bipolar clients.

7.3 Psychotherapists Will Recognize and Manage More Bipolar Clients

Bipolar is under-recognized and misdiagnosed—and therefore many are not most effectively treated. Despite the fact that its etiology remains uncertain and there is no physical test for it, the signs and symptoms for classic Bipolar are disease specific and unique. Bipolar can be accurately recognized and diagnosed by Bipolar-knowledgeable therapists now because of its unique signs and symptoms. Fortunately, according to Harrison et al. (2018), new technologies in neuroscience, genetics, and digitization are making important advances toward a diagnostic laboratory test.

This situation presents psychotherapists with an opportunity once they *understand Bipolar*. Psychotherapists will realize that the Bipolar population presents a substantial opportunity to grow their client base and to help these clients as well. Bipolar requires long-term psychotherapy treatment. Undiagnosed Bipolar II and Cyclothymic clients are more likely to initially seek psychotherapy rather than a psychiatrist. Some of these clients are likely already under treatment.

Improved treatment including psychotherapy begins with the correct diagnosis; with some intuition, Bipolar II and Cyclothymia cases will be recognized among those misdiagnosed with personality disorders, ADHD, ODD, and IED, as well as MDD and DMDD. Psychotic Mood Disorders will be accepted in cases previously diagnosed with "Schizophrenia" or "Schizoaffective Disorder." Some Bipolar I clients will also seek therapists for help with the chaos in their lives, unaware that Bipolar may be involved. These disorders can present a diagnostic challenge as their Bipolar symptoms can be subtle or extreme and require detailed questions that will only be asked if there is a high index of suspicion and knowledge of Bipolar.

Psychotherapists are in a better position to recognize and manage Bipolar clients than the traditional psychiatrist or PCP once therapists are knowledgeable about Bipolar cycling including persistent mood instability. Psychiatrists are trained to prescribe medicines and usually do this in 10- to 15-minute sessions with follow-ups every one to six months. Significant mood changes can occur monthly so that with one-to-six-month follow-ups, psychiatrists may not recognize such cycling, and the disorder gets worse. Weekly meetings allow Bipolar-educated psychotherapists to identify and manage such cycles.

Psychiatrists have typically seen Bipolar clients when they present for treatment in the midst of a major episode, not at early stages. Current strategy is to follow closely enough to initiate treatment intensification in order to postpone the next episode, make it milder, or maybe to prevent the next episode altogether. Preventative measures are increased psychotherapy and medication adjustments (Sects. 6.2 and 6.4). Frequent contact is necessary to do this.

Managed care is surely responsible for the change away from psychiatrists prescribing and doing weekly therapy; the demise of many Bipolar clients has resulted. Psychotherapists can fill this gap with the proper training about Bipolar.

Since they cannot prescribe, therapists will routinely vet and recruit a psychiatrist or PCP who is knowledgeable about Bipolar as a common diagnosis and who uses the mood-stabilizing medicines frequently. The therapist maintains management of the client. In the future, psychotherapists will more commonly collaborate with such a Bipolar-knowledgeable psychiatrist or PCP. There will be mutual cross-referrals and agreements to tend to one another's calls or texts concerning current client issues or new clients. The lives of Bipolar clients and their families will fare better under this system.

7.4 Our Justice System Will Adopt Psychology's Definition of Psychosis and Insanity

It is unfortunate that in the US judicial system the fact that violence was committed during a psychotic episode does not necessarily entitle that person to an insanity defense. The legal and psychological definitions of insanity are different, and these definitions can mean the difference between life or death or at least long-term prison time versus inpatient mental health treatment and rehabilitation. In the current legal system, psychosis does not equal insanity and a psychologist is merely an expert witness. Moreover, unfortunately, experts' opinions of the presence of psychosis can differ. Ultimately, the judge and/or jury will make the insanity determination.

From a psychological standpoint, *psychosis is insanity*, and psychotic perpetrators of violence are not guilty by reason of insanity, even if they planned ahead, knew that their act was illegal, and had some clear thinking. Psychotic killers can usually be identified by the characteristics of their attacks (Sect. 4.7).

The most tragic violence, filicide, is usually committed by psychotic mothers (Sect. 4.6). The situation gets worse when these psychotic killers are *deemed legally sane*. They sincerely believe that they are saving their children from the devil or further torture on earth by killing them. They usually attempt to kill themselves in order to join their children in a better place. When they survive and it is shown in court that they planned ahead, their chances for being found not guilty by reason of insanity are reduced if not eliminated. Psychotic defendants are frequently imprisoned and occasionally executed, both at great expense, when the better outcome for both defendants and society would be appropriate locked-down mental health rehabilitation.

Examples of psychotic mothers are Ms. Andrea Yates, a 37-year-old nurse, Ms. Marilyn Lemak, a 41-year-old surgical nurse, and Ms. Christina Riggs. Having killed their children, all of these mothers were found sane and convicted of murder. Ms. Yates and Ms. Lemak were sentenced to life in prison. Ms. Yates' sentence was reversed four years later to not guilty by reason of insanity but she remains incarcerated in a TX mental hospital. Ms. Lemak remains in prison. Ms. Riggs was executed.

It is logical that the field of psychology that studies mental health should have more input for setting the standards for insanity versus sanity. *Detailed planning ahead does not rule out psychosis or insanity.*

This is another aspect of improper treatment of Bipolar clients who have found themselves in the judicial system. Some of these are innocent people who were likely in the throes of a manic or depressive episode that was severe with psychotic features. Equating planning ahead with sanity is a tragic and irrational state of affairs in much need of correction. It could get worse if the former Vice President of the United States has his way. Instead of supporting gun control, Pence is apparently promoting a national law mandating execution of mass killers likely in a bid for votes for the 2024 Republican nomination. Some of these killers suffer with a severe mental illness. Such a law would return us to the Dark Ages when the mentally ill were burned to death at the stake as witches (Sect. 2.1).

It is hoped that the justice system will adopt psychology's definition of psychosis/insanity, spare psychotic perpetrators of violence from inappropriate sentencing, and instead offer opportunities for treatment and rehabilitation. Mental health professionals should take every opportunity to educate legislators and lawyers.

7.5 Diagnoses of "Schizophrenia" and "Schizoaffective Disorder" Will Be Dropped from the DSM and Other Mental Health Nomenclature

The psychotic Mood Disorders explain all symptoms attributed to "Schizophrenia" and "Schizoaffective Disorder" (Sect. 3.9). That these latter two disorders are not valid diagnoses has been documented by many respected neuroscientists, especially from the United Kingdom and the United States (Lake 2012). The DSM has downgraded "Schizophrenia" for decades, most recently with the DSM that eliminated all the subtypes and Schneider's "pathognomonic" delusions previously required for the diagnosis. Nevertheless, "Schizophrenia" and "Schizoaffective Disorder" remain in the DSM-5 and the DSM-5-TR, reflecting poorly on the scientific grounding of psychology and psychiatry. These psychotic clients have a psychotic Mood Disorder: Bipolar, manic, or depressed; MDD; PPD. Clients so misdiagnosed are poorly served. They do not get the proper focus in therapy nor the right medications. By the publication of the DSM-6, it will be in the best interest of the mental health professions, and even more beneficial for psychotic clients, to eliminate these two diagnoses from the nomenclature; using such diagnoses falls below standard of care.

A summary of take-home messages is given in Table 7.1.

Table 7.1 Take-home messages for your clients

1. BP is a physical, neurological disease of the brain
2. BP is a severe life-long mental illness yet associates with intelligence, success, and fame
3. BP has a history of consistent symptoms for over 2,000 years
4. BP is under-recognized and misdiagnosed
5. Management of BP requires early recognition, accurate diagnosis, acceptance, weekly therapy, and correct medications
6. Three mood-stabilizing drugs at once are treatments of choice for manic and depressed clients (concomitant with a short-term SGA if psychotic)
7. SGAs alone in functionally psychotic clients falls below standard of care
8. The primary goal of managing BP is to postpone or prevent the next episode
9. For BP, the more episodes, in general, the faster they come and the worse they get
10. Delusional paranoia means a psychotic Mood Disorder
11. Clients misdiagnosed with SZ or SAD have a psychotic Mood Disorder, BP, or MDD; diagnoses of SZ and SAD fall below standard of care
12. Seek mood symptoms in the initial diagnostic interview of a functionally psychotic, paranoid patient.
13. Non-manic indicators of BP convert MDD to BP (Table 3.11)
14. Mood-stabilizing drugs are equally effective in MDD and BP
15. Avoid antidepressant drugs in Mood Disorders
16. Children diagnosed with ADHD, IED, or ODD are likely BP

References

Harrison PJ, Geddes JR, Tunbridge EM. The emerging neurobiology of bipolar disorder. Trends Neurosci. 2018;41(1):18–30.
Lake CR. Schizophrenia is a misdiagnosis. New York: Springer; 2012.
Pignone MP, Gaynes BN, Rushton JL, Burchell CM, Orleans CT, Mulrow CD, Lohr KN. Screening for depression in adults: a summary of the evidence for the US Preventive Services Task Force. Ann Intern Med. 2002;136:765–76.
Prestidge BR, Lake CR. The prevalence and recognition of depression among primary care outpatients. J Fam Pract. 1987;25:67–72.

Index

C. R. Lake, *Bipolar for Psychotherapists and Their Clients*,
https://doi.org/10.1007/978-3-031-38750-0